From Clinic to
Concentration Camp

Representing a new wave of research and analysis on Nazi human experiments and coerced research, the chapters in this volume deliberately break from a top-down history limited to concentration camp experiments under the control of Himmler and the SS. Instead the collection positions extreme experiments (where research subjects were taken to the point of death) within a far wider spectrum of abusive coerced research. The book considers the experiments not in isolation but as integrated within wider aspects of medical provision as it became caught up in the Nazi war economy, revealing that researchers were opportunistic and retained considerable autonomy. The sacrifice of so many prisoners, patients and otherwise healthy people rounded up as detainees raises important issues about the identities of the research subjects: who were they, how did they feel, how many research subjects were there and how many survived? This underworld of the victims of the elite science of German medical institutes and clinics has until now remained a marginal historical concern. Jews were a target group, but so were gypsies/Sinti and Roma, the mentally ill, prisoners of war and partisans. By exploring when and in what numbers scientists selected one group rather than another, the book provides an important record of the research subjects having agency, reconstructing responses and experiential narratives, and recording how these experiments – iconic of extreme racial torture – represent one of the worst excesses of Nazism.

Paul Weindling is Research Professor in the History of Medicine at Oxford Brookes University, UK. His research covers evolution and society, public health, and human experimentation post-1800. He has especial interests in eugenics, human experiments, corporate philanthropies in the field of international health, and medical refugees from Nazi Germany. He has published on victims and survivors of Nazi experiments and develops research on the thousands of victims and their body parts.

The History of Medicine in Context

Series Editors: Andrew Cunningham and
Ole Peter Grell

Department of History and Philosophy of Science,
University of Cambridge
Department of History, Open University

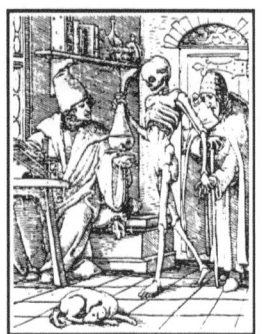

A full list of titles in this series is available at
https://www.routledge.com/history/series/HMC

Titles in the series include:

From Clinic to Concentration Camp

Reassessing Nazi Medical and Racial Research, 1933–1945
Edited by Paul Weindling

Medicine, Natural Philosophy and Religion in Post-Reformation Scandinavia

Edited by Ole Peter Grell and Andrew Cunningham

Medicine, Trade and Empire

Garcia de Orta's Colloquies on the Simples and Drugs of India (1563)
in Context
Palmira Fontes da Costa

The Political and Social Dynamics of Poverty, Poor Relief and Health Care in Early-Modern Portugal

Laurinda Abreu

The World of Plants in Renaissance Tuscany

Medicine and Botany
Cristina Bellorini

From Clinic to Concentration Camp

Reassessing Nazi Medical and Racial Research, 1933–1945

**Edited by
Paul Weindling**

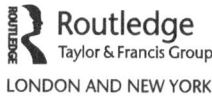
Routledge
Taylor & Francis Group

LONDON AND NEW YORK

First published 2017
by Routledge
2 Park Square, Milton Park, Abingdon, Oxon OX14 4RN

and by Routledge
605 Third Avenue, New York, NY 10017

First issued in paperback 2021

Routledge is an imprint of the Taylor & Francis Group, an informa business

Publisher's Note
The publisher has gone to great lengths to ensure the quality of this reprint but
points out that some imperfections in the original copies may be apparent.

British Library Cataloguing in Publication Data
A catalogue record for this book is available from the British Library

Library of Congress Cataloging in Publication Data
Names: Weindling, Paul, editor of compilation.
Title: From clinic to concentration camp : reassessing Nazi medical and racial
research, 1933–1945 / edited by Paul Weindling.
Description: Milton Park, Abingdon, Oxon ; New York, NY : Routledge, 2017. |
Series: The history of medicine in context | Includes bibliographical references
and index.
Identifiers: LCCN 2016053650| ISBN 9781472484611 (hardback : alkaline paper) |
ISBN 9781315583310 (ebook)
Subjects: LCSH: Human experimentation in medicine – Germany – History –
20th century. | Medicine – Research – Germany – History – 20th century. |
Medicine – Research – Moral and ethical aspects – Germany – History –
20th century. | Involuntary treatment – Germany – History – 20th century. |
Clinics – Germany – History – 20th century. | Prisoners of war – Medical
care – Germany – History – 20th century. | Concentration camp inmates –
Medical care – Germany – History – 20th century. | Racism in medicine –
Germany – History – 20th century. | National socialism and medicine – History. |
World War, 1939-1945 – Atrocities – Germany.
Classification: LCC R853.H8 F76 2017 | DDC 610.72 – dc23
LC record available at https://lccn.loc.gov/2016053650

ISBN 13: 978-1-03-209693-3 (pbk)
ISBN 13: 978-1-4724-8461-1 (hbk)

Typeset in Bembo
by Florence Production Ltd, Stoodleigh, Devon, UK

Contents

Figures

Contributors

Margit Berner, PhD, born in Vienna, studied Physical Anthropology at the University of Vienna, curator of the cast collection at the Department of Anthropology, Museum of Natural History Vienna, research and publication in History of Anthropology and Physical Anthropology, cooperation in various scientific projects and participation in exhibitions.

Christian Bonah, MD, PhD is professor for the history of medical and health sciences and member of the Institute of Advanced Studies of the University Strasbourg. He has worked on comparative history of medical education, social and cultural studies of science and technology including notably the history of medicaments and the history of human experimentation. Recent works include research on risk perception and management in drug scandals and courtroom trials as well as studies on medical/health film.

Gabriele Czarnowski, Dr. phil., Institute of Social Medicine and Epidemiology, Medical University Graz, Austria. Fields of study: social history of gender relations, medicine and public health in National Socialism, history of gynaecology and obstetrics. Publications include: ' "Das unheilbar Erkrankte aus dem Volkswachstum ausschalten": Politische Gynäkologie an den Berliner Universitätsfrauenkliniken im Nationalsozialismus', in Sabine Schleiermacher and Udo Schagen (eds), *Die Charite im Dritten Reich. Zur Dienstbarkeit medizinischer Wissenschaft im Nationalsozialismus*, Paderborn: Ferdinand Schöningh 2008, pp. 133–150. 'Women's crimes, state crimes: abortion in Nazi Germany', in Margaret L. Arnot and Cornelie Usborne (eds), *Gender and crime in modern Europe*, London: UCL Press, 1999, pp. 238–256.

Herwig Czech, Research fellow at the Documentation Centre of the Austrian Resistance and lecturer at the Medical University Vienna. Studied history at the Universities of Graz, Vienna, Paris VII and Duke. 2003/04 Gedenkdienst (voluntary service) at the Centre de Documentation Juive Contemporaine in Paris. 2007 PhD from Vienna University with a thesis on Medicine in National Socialist Vienna. Teaching assignments at the

Universities of Wroclaw, Newcastle and Vienna. In 2006, 2012/13 and 2014 Visiting Fellow at the Institute for Human Sciences, Vienna. In 2011 to 2014 recipient of an APART-fellowship of the Austrian Academy of Sciences for a project on social and medical conditions in Vienna, 1944 to 1948.

Nichola Farron graduated from Royal Holloway College, University of London with an honours degree in history and a Master's degree in Holocaust Studies. Studentship on the AHRC funded project "Victims of Human Experiments and Coercive Research under National Socialism", where her research focused on the under explored aspect of Soviet victims, the subject of her thesis, *The Soviet Experience of Nazi Medicine: Statistics, Stories and Stereotypes*, Oxford Brookes MPhil, 2011. Now resident in Portland, Oregon she continues to contribute to academic conferences and co-authored publications, as well as maintaining an active involvement in the area of Holocaust studies including previous work with the Oregon Holocaust Resource Center.

Sabine Hildebrandt is Assistant Professor in the Division of General Pediatrics, Department of Medicine at Boston Children's Hospital and Lecturer on Global Health and Social Medicine at Harvard Medical School. Her research focuses on the history and ethics of anatomy. She published: *The Anatomy of Murder. Ethical Transgressions and Anatomical Science during the Third Reich*, 2016.

Gerrit Hohendorf, MD is titular professor at the Technical University Munich. He lectures on the history and ethics of medicine, and is a clinical psychiatrist. He developed the new memorial exhibition at the former "T4" site in Berlin, and is author of a major study on the history and ethics of "euthanasia" under National Socialism. He published: *Der Tod als Erlösung vom Leiden – Geschichte und Ethik der Sterbehilfe seit dem Ende des 19. Jahrhunderts in Deutschland*, Göttingen, Wallstein, 2013. He co-edited with Petra Fuchs, Maike Rotzoll, Ulrich Müller and Paul Richter, *"Das Vergessen der Vernichtung ist Teil der Vernichtung selbst". Lebensgeschichten von Opfern der nationalsozialistischen "Euthanasie"*, 3rd ed., Göttingen: Wallstein, 2014.

Astrid Ley, PhD, deputy head of Sachsenhausen memorial and museum, Oranienburg (Germany). Historical degree at Erlangen university, research associate at the institute of the history of medicine at Erlangen university, 2003 dissertation on the involvement of German doctors in the Nazi sterilisation programme. Since 2003 at Sachsenhausen memorial, permanent exhibitions "Medicine and Crime" (2004), "Sachsenhausen Concentration Camp" (2008), "The Euthanasia Institution at Brandenburg an der Havel" (2012).

Aleksandra Loewenau, PhD (University of Calgary) Aleksandra graduated with a PhD in History of Medicine from Oxford Brookes University in 2012. After the successful completion of her thesis entitled *The Impact of Nazi Medical Experiments on Polish Inmates at Dachau, Auschwitz and Ravensbrück*, Aleksandra worked as a Post-Doctoral Research Assistant on the Wellcome Trust funded Programme Grant investigating "Disputed Bodies: Research Subjects' Narratives of Medical Research in Europe, 1940–2001" lead by Professor Paul Weindling. Currently she holds a Postdoctoral Fellow position at University of Calgary where she works on "The Impact of German-speaking neuroscientists on development of neuroscience in North America" project led by Dr Frank Stahnisch.

Volker Roelcke, MD, PhD is director of the Institute of the History of Medicine, Giessen University, Germany. His publications include *Silence, Scapegoats, Self-Reflection: The Shadow of Nazi Medical Crimes on Medicine and Bioethics*, Göttingen: 2014 (editor, together with Sascha Topp and Etienne Lepicard); *International Relations in Psychiatry: Britain, Germany, and the United States to World War II*, Rochester, NY: 2010 (editor, together with Paul Weindling and Louise Westwood); *La médecine expérimentale au tribunal. Implications éthiques de quelques procès médicaux du XXe siècle européen*, Paris: 2003 (editor, together with Christian Bonah and Etienne Lepicard).

Maike Rotzoll, PD Dr. med., is psychiatrist and medical historian. Currently she is working as research fellow at the Institute for the History and Ethics of Medicine, Heidelberg. Her main focuses are medicine in the early modern period and psychiatry in the late nineteenth and twentieth centuries with a special interest in patient history.

Florian Schmaltz, Diss. phil., studied history, philosophy and literature at the University Hamburg and the FU Berlin. Project Director of the Research Programme "History of the Max-Planck-Society" at the Max Planck Institute for the History of Science, Berlin. Research and publications on the history of science and technology, the Nazi era, human experimentation and the history of chemical warfare.

Hans-Walter Schmuhl, born 1957. Assistant lecturer Department of History, Philosophy and Theology, Bielefeld University (1984–85). Doctorate (1986). Assistant lecturer for special research programme "Social history of the modern bourgeoisie: Germany in international perspective" (1986–91). Postdoctoral thesis required for professorship (1995). Independent historian (1999). Aplied Professor (2005). Guest researcher in the research programme "The history of the Kaiser-Wilhelm-Society under National Socialism" and "The Society of German Neurologists and Psychiatrists under National Socialism". Research areas: National Socialism, comparative genocide, history of science, history of psychiatry, history of social welfare work.

Publications: *Grenzüberschreitungen. Das Kaiser-Wilhelm-Institut für Anthropologie, menschliche Erblehre und Eugenik, 1927–1945*, Göttingen: 2005; Engl. edition as: *The Kaiser Wilhelm Institute for Anthropology, Human Heredity and Eugenics, 1927–1945. Crossing Boundaries*, Dordrecht: 2008; *Die Gesellschaft Deutscher Neurologen und Psychiater im Nationalsozialismus*, Berlin and Heidelberg: 2016.

Michal V. Simunek, Institute of Contemporary History of the Academy of Sciences, Prague, maintains research interests in the history of eugenics, with a particular focus on its role in modern racism and its application in the Czech lands and in the history of biopolitics.

Raphael Toledano, born in 1980, studied medicine at the University of Strasbourg. He earned his medical degree in 2010 with his thesis titled *Medical experiments of Pr. Eugen Haagen of the Reichsuniversität Strassburg*, which received the Auschwitz Foundation Price in 2011. Since 2012, he has been a member of the scientific council of the Centre Européen du Résistant Déporté (Struthof-Natzweiler Museum). In 2014, he co-directed *Le nom des 86*, a documentary about the "Jewish skeleton collection" project of August Hirt. In 2015, he discovered remains of Jewish victims of the Nazi doctor August Hirt at the Forensic institute of Strasbourg. His main field of research is the medical experiments conducted in Alsace during the Second World War.

Kamila Uzarczyk studied at the University of Wrocław in Poland and, within the Socrates-Erasmus Program, at the University of Ghent in Belgium. In 2001 she obtained her PhD from the University of Wrocław for the dissertation on the history of race hygiene movement (K. Uzarczyk, *The concept of race hygiene and implementation of race hygienic legislation in German province of Lower Silesia*, Toruń: Marszałek, 2002, pp. 363). From 2000 affiliated at the Medical University of Wrocław, since 2003 as an assistant professor at the Department of Medical Humanities and Social Sciences in Medicine. Research interests include history of eugenics and implementation of eugenic policies in interwar years, extermination of mentally ill and disabled individuals in the Third Reich, Nazi medical experiments and brain research on euthanasia victims (associate of the project "Victims of medical experiments under National Socialism" directed by Prof. Paul Weindling).

Anna von Villiez holds a PhD in German History from the University of Hamburg. After working at Oxford Brookes University since 2007 in the "Victims of medical experiments under National Socialism" project as a research officer she took a post at the State and University Library Hamburg at the unit for provenance research in 2015. She also teaches at the University of Hamburg. Her research interests include: medicine under National Socialism, Jewish medical refugees and concepts of race in history. Her monograph *Mit aller Kraft verdrängt. Entrechtung und Verfolgung "nicht arischer" Ärzte in Hamburg 1933 bis 1945* was published in 2009 by Dölling & Galitz.

Paul Weindling, MA, PhD, ML is Research Professor in the History of Medicine, Oxford Brookes University. His research covers medical refugees 1930–45, eugenics, international health organisations, and the victims of Nazi coerced experimentation. He is a Trustee of CARA, the Council for At-Risk Academics. He was awarded the Anneliese Maier Prize, which he holds at the German National Academy of Sciences, Leopoldina in Halle, Germany, and elected an Honorary Member of the German Association of Psychiatry (DGPPN) for investigating its role under Nazism. His books include: *Health, Race and German Politics* (1989), *Epidemics and Genocide in Eastern Europe* (2000), *Victims and Survivors of Nazi Human Experiments* (2014).

Acknowledgements

I am immensely grateful to Dr Michał Palacz for his skilled assistance with the final stages of seeing the collection to publication.

I gratefully acknowledge support leading to this collection from:

- Wellcome Trust Grant No 096580/Z/11/A on research subject narratives.
- AHRC GRANT AH/E509398/1 Human Experiments under National Socialism.
- Conference for Jewish Material Claims Against Germany Application 8229/Fund SO 29
- Humboldt Foundation Anneliese Maier Prize funds

The book derives from a conference: "Reassessing Nazi human experiments and coerced research, 1933–1945: new findings, interpretations and problems", 4–7 July 2013 in Oxford. The conference was organised by Oxford Brookes University with support from the University of Giessen. The presentations are available on www.pulse-project.org/node/572 (accessed 16 July 2016).

Part One

Contexts

1 Introduction

A new historiography of the Nazi medical experiments and coerced research

Paul Weindling

There has long been public nervousness about abuse of patients and other vulnerable persons in clinics and custodial institutions as human guinea pigs. These anxieties stretch back to the rise of experimental medicine in the seventeenth century, and especially to the bacteriological and surgical breakthroughs in the later nineteenth century.[1] Nazi Germany was heir to a highly scientised system of medicine, and saw a colossal rise in coerced medical experiments and other forms of exploitative, non-consensual research. The experiments and coerced research took multiple forms, but the scale under Nazism was unprecedented, finding a parallel only in the more centralised organisation of Japanese military medical experiments on Chinese civilians and Allied prisoners of war.[2] At the end of the Second World War a shocked world learned of the German medical experiments and coerced research in concentration camps and clinics on a monstrous scale.[3]

The experiments and associated forms of coerced research have remained in public understanding as among the worst Nazi atrocities. Yet for many years they were marginalised as "pseudo-science", so that they were disconnected from mainstream German medical science and academia.[4] The purpose of this collection is to examine not only rationales and motivations of the perpetrators, but also the identities and responses of victims. The extent of experiments and the collecting of body parts have been greatly underrated, and hitherto unknown instances are still being uncovered by determined historical researchers. The coercive institutional structures, distinctive intellectual and academic agendas, the extent of the experiments and victim responses provide important insight into the dynamics of power and persecution in Nazi Germany and the Holocaust. Rather than random and marginal, the experiments, their perpetrators and the victims can be understood in structural terms as well as located in coherent historical processes. The experiments, their resourcing and their corralled victims reflect the twists and turns of Nazi racial policies, and the medical aspects of "total war", and the "final solutions" of the Jewish, Roma and psychiatric "problems". Nazi doctors stockpiled bodies, body fluids, brain tissues, skulls and bones on a massive scale. The scale of the coerced research on living persons was unprecedented; after the war ended, the outcomes in terms of death, survival and injury reached deep into the Federal Republic and Austria as regards the stored corpses and brain tissues of the dead.[5] To take one example, the Auschwitz camp doctor Josef Mengele's collecting of twins is well known to a wider public, and yet the twins remain poorly understood in terms of their identities and numbers, what happened to them and why, and they achieved belated compensation only in the 1980s. The massive use of brain tissues for research from "euthanasia" victims during and after the war has – despite pioneering research by the historian and political scientist Götz Aly – been largely overlooked.[6]

Why then should medical experiments under National Socialism be reinstated in the narrative of Nazism, racial war, and the Holocaust, and their aftermath? Beyond compassion for the victims is that the experiments were specially resourced and administered, and that specialist knowledge was involved. The survival of the German *Volk* and National Socialist Reich was deemed to be at stake. Who initiated the experiments? Hitler, only once for "N-Stoff", and Hitler's Chancellery once – for X-ray sterilisation in Auschwitz; Himmler on multiple occasions but he did not have a controlling monopoly; often the scientists themselves took the initiative of requesting resources for concentration camp experiments.[7] Most experiments were commissioned by industry, or were initiated by the scientists themselves. The victims – long underestimated in terms of numbers, and largely unknown in terms of their identities – reflect the wider phases of the unfolding of racial war and the Holocaust. Often isolated in special compounds, victims responded to the exercise of medical power in ways that were distinctive. Yes, the victims faced manifold forms of brutality widespread in any concentration camp; but additionally they were subjected to violence, which was delivered in specially calibrated scientific doses and forms.[8] Confidentiality restrictions have further compounded the marginalisation of the experiments and their victims.

The coerced experiments can be seen in a wider context of clinical medical research, which was strong in the German tradition of rigorously scientised medicine: it was necessary to produce a thesis to gain the title of "Dr med". Advanced research for a higher thesis, known as a Habilitation was required to make an academic career. The experiments were linked to the harnessing of science and technology for National Socialist racial and military aims, as well as providing an opportunity to resource scientists' gargantuan appetites for "research-material". Experimenting on racial "undesirables" was to advance strategic issues such as survival in extremes of cold, or the toxicity of explosives and poison gas. The problem thereby changes from one of the experiments as "pseudo-science" (a concept now redundant) to how did Nazi ideology and the Nazi elite form strategic alliances with the experimentally oriented experts, intent on driving forward military and ultimately racial aims.

"Medical experiments" occurred in a variety of clinics and other medical locations in addition to large-scale concentration camp experiments and the plethora of small-scale experiments in camps and clinics. The shorthand label of "Nazi medical experiments" covers research on the living – at times to the point of death – and research on the dead, often stockpiled on an immense scale. The "experiments" span taking anthropological and physiological measurements, and dissecting the brains and bodies of those who were killed, some selected when living as of scientific interest, and many channelled from execution chambers to the dissection slab. We find instances of dietary experiments, the testing of vaccines, deliberate infection, the taking of brains and other internal organs for dissection, and the stripping away of flesh to obtain skeletal bones. In short, German scientists mobilised to conduct a wide variety of scientific procedures in specially segregated spaces such as compounds within camps, and in special wards and clinics.

The experiments were variously driven by economic exploitation, racial policy, total war and the Holocaust. Similarly, the responsible scientists varied to the extent that they were members of the NSDAP (if at all), SA or SS, and of university medical faculties. The coerced experiments indicate the importance of science in sustaining Nazi power. Just as research institutes, field stations and clinics functioned on the basis of forced and slave labour, the coerced research drew on stockpiles of Nazi victims. Resources came from special military and racial measures, and the experiments channelled human "material" into a realm of holding compounds. The research subjects did not know whether a temporary reprieve from forced labour and improved diet available in an experimental compound would enhance their chances of survival or lead to their maiming (often permanently) or death. The transfers and holding of bodies and brains means that a disjunction and displacement has occurred from the place of killing to where and when (often decades later) body parts were finally disposed of. To the life history of the victim, there needs to be a "death history" of documenting their body parts on into post-war Germany, Austria and former occupied territories.

Medical researchers sustained the momentum of research through and beyond the death throes of the Third Reich: even when the war was clearly lost, German scientists frenetically continued their endeavours. Long running experiments by Claus Schilling on malaria in Dachau concentration camp continued right up to liberation (he asked the American military whether the experiments could continue on a voluntary basis), as did the shoe testing track (where high performance amphetamines were sporadically used) in Sachsenhausen concentration camp. Remarkably, several new sets of experiments began in early 1945 raising questions about the mind-set of the involved scientists. Scientists saw a unique opportunity to lay foundations for their post-war careers. From June 1944 (a year after Mengele visited the racial geneticist Otmar von Verschuer, who then mentioned Mengele in a research report to the *Deutsche Forschungsgemeinschaft*, DFG) the Auschwitz camp doctor Josef Mengele surveyed streams of arrivals, mainly from Hungary, with a genetically trained eye to select twins and dwarves to conduct measurements and tests: his intention was to use his copious "material" for a Habilitation thesis. Others saw the experiments as staging posts towards establishing new research installations – here the ambitious orthopaedic surgeon Karl Gebhardt supported human subject research in the concentration camps of Ravensbrück and Neuengamme. Gebhardt at his tuberculosis and orthopaedic sanatoria at Hohenlychen (a rambling neo-Gothic complex) absorbed laboratory installations evacuated from nearby Berlin, such as the pathology laboratories from the Virchow Hospital where body parts from Wittenau psychiatric hospital were being processed.[9] (Indeed, the decanting of scientific institutes from Berlin presaged the decentralised structures of research in the Federal Republic.) Another instance is that the SS sponsored research by the gynaecologist Carl Clauberg holding victims in a special Block 10 in the Auschwitz main camp: Clauberg envisaged his Auschwitz research as a prelude for a new City of Mothers at Bad Königsdorff established late in the war for infertility treatment. Clauberg secured the services of the Polish prisoner surgeon, Władysław Dering from Auschwitz for his clinic at Königshütte (Chorzów) as well as for launching his ill-fated venture.[10]

The experiments gain further importance once one moves away from overly schematised historical conceptualisations of Germany under National Socialism as consisting of the *Führer* and *Volk*. It is necessary to recognise the importance of science-based professions, which aligned themselves with Nazi aims and purged their memberships, and of knowledge-production for the German economy, military and medicine in the cataclysmic twelve-year Reich. Science-based expertise had a key role in delivering on strategically important issues such as health, race and population policies, as well as in formulating racial ideology and imposing the categorisation of who belonged in what racial group. The Nazi state clung to its racial priorities through its colossal expansion as scientific energies were expended in exploiting and exterminating Jews, Sinti and Roma, and the mentally ill and disabled. Nazi Germany as a "Racial State" (or in its original more culturally-oriented conceptualisation of the French political scientist Henri Lichtenberger of an *état raciale*) involved not just imposition of racial policy and an immense sifting of the population by multiple and competing agencies, but also a research dynamic, encompassing bodies, body fluids, bones and organs.[11] While "race" provided over-arching social cohesion, defining race was contested by a plurality of scientists and agencies. Researching race and arising issues of human growth and variation required substantial resources. Once this is recognised, the coerced experiments move from the margins of history towards the mainstream of historical concerns with the defining of the racial community or *Volksgemeinschaft*, and become an essential component of the war economy. At the same time the research endeavours reveal the efforts to sustain the power and drive forward policy of key groups – notably within the SS, but other interests were also involved – in crucial sectors of the Nazi system of power. While the research was carried out by specialist experts, *Reichsführer SS* Heinrich Himmler saw the potential for the SS in gaining power over the academic sphere by means of a radicalised form of medical research, which involved ruthless exploitation of persons demonised as racial enemies, criminals and social parasites. Himmler's backing of the young air force doctor Sigmund Rascher represented the hope of pioneering a Nazified form of medical science oriented to homoeopathy and deadly experiments.[12]

Towards historical accountability

Historiographically, the new wave of historians of German eugenics since the mid-1980s raised the issue of technocratic elites in Nazi society, and of transitions in health and population structures.[13] Smaller families, lengthening life expectancy and female education and participation in the labour force were viewed ambivalently by professional and political elites from the 1900s. The new interest in gender and the social history of everyday life (*Alltagsgeschichte*) challenged the elitist political approach, but professionalisation and the history of the ideological manipulation of research structures were regarded as minor curiosities. The work by Michael Burleigh and Wolfgang Wippermann on the "Racial State" represented a breakthrough in providing a new synthesis, in which race rather than class had pre-eminence.[14] Race remained motivating ideology rather than defining scientific practices. The insertion of categories of expertise into the social structures and the mentalities, as well as scientised definition of victim groups continued to meet with considerable scepticism and resistance from the historical mainstream. In a breath of fresh air challenging elitist conventions, Karl Heinz Roth, and Götz Aly and Susanne Heim took forward the agenda of an expert-driven and technocratic racial policy onto a wider historical canvas of total war and the Holocaust.[15] A change eventually came about, although the preoccupation continued to be the power structures of ruling elites and continuities into the post-war era rather than the victims themselves, or any evaluation of the after-effects inflicted by the Nazified medical profession.

Large-scale projects have examined funding of the German Research Foundation, and of a number of scientific institutions, most notably the Kaiser Wilhelm Society. These reveal complex patterns of representation by leading Nazi figures on governing committees, and the funding of SS agencies by the German Research Fund.[16] Nazi Germany continued to invest massively in research until its final death-throes. Many victim groups remained unidentified until recently (here the contributors to this volume have taken the lead in identification and historical reconstruction). Unravelling the intricate rationales of research requires attention to specificities of science and the complexities of prisoner holding, transfer and resourcing: only once this dual scientific and prisoner/patient related research is carried out can an evidence-based general picture be established. Linking the victims to institutions offers a form of accountability: this was not undertaken comprehensively in the projects on the German Research Society, the Robert Koch Institute and the Kaiser Wilhelm Society under National Socialism.

The combination of Nazi ideology and science poses problems to conceptualise what was going on. Recognising the role of research funding and leading scientists challenged the idea of the coerced experiments as debased "pseudo-science". Among the current conceptualisations are that of "resources for another" and "a Faustian pact".[17] The difficulty of the "resources" concept is that the victims of coerced experiments are lumped together as an anonymised resource, denying agency and identity. The Faustian conceptualisation has the pitfall that it places so much emphasis on the motive and situation that it becomes a form of apologetics. Volker Roelcke has argued that normal science – involving a high degree of coercion and non-consensual practices – prevailed under National Socialism.[18] Nazism released ethical restrictions and inhibitions, allowing unrestrained science.[19]

Most notoriously some experiments took the research subject to the point of death with the aim of scientifically defining an amount of cold, air pressure or poison gas causing death and the physiology of the onset of mortality. Other "experiments" involved holding a group selected for their scientific interest such as twins or dwarves, and systematically studying physical characteristics in minute detail. The harvesting of brains and nerve tissue, and other body parts such as eyes and internal organs, was not as such an experiment (in the sense of a scientifically measured series of interventions), but can be grouped with the experiments as scientific exploitation of bodies. On occasions researchers selected the living for clinical study and then killed them to order. Denoting all these investigations as "experiments" admittedly stretches the term, but it is reasonable to see "experiments" as standing for a range of coerced medical interventions motivated by research aims. There is now quantitative analysis of the various victims for these different types of grotesque experiments.[20]

The experiments and racial anthropological surveys took place to an uneven extent in the camps only from 1939. The historian Michael Kater devoted primary attention to the *Ahnenerbe*'s studies of pre-history but he gave only limited attention to the medical experiments, whether in the *Ahnenerbe* or – as pointed out by Reitzenstein – in the spun-off Institute for Applied Military Research.[21] Moreover, Kater has taken no interest whatsoever in the victims. Michael Burleigh describes the "euthanasia" and poison gas killings as "pseudo-medical" to convey the medical deception of hygienic routines. He places "experimentation" in inverted commas to question the scientific integrity, and quotes a leading Nazi medical official that "One may hang a copy of the Oath of Hippocrates in one's office but nobody pays any attention it", and in any case noting the shift from the individual to the collective.[22] Klee depicted telling examples, but his narratives lack structure. Other histories overlook "euthanasia" as a research opportunity, and fail to examine research victims to any meaningful extent, as well as the resourcing and the power structures surrounding research.[23]

Rather than approaching the experiments as random incidents of cruelty (often occurring), there was intensification of exploitative experimental research during the war for strategic, ideological and intrinsic scientific reasons. The studies presented here represent a collective endeavour to provide an evidence-based reconstruction of the victims of Nazi research. A victim-related reconstruction shows a minimum of 15,738 persons; whereas an additional "pending" group of claimants requires further linkage to documentation. Taking a wider view of large groups used for research – such as on racial identity (some 20,000 Sinti and Roma were identified), vaccine trials or an experimental diet – in all 98,000 persons fell victim to some sort of experimental or coerced medical intervention.[24] The documented group of 15,738 individuals represents persons held as human laboratory animals (so to speak – victims sometimes referring to themselves as "Rabbits") in special compounds or whose lives were destroyed by research interventions. Overall these victims represent a sizeable but generally overlooked group among the numerous categories of victims of National Socialism. As the studies in this volume indicate, historical research on clinical records, brain anatomy and anatomical victims shows that further instances are still coming to light. Overall numbers are set to rise further, as the research in this area identifies hitherto overlooked victim clusters.

From the late 1990s there has been a shift away from regarding the experiments as "pseudo-science" and examining their rationales and institutional settings. This effort to establish a cultural history of the coerced research has been fruitful in elucidating whole areas such as sulphonamide research. It became fixated on perpetrators and perpetrating institutions to the cost of marginalising, or completely overlooking victims, who should have been figured in as part of the historical accountability. The Kaiser Wilhelm Society was reconstructed mainly on the basis of case studies of certain institutes – the apology to victims was to a select group and no attempt was made to reconstruct Mengele's research victims as named individuals. The historical project on the German Research Fund directed by Rudiger vom Bruch and Ulrich Herbert crucially neglected a full evaluation of the proportion of the research grants identifying those grants that involved coercive and physically damaging research. The DFG gave funding to lethal brain research or formalised a crucial link to Mengele's researches in Auschwitz. Similarly the Robert Koch Institute did not identify the names and numbers of the victims of its research.[25] A victim oriented perspective exposes clear deficiencies in these high prestige projects, concerned primarily with administering structures and the scientists themselves. These high prestige German projects show a conspicuous blind spot as regards assessing the physical damage to coerced research subjects inflicted by scientists in the context of the Holocaust. In turn the resource-oriented approach has inhibited the idea of public apology and disclosure. The German Chamber of Physicians appears to think that it can give a public apology without any historical research validating the apology.[26] Other organisations, notably the German Association of Psychiatry have commissioned substantial research – here Hans Walter Schmuhl reconstructs ambitious schemes of psychiatrists and neurologists. The victims were at best an incidental, anonymised "resource" – to cite a term that has been much in vogue among historians.[27]

Forging a new historiography

The new historiography to this area links the social and cultural history of science and medicine to the history of euthanasia and racial policy. There are a number of crucial features:

First, figuring in the victims as named and identified historical actors in their own right is the fundamental element of the new historiography. Here a life history approach to the thousands of overlooked victim lives has required large-scale reconstruction. Age, religion and ethnicity could all be factors in the selection of victims. This new approach to the victims coincided with an effort in the history of anatomy to identify the ca. 20,000 executed persons channelled to anatomical institutes.[28] Just as with euthanasia, in a proportion of cases – more pronounced in certain locations – there was a definite research element, again something to be captured in terms of motives, structures and material history.

Second, recovering victim narratives opens the door to understanding the conduct of experiments. Victims recorded experiences in terms of procedures, and how they came to be selected as suitable "material". Research subjects narrated incidents of coercive terror: the drawing of a pistol when a selected research subject protested against inclusion for a third set of experiments after surviving freezing water and malaria infection.[29] There were some false sets of twins, measuring equipment was tampered with and bacterial cultures were weakened to make them less harmful. Indeed, the saving of research records when they were meant to be destroyed was a form of resistance. Given all the evasion and sabotage, questions arise about the accuracy and scientific quality of results.

Third, there is a need to determine the outcomes of experiments from the victims' point of view. Exactly how many of the experiments were fatal, how many victims survived, how many victims were used for not just one but for two or three different experiments? What was not known about the coerced medical experiments and other forms of coerced research was their overall extent, and the numbers and identities of victims. Until now historians have focused on perpetrators and certain organisational aspects, with the victim seen as incidental and insignificant. The life histories of those caught up in the experiments appeared to contribute neither to the history of the organisation of experiments, nor to the wider history of the persons experimented on – Jews, Roma, Russians, the sick and disabled, etc. Such a basic issue has been left unanswered in the work of such as Kater on the *SS-Ahnenerbe*. Institutions with a continuing history in the Federal Republic of Germany have stopped short of transparency as to the victims of research that they sponsored. The research project directed by Rüdiger vom Bruch and Ulrich Herbert on the DFG did not analyse the extent that DFG (and associated *Reichsforschungsrat* projects) involved coercion and resulted in injuries and deaths of research subjects. Its memorial to victims was abstract and opaque. Quite exceptionally the Max Planck Society (MPG) President, Hubert Markl in June 2001 did apologise to a small group of surviving experimental victims, mainly Mengele twins. The inclusion of some other survivors gave the momentous occasion status as a general apology made by German science – just that other institutions did not take the opportunity to validate a magnanimous and significant gesture by full historical disclosure. The MPG itself did not reconstruct the totality of research victims: whether as regards the Mengele twins, or as regards its own stockpiling of brain sections in terms of the overall extent and the identities of victims. The brain pathologist Hugo Spatz received brains from Sigmund

Rascher's low-pressure experiments at Dachau concentration camp. Other institutions – for example the Robert Koch Institute (RKI) – did not seek a full disclosure regarding the identities of its experimental victims. In short the priority remained the perpetrators with the victims as incidental and anonymised. At the inaugurating of the RKI memorial, one victim received symbolic mention – but what should have been provided was a full reconstruction of the totality of victims.[30]

Fourth, it becomes necessary to rescue the experiments from their marginalised status in the historiography of National Socialism. For many years the coerced experiments have been at best accorded an incidental role by general historians interested in a grand narrative of the Holocaust. Attention shifted from medical experiments to the killings of psychiatric patients, euphemistically referred to by the Nazis as "euthanasia", as offering evidence of the first poison gassings of racial undesirables, the first occasion when Jews were killed by poison gas, and ultimately for transfer to staff and technology to the *Aktion Reinhardt* extermination camps in the east.[31] This left euthanasia as less a phenomenon to be investigated in its own right, than as a significant but also transitory phase in the shaping of the Holocaust. But the experiments receded to having a very minor element in the maelstrom of the violence and executions inflicted in concentration camps. Similarly, accounts of Nazi "euthanasia" all too often ignored the retention of brains for research.

Fifth, the gathering of basic biographical data allows the development of a structural approach to the coerced experiments, by aggregating the life history data on victims and perpetrators. This enables the overall placing of the experiments within wider events such as war – for example its radicalisation in the wake of the "Operation Barbarossa" campaign against the Soviet Union, pursuit of experiments to the end of the war, and the imposition of racial policy. On the perpetrator side, identifying those who had status on university faculties, and the extent of membership in the NSDAP, SA and SS answers very basic issues, correcting misconceptions in the historiography. Researchers gained access to the bodies arguing for an ulterior purpose – for example in terms of war aims such as night vision studies, or to complete an MD or Habilitation thesis. They claimed that they were allowing bodies not to go to waste, but that they were innocent of the actual killings. Against this, researchers actively selected victims for killing, such as the anatomist Kremer in Auschwitz delivering lethal injections. Russians, Jews and Sinti and Roma ("gypsies") were especially vulnerable.

Sixth, an overlooked dimension is that a counterpart and extension of any "life history" approach was what might be called "a death history" of the circumstances of killing in fatal experiments and the subsequent stockpiling and use of victim body parts. For others, the experiments – such as for the sterilisation victims in Block 10 or Mengele's twins in Auschwitz concentration camp – defined their incarceration, and for the executed persons such as the 86 "Jewish skeleton" victims killed by poison gas at the concentration camp of Natzweiler, their fate.

For "euthanasia" victims, it is necessary to reconstruct whose brains were retained for research, and the full history of the usage of body parts and tissues. The percentage of those whose brains were retained for research and their identities has still to be established. What emerges is a variety of locations and schemes, which need to be understood within a wider historical dynamic. Nazi "euthanasia" had various phases and elements with the development of a separate "child euthanasia" programme in special *Kinderfachabteilungen*. The extent that these "special children's units" had a research role has to be fully reconstructed. Moving from episodic studies – here Ernst Klee's eloquent but impressionistic historical writings are notable – to systematic reconstructions allowing a structural analysis.[32] The individual victim life history can be a telling and moving instance of the wider human exploitation for research. But the individual is not an endpoint in itself: what is required is a full reconstruction of all victims.

There are instances of supply of body parts like heterochromic (i.e., different coloured) Sinti eyes or fluids such as blood samples from Auschwitz to the Kaiser Wilhelm Institute for Anthropology. Such an analysis gives the individual life history additional significance by enabling reconstruction of timing, location, age, gender, religion and ethnicity. This allows identification of victims and in turn reveals multiple intersections with the Nazi pursuit of total war and the imposition of the Holocaust.

Seventh, it is necessary to recognise how a key role is taken by prisoners in intermediate positions such as in administration, research assistance and as prisoner nurses or prisoner doctors in the camp clinics, or *Krankenrevier*. The Revier were complex locations, and the extent to which research was conducted varied greatly, but needs to be figured in. There were high numbers of prisoner physicians in Auschwitz who had difficult tasks imposed on them: various categories of analysis such as of a "grey zone" have been applied.

Finally (and eighth), a key issue concerns location: post-war prosecutions as at the Nuremberg Medical Trial focused on criminal proceedings in con-centration camps. This was a pragmatic decision made by the Allies so as not to disrupt medical provision under occupation. But clinics (particularly in psychiatry) and also hospital clinics were major locations of experiments. Other locations were ghettoes and a wide variety of holding camps, which were all on occasion locations of experiments. It is also necessary to recognise that the experiments occurred unevenly in concentration camps, again due to the types of prisoners and the successive phases of the Holocaust.

The studies presented here indicate that there were higher numbers of victims than hitherto recognised, in diverse locations and circumstances. It is also necessary to look beyond the war's end in May 1945, when disclosures to the Allied occupation powers were only very partial, and the stockpiled body parts continued to be used for research. Researchers disconnected the circumstances of killing from their research, denying any link to the point that a researcher could be present at an execution and extract "fresh material" from the killed person: brains, eyes, spleens and ovaries were among the body parts collected for dissection or physiological or neuro-pathological research. In short, body parts were retained and were used for research from 1945 on into the 1980s.

A flawed historical narrative

Eugenics and "euthanasia" killings – both marginalised until the 1990s – have since then rightfully been given sustained historical attention, such as showing how the German medical profession mobilised for mass murder of the mentally ill, disabled and the elderly infirm. In part, this is part of a revised narrative of the origins of the Holocaust, which itself gained in historical recognition, as well as of power structures and categories of persons deemed undesirable from a reconstructed new Germany. "Expert" groups such as physicians attempted to extend their power in the spheres of race and gender, and on the other hand, the categories of groups deemed to be an undesirable burden on the racially "fit".

The outcomes included the first killings of Jews by poison gas. At first, the Allies sifting through the vast heaps of Third Reich documents thought the medical experiments were pilot studies for the mass killing by poison gas, but this was evidently not the case. Although there were momentous test gassings at the Brandenburg prison in January 1940 with 15 observers, at Auschwitz on 3 September 1941 and at Belzec in August 1942 and to trial the efficacy of poison gases. These tests were conducted without careful study of the metabolic effects of the gas apart from the quantity of the gas, number of victims and time taken. In this sense these were crude empirical tests rather than full-scale experiments involving multiple variables and calculations. At Brandenburg (witnesses included Karl Brandt, Leonardo Conti, Eberl) and Belzec (witnessed by the professor of hygiene Wilhelm Pfannenstiel and the technical expert Kurt Gerstein), medical experts were present, and details of the Auschwitz test are only that this happened, so that whether a camp doctor observed is not known. A distinction needs to be drawn between these rough and ready tests – certainly of significance – and the systemised requirements of a scientific experiment. Here additional resources were necessary in terms of camp compounds that were sometimes erected, instrumentation and staffing.

Grand narratives of Nazi Germany perfunctorily mention experiments, mainly by reference to Mengele, and similarly biographies of leading Nazis – notably Himmler – mention the experiments. Clearly Mengele had a key role in the implementation of the Holocaust in Auschwitz by selecting arrivals for (mostly) death rather or forced labour (effectively being worked to death). But his use of his gatekeeper role to sift out twins, dwarves and others of human genetic interest requires a more judicious interpretation than the incidental role in the narratives allows. What is missing is substantive evidence for centrally resourcing Mengele's research activities by Himmler and the SS. That the majority of Mengele's twins were Hungarian – arriving in Auschwitz only from mid-May 1944 – indicates that it was only a year after his arrival that his twin research could begin in earnest. Similarly, evidence from the sending of body parts derives from the pathologist, Miklós Nyiszli, who arrived in Auschwitz in June 1944. Only by resolving such intricacies can one then address basic historical issues such as structure, extent and motive. Here the experiments become a distinctive feature within the complex histories of the multi-functional camps denoted as "Auschwitz".

While most experiment victims were in Auschwitz between 1942 and 1944, the experiments occurred not only in concentration camps but also in clinics, prisoner of war camps and improvised detention centres (such as the Prater Sports Stadium in Vienna). The aim of this collection is to rescue the experiments and coerced research from marginalisation, and to investigate them as a wider ranging set of atrocities, involving policies, resources and people to a hitherto underestimated extent.

From 1945 to around 2000 the experiments were marginalised as "pseudo-science", and thereby disconnected from mainstream scientific and medical research structures under National Socialism. The experiments were associated with the idea of medicine "going mad", and disconnected from mainstream research and professional structures.[33] From 1951 German compensation authorities referred to "pseudo-science". This implied that the experiments were carried out by rabid Nazi fanatics, and that mainstream agencies and institutions were somehow immune. The successive phases of compensation with decentralised organisations in countries like Poland continued to use the phraseology of "pseudo-science". The idea that the experiments were a type of "pseudo-science" disconnected from mainstream medicine also came to pervade post-war prosecutions. The irony was that compensation agencies looked for structured analytical procedures in determining whether an intervention was an experiment.

Matters improved at the end of the 1990s in the shape of new projects on Nazi science. These dealt with how science intersected with racial policy. A major project was on the Kaiser Wilhelm Society under National Socialism. This achieved a colossal amount in terms of unravelling the perpetrating structures. It also published on the biographies of the dismissed and persecuted scientists. The MPG President offered an apology to victims, mainly surviving twins from Auschwitz.[34] But what this project failed to do was a full-scale reconstruction of the totality of twins let alone all victims of the experiments and coerced research conducted by the Kaiser Wilhelm Society and then on body parts retained by the MPG. Issues concerning brain research and other forms of research are explored in the final chapter, not least as taking the history forward into post-war Germany. Other projects that achieved much in terms of reconstructing administrative structures and scientific careers, also failed to identify fully victims. This dark spot was apparent in the failure of the DFG history project (*Forschungsgruppe zur Geschichte der DFG 1920–1970*) to reconstruct the extent that its extensive funding of human research involved coercion. It is not enough to simply identify whether Mengele or another concentration camp doctor was mentioned in one or another application, or to assess research in a sensitive area such as hereditary biology: all clinical and human research needed to be evaluated as coercive research at times took place in clinics. The DFG project left open the issue as to what extent the DFG funded ethical research within the guidelines of the period, and to what extent the research was exploitative. Similar blind spots can be seen with the project on the Robert Koch Institute under National Socialism when the coerced experiments were fully reconstructed as regards the involved scientists and institutional support, and yet not linked to identification of victims. Again, much was achieved in terms of reconstructing experiments and the perpetrating structures, but the victims were left an open issue, and seen as incidental. Similar efforts to assess "normal science" in dissertations show that a high degree of coercion was involved in normal research.[35]

Forensic investigations

Multiple types of unethical human subject research occurred under National Socialism. At first the coerced research was linked to the Nazi compulsory sterilization measures which began in 1934. The anthropologists Wolfgang Abel and Eugen Fischer were involved in the sterilisation of the mixed-race African and Asian German adolescents, stigmatised as the *Rheinlandbastarden* – a racial measure going beyond the law, and the children were held together and used as research objects. Some research was undertaken in psychiatric hospitals: a noted series of experiments was by the neurologist Schaltenbrand who tried to prove that multiple sclerosis was an infectious disease by cross injecting blood from psychiatric patients to apes. Research in concentration camps began only in 1939. Just prior to the war Sinti and Roma research increased enormously including studies in concentration camps. During the Second World War experiments rose immensely in 1942, prompted by military needs such as survival at sea, and epidemic problems on the Eastern Front. Prisoners clandestinely documented the coerced experiments, and (as at Auschwitz, Buchenwald and Dachau) saved records. On liberation former prisoners documented the effects of experiments. These included the sulphonamide experiments on 74 Polish women at Ravensbrück: many of these women resisted and evaded, and the camp prisoners showed solidarity and support.[36]

These efforts to document Nazi medical experiments had a profound impact on the Allied scientific intelligence and war crimes investigation teams during the immediate post-war aftermath. The British liberators of Bergen-Belsen encountered survivors of Auschwitz experiments. The Scientific Intelligence officer John W. Thompson conceived the idea of an inter-allied Scientific Commission to document all "Medical War Crimes" (he was the first to use the phrase), because he realised many perpetrators were either no longer alive or not in Allied hands. This documentation made possible The Medical Trial as the first of the US-administered successor trials at Nuremberg.[37] This was the only one of the successor trials at Nuremberg which relied extensively on victims' evidence.[38] At the same time, the scientific intelligence officer Thompson set out to document all coerced Nazi experiments as "medical war crimes" in an International Scientific Commission. The aim of fully documenting the experiments has been carried out by a comprehensive project reconstructing the life histories of victims. It is necessary to analyse the distinctive characteristics of each episode of coerced research, while placing them in a wider context.

Thompson alleged in November 1945 that the "sacrifice of humans as experimental subjects" was widespread, and "something like 90 per cent of the members of the medical profession at the highest level were involved . . .". [39] The idea of the experiments as arising from modern research procedures was stated by the head of the German medical delegation to the Medical Trial, Alexander Mitscherlich.[40] More recently, Volker Roelcke has articulated this potential of modern medical research.[41]

Identifying victims

After 1945 the voice of survivors continued to be heard. The surviving Ravensbrück "Rabbits" (a self-designation) were vociferous in defending their rights. Their name was a self-designation creating solidarity among themselves and with their fellow prisoners.[42] The suggestion that the term was imposed by the experimenters and is derogatory is a distortion arising from the one sided perpetrator oriented approach. Caroline Ferriday and the former Nuremberg Trials lawyer, Ben Ferencz took up their demands for obtaining financial compensation and access to surgical rehabilitation. This represented a noted solidarity between a Catholic and a Jewish lobby. As the Mengele victims grew up, the twins gained a voice with the Candles representative organisation, founded in 1985. The twins gained the interest of journalists, and it was only in the mid-1980s that 79 of the twins were eventually awarded compensation from the Federal German government, which set aside a million DM.[43] While it appeared at the time that this was the reward offered by the German government for finding Mengele (who by then was dead), it was just a normal amount offered in a long running compensation scheme.[44]

Journalists have written about survivor groups, bringing their identities into the open. Guenther Schwarberg of the *Stern* illustrated magazine identified the 20 children killed in the night of 20–21 April 1945.[45] The Tübingen journalist Hans-Joachim Lang also achieved notable documentation with the 86 "Jewish" (at least one was a baptised Protestant) skeleton victims.[46]

Their achievement in restoring identity stands in sharp contrast to anonymisation policies in Germany. From the 1980s documents have had names blanked out. Archives vary greatly in their procedures and in their interpretations of German archival law. Exhibitions have been unsystematic in displaying blacked out and named documents – such as the "Deadly Medicine" exhibition, mounted to much acclaim by the United States Holocaust Memorial Museum (USHMM).[47] There has been use of digitised documents so that the anonymisation is not visible.[48] There has also been the idea that the names of killed victims somehow needed to be protected. The policy in this collection is that if a name is anonymised, the reason – generally a requirement by the holding archive – is stated.

There is a clash of ethics. On the one hand, the ethic in Holocaust history since the 1990s has been the naming of victims. On the other, experiment and euthanasia victims have been commemorated only partially. From the 1990s many institutions sought to commemorate victims by erecting anonymised collective memorials, representing an achievement in disclosure of atrocity, albeit not taking matters to the level of the individual lives lost. The MPG in 1990 provided a collective memorial for victims, but sentiment is growing that victims should be individually named. The background is examined in the final chapter.

The historian has to weigh a range of problems. Injuries from the Nazi experiments vary in their severity. Given that victims were healthy, one can question whether it would be legitimate to regard the injuries as medical and so dictate a 75-year closure. It would be better to regard the injuries as a form of Nazi violence, and remove the anonymisation. Many victims have themselves spoken publicly of their experiences and injuries. In contrast to Holocaust victims, there is no collective public listing of "euthanasia" victims in Germany or Austria.[49] Indeed, placing such a listing in the public domain has been regarded as "illegal" in the German context, although at long last this situation appears to be changing.[50] Clearly, there is a difference between a living and killed victim, but why there has been such intense protectiveness around victims raises many issues. Important is a stigma of mental illness, which would mean that families of victims should understand that it is no shame to have had a relative killed in the context of Nazi "euthanasia" and that the victim's identity should be recognised rather than suppressed. It needs to be understood that diagnoses from the time were associated with much in the way of conjectures and suppositions, not least whether there was a hereditary component.

Naming is a considerable responsibility, and has to be done with meticulous attention to accuracy. The case of "Child K." is instructive. The historian of "euthanasia", Udo Benzenhöfer, made an identification of the child as disabled and dying at the time that parents appealed to Hitler. Benzenhöfer refrained from naming this supposed case as the initial cause of the Nazi decision to impose "euthanasia" measures. Based on Benzenhöfer's research (the latter has referred to this as "academic piracy") the victim was named (at first the name was according to Benzenhöfer incorrectly transcribed). However, the naming prompted the sister of the supposed first victim to point out a number of facts indicating that her brother could not have been the child in question. Benzenhöfer has then retracted the identification: one fact being that in the sister's opinion, her anti-Nazi parents would not have written to Hitler requesting that her brother be killed.[51] The situation is now that Benzenhöfer has retracted his initial "discovery", although for others the refuted naming and the associated identification still stands. More constructively, one might hope that accurate naming could open the door to a new generation of naming victims and memorialisation.

The rationale of the volume

These chapters represent a new wave of research and analysis concerning Nazi human experiments and coerced research.[52] For many years accounts of the experiments drew on the standard summary of the Nuremberg Medical Trial of 1946–47. This view was that the criminal experiments were limited to research in concentration camps, and carried out by SS doctors. The significance of the Medical Trial and its evidence was reasserted by the Annas and Grodin landmark collection on the Nuremberg Medical Trial, and a comprehensive edition of Trial documents published as a microfiche edition by the Saur Verlag.[53] Given that only 20 doctors and three SS officials could be prosecuted, the Medical Trial left many questions open and unresolved. In 1946 – at the prompting of the Royal Canadian Airforce scientific intelligence officer Squadron Leader (later Wing Commander) John Thompson – the British and French war crimes divisions established an International Scientific Commission to fully document all Nazi medical experiments.[54]

In the two decades since 1990 new areas of victim history have opened up: the history of the killings of psychiatric patients, and the persecution of the "gypsies" (Sinti and Roma), and the persecution of homosexuals. The experiences and significance of forced labourers have gained recognition in the Nazi war economy and human exploitation in occupation policies. Most recently, the history of anatomy has opened up questions concerning the rapid rise in executions and floods of bodies exploited for research and teaching. Experiments and coerced research were involved in the wide spectrum of victim groups, and add immensely to an understanding of what these groups underwent. We find for example research on foetuses obtained after forced abortions on slave labourers. These developments in understanding the extent that the Nazi "racial state" persecuted so many diverse groups has meant that the history of the coerced experiments greatly expanded.

The chapters in this book deliberately break with a top-down and institutionally restricted history of the experiments as limited to concentration camp experiments under the control of Himmler and the SS, as well as looking for implications beyond the collapse of Nazi Germany. The deadly experiments when research subjects were taken to the point of death indeed occurred. I have identified 554 such instances. These were part of a far wider spectrum of abusive coerced research. As John Thompson alleged in 1945, 95 per cent of the research by leading clinicians during the Second World War was criminal. The chapters here consider the experiments not in isolation but as involved with wider aspects of medical provision as it became caught up in the Nazi war economy. Some chapters indicate that even when experiments were authorised by the SS, researchers were opportunistic and retained considerable autonomy. The chapters as a whole show how the research took a variety of forms, and often was conducted autonomously outside the centralised structures of the SS.

The sacrifice of so many prisoners, patients and otherwise healthy people who were rounded up as detainees raises the wider issue of the identities of the research subjects: who were they, how did they feel, how many research subjects were there, and how many survived? This underworld of the victims of the elite science of German medical institutes and clinics has hardly been a historical concern. Jews were a target group, but so were "gypsies" (Sinti and Roma), the mentally ill, prisoners of war and partisans. Why, when and in what numbers did the scientists select one group rather than another? It is important to accord the research subject agency, and to reconstruct responses and experiential narratives. The Nazi experiments became iconic of the extreme of racial torture, representing one of the worst excesses under National Socialism.

The first section of the book deals with the parameters and rationales of the experiments. Volker Roelcke provides an ethical perspective as regards the codes of medical ethics prevailing in the period 1930–45. He focuses on the Reich Guidelines Concerning Human Experimentation of 1931. Significantly these guidelines (importantly falling short of being a law) required that non-therapeutic research be rendered impossible without consent. Although it has been suggested that the guidelines were not known, they were legally in force through the Nazi period, and even published in several major medical journals during the war. The chapter adds greatly to the documented instances of doctors referring to these guidelines. The conclusion is drawn that while there was clear awareness of the guidelines they were only erratically implemented.

Hans-Walter Schmuhl demonstrates in Chapter 3 how Nazi coerced sterilisation had implications for research, particularly in the field of psychiatry. The psychiatrist and advocate of racial hygiene, Ernst Rüdin forged strong linkages both to the Nazified public health structures, and to the psychiatric profession. This provided a basis not only for the implementing of coerced sterilisation but also for exploiting the new procedures for research ends. There was at the same time instability, as rival academic factions forged opposing alliances with feuding health officials. It was in this context that Rüdin saw euthanasia as a research opportunity. This can be seen in his 17-point research plan of 23 October 1942, which is analysed here. This was aimed to cultivate the fertility of "eternal Germany" by implementing ambitious programmes of both animal and human experiments to boost the nation's fertility. His aim was that a genetically based psychiatry and racial hygiene should determine which children should be eliminated. This manifesto indicated how euthanasia was regarded as a research opportunity.

Part Two examines how clinics became locations of coerced and exploitative research. Gabriele Czarnowski and Sabine Hildebrandt examine in Chapter 4 how victims of National Socialism became subject to coercive medical experiments not only in life, but their bodies were also used for *post-mortem* experiments. Collaborative experiments by the gynaecologist Karl Ehrhardt, chairman of gynaecology at the University Graz, and the anatomist Alfred Pischinger, chairman of embryology and histology there, were situated on the boundary of life and death. In 1941 both researchers published results on experiments performed on at least five 4- to 6-month foetuses, which had been surgically removed from the uteri of women undergoing a termination of pregnancy and sterilisation for medical or so-called "eugenic" reasons. These were forced procedures following verdicts by "Genetic Health Courts" based on the 1933 "Law for the Prevention of Hereditarily Diseased Offspring". One to three days before the planned surgery, Ehrhardt injected radiographic contrast media through the abdominal wall of the pregnant women for foetography. This method allowed him to visualise foetal organs and study their function via radiography in the women's womb and after removal of the foetus from the uterus. He concluded that foetuses were capable of breathing and drinking. Pischinger performed histological studies on the same foetuses but came to different conclusions. While confirming the drinking function, he found no clear evidence for foetal breathing, and suggested additional experiments on foetuses with intra-amnial injection of India ink, an experiment that had only been performed on animals before. Pischinger initiated a new set of human experiments, which were then performed by Ehrhardt in four further cases. However, the results were the same and Pischinger still found no definite proof for regular foetal breathing. This experiment on the physiology of human foetuses was unique among Pischinger's published work, as his true expertise was in the field of histochemistry. The foetal study is not listed in his official bibliography. For Ehrhardt, this human experiment was one among many other coercive studies performed on women during the Second World War. Pischinger and Ehrhardt made the planned death of the study- "subjects" part of their experimental design. The clinician Ehrhardt, whose traditional work was with the living, crossed the boundary to work with the dead, while the anatomist and embryologist Pischinger, whose traditional work was with the dead, crossed this boundary to work with the living. Under the conditions set by the National Socialist regime all manner of ethical transgressions became possible.

Raphael Toledano in Chapter 5 on the delivery of corpses examines the hitherto overlooked use of Russian prisoners for anatomical research. This study is focused on the anatomy institute at Strasbourg, which also had 86 Jews transported from Auschwitz and killed. The large numbers of Russian anatomical cadavers raises issues of the rationales for killing and the identities of the victims. Here important Russian sources are drawn on. The chapter shows how an academic department was inextricably involved in killing procedures.

Margit Berner in Chapter 6 deals with the role of Vienna anthropologists in taking facemasks of Jews. On 10 and 11 September 1939, directly after the start of the war, stateless and Polish Jews were arrested in Vienna following an order by the Chief of the Security Police, Reinhard Heydrich, within the framework of a Reich-wide action. Because the prisons were overcrowded, more than 1,000 men were interned in the Vienna Stadium. An eight-member anthropological commission led by Josef Wastl came from the Natural History Museum to the stadium and took the measurements of 440 men. Almost all of the men were photographed; the anthropologists took hair samples from

105, and made facemasks of 19. The numerous personal conversations, letters and telephone calls, but also documents such as postcards from the stadium, as well as personal chronicles, offer a glimpse into the stories of persecution, imprisonment and the measuring that took. This important information about the survivors and their relatives enabled Berner to partially reconstruct the events, and at the same time it informed discussions about how the museum collections could be dealt with in future. For survivors and their relatives, the documents and artefacts found in the Natural History Museum are personal memories. One survivor was Gershon Evan, formally Gustav Pimselstein. He was sixteen years old when he was picked as a research subject in the stadium by the anthropological commission. He still remembers being measured and having his facemask made. In his autobiography, which was published in 2000, he describes his feelings as an involuntary "scientific research object".

Herwig Czech in Chapter 7 considers the wider context of Vienna: to date, the only large-scale effort to shed light on unethical research practices at Vienna's Medical Faculty during National Socialism was a research project initiated by the university in 1997, after publicly voiced concerns that anatomist and former dean Eduard Pernkopf had used body parts of Nazi victims to create his famous topographical atlas. Although the commissioned report contained detailed studies of the use of victims' body parts at various university clinics and departments during and after the war, it was never published and the affair was quickly forgotten by the public. Furthermore, the mandate of the commission was limited to the question of the (mis-) use of human remains, so that the broader question of human experiments and coerced research was never properly addressed. Regarding other instances of unethical research practices documented in the literature, the involvement of Hans Eppinger and Wilhelm Beiglböck in the desalination experiments in Dachau is the most important example, along with the tuberculosis experiments on mentally handicapped children carried out at the Paediatric University Clinic. This chapter provides an overview of the current state of research, including recent findings on hitherto unknown experiments at various university clinics on methods of shock treatment, hypothermia and others.

Maike Rotzoll and Gerrit Hohendorf in Chapter 8 examine the Heidelberg "research department" of the "T-4" Nazi "euthanasia" agency. Here Rüdin arranged for his assistant Deussen to take charge of a clinical research programme on so-called "idiot" children. This was an exercise in "euthanasia"-related patient research. The Heidelberg professor of psychiatry Carl Schneider was deeply involved. The complete set of extensive patient records allows in-depth study of research aims, and also of the feelings and condition of the research subjects. The biography of the Heidelberg Professor of Psychiatry Carl Schneider (1891–1946) represents a combination of a quest for psychiatric reform, pronounced interest in brain research, and commitment to the first systematic extermination of a minority during the Nazi era, the murder of psychiatric patients. Guided by a biological concept that included the individual and his environment and thus interpreting the interactive and social sphere from a purely biological viewpoint, Schneider considered cure and extermination as two sides of the same coin. Psychiatric patients should receive intensive "biological" therapy, but if they were incurable and could not be integrated into society, they would lose their reason for existence also in the biological sense. This can be illustrated by Schneider's research department in Heidelberg (1943/1944) where 52 children and adolescents were subjected to an extensive diagnostic programme. At least 21 of these children were murdered in the name of research at the Eichberg psychiatric asylum.

Kamila Uzarczyk in Chapter 9 provides a case study of research at the Silesian psychiatric hospital of Loben. Psychiatrists (notably Buchalik) undertook phenol experiments on large numbers of children and adolescents. The patient records allow the research to be assessed, and linked to the testimonies of the very few children who survived. Psychological evaluation of children reported by various care institutions, orphanages and psychiatric clinics constituted an important field of investigation among Nazi medical researchers. Depending on the results of these coercive examinations, children were transferred either to the children's special care units (*Kinderfachabteilungen*), correctional institutions and juvenile reform schools, or recommended for *NS-Jugendheimstätten* and family care. The chapter focuses on the psychiatric-psychological evaluation of the children admitted to the *Jugendpsychiatrische Klinik* in Loben. It analyses examples of medical reports containing information on family background, intelligence tests and diagnostic tools used in the course of observation of the children.

The third section considers concentration camps. Astrid Ley in Chapter 10 considers how, as the war progressed, children increasingly became targets for infectious disease experiments, especially for hepatitis. Mengele was involved in selecting batches of children to be used for experiments on both hepatitis and tuberculosis. The chapter provides detailed consideration of how in Sachsenhausen in September 1944 experiments were conducted by Dohmen of the Robert Koch Institute, Berlin. The chapter brings together research records (notably of Dohmen), camp records and the recollections of the victims.

Aleksandra Loewenau in Chapter 11 focuses on a series of photographs of the Ravensbrück "Rabbits", the 74 Polish women used as coerced subjects for wound infection experiments as well as for deliberate leg fractures. The different contexts and aims of the photographs are reconstructed. These photos include a set of covert photos taken on 1 October 1944 of five of the "Rabbits" in the camp. In November 1945, 54 of the "Rabbits" were invited to the Gdańsk Medical Academy. The results were X-ray photos of a series of victim legs, and the chapter considers the cases of some of the bone experiment victims and the intention and context of the X-rays. On 17 December 1946, four of the surviving "Rabbits" were photographed in Nuremberg by the representative of the prosecution team. Two types of photographs were taken. The first technique used was the medical photography, when the focus was only on scarred limbs. In the second type of image, Dzido, Broel-Plater, Kuśmierczuk and Karolewska were presented in a more personal way. In other words, the "Rabbits" were facing the camera regardless if it was a front or a profile photo, which could be understood as giving the victims the face and the voice rather than presenting them as nameless statistics. Moreover, they were dressed only in white sheets, which covered just the private parts of their body. In addition, details, such as long hair, jewellery and slightly shy smile, regardless if it was intentional or not, gave these images a gender character. Strictly speaking, the "Rabbits" were not only presented as victims and witnesses but also as attractive, young and physically fragile. Here the outfit and body posture indicated the victim's relatively high social background and brought from family home good manners. These contexts are compared and considered as regards the image of the medical victim, as the "Rabbits" took on iconic status among the survivors.

Nichola Farron in Chapter 12 takes as her focus "Russian" or Soviet prisoners as research objects. This category covered a range of victims in terms of ethnic identity and status as prisoner of war, forced labourer or civilian. The central argument of this chapter is based on the starting point that, despite persistent neglect by scholars, there is substantial evidence and material to support research into this field. Further, the chapter demonstrates that the Soviet experience of Nazi medicine was not confined to concentration camps, but was geographically and institutionally spread across a wide spectrum of facilities both in the Reich and the occupied territories. An argument is presented to demonstrate that the Soviet experience of Nazi medicine was defined by the twin concepts of Robbery and Ruin. The chapter draws on records of the International Tracing Service and the Soviet Extraordinary Commission for Nazi Crimes.

Anna von Villiez in Chapter 13 focuses on the chest specialist Kurt Heißmeyer who conducted coerced and deadly experiments on tuberculosis in Neuengamme from summer 1944 to January 1945. While the story of his 20 child victims – known as the children of the Bullenhuser Damm – who had been transferred for him especially from Auschwitz and who were killed in April 1945 to disguise his doings have been extremely well documented, there has been next to nothing known about his adult victims. This chapter presents the results of a research project on this victim group, which reconstructed the biographies of the 34 victims known by name. The fact the adult victims of Heißmeyer have been neglected both in the public memory as well as in academic research is puzzling given the excellent source base. The rare case of original documentation from the experiments put together by Heißmeyer including case files on the victims with full medical documentation and even photographs make it even harder to grasp that these victims have never been named. The chapter explores three dimensions: a) Heißmeyer's research on tuberculosis in the context of Nazi medicine, b) the biographical research into the victims' lives and suffering during the experiments and c) the post-war history of Heißmeyer and history of remembrance of Heißmeyer's victims.

The fourth part of the volume opens up issues surrounding post-war prosecutions and legacies. Christian Bonah and Florian Schmaltz in Chapter 14 examine post-war prosecutions of medical war crimes. The chapter examines links between the Strasbourg Medical Faculty and the concentration camp of Natzweiler-Struthof in Alsace. The chapter reconstructs and analyses the convoluted efforts to prosecute the virologist Eugen Haagen for experiments on yellow fever and epidemic typhus, involving mainly Roma, deported from Auschwitz. The analysis is based on in-depth reconstruction of interrogations and court proceedings. It is shown how the French prosecutors' aims evolved, and how the Federal German agencies aimed to secure acquittal. The case became important for the defence of having acted on a scientifically rational basis, irrespective of ethical boundaries.

Michal Simunek in Chapter 15 examines post-war Czechoslovakia. Despite the high number of victims of the Nazi regime, who came from Czechoslovakia and were murdered in the concentration and death camps, relatively few witness reports and affidavits by imprisoned physicians were delivered for investigation purposes after the war. The aim of this contribution is to summarise the main characteristics of these reports and to set them in a proper context. Special attention is paid to links with the International Military Tribunal and to the limited possibilities of investigation, which Czechoslovak authorities faced in the immediately post-war period. Finally, the contribution describes a previously overlooked group of SS-physicians from Sudetenland who worked in the camps and some of whom participated in carrying out the medical experiments.

Chapter 16 examines the problematic legacies as regards victims of the experiments in the Federal Republic of Germany. Most victims survived but in a severely damaged state. From 1951 there was an entitlement to compensation, but the compensation procedures became traumatising as they involved renewed subjugation to German medical evaluation. Small sums of compensation, hardly enough for medical costs arising from the experiments, have been grudgingly doled out to victims by the Federal Republic. The compensation was never evidence-based in that German officials relied on highly selective prosecutions conducted by the Allies at Nuremberg. As a result, Mengele twins, who were intensively subjected to abusive and invasive research, were denied compensation by the Federal German Ministry of Finance on the basis that Mengele was not prosecuted at the International Criminal Tribunal at Nuremberg, and that his researches were anthropological rather than medical. The experiments were classified as "pseudo-science" of Nazi fanatics and the SS so obscuring links to mainstream German academia. A second set of issues relates to the stockpiled brains and bodies in German research institutes and medical departments. The continuing research on the bodies will be outlined. In 1989–90 an intense debate erupted in the Federal Republic of Germany over the status of anatomical specimens from the period of National Socialism. Pressure was brought on the German universities and research institutes to remove body parts. The solution was deemed rapid burial of all specimens whose provenance was in doubt. A range of options was considered, and the eventual decision to bury cremated remains was deemed the best way to draw a line under an uncomfortable past of Nazi medical atrocities. The aim was to achieve closure on this issue by a rapid "cleansing" of collections. However, identification of victims was left unresolved amidst the heated debates at the time.

Conclusions

There is much still to do in the fine analysis of reconstructing research atrocities, piecing together a structural analysis and in developing wider implications. The studies are stepping stones towards a more comprehensive analysis. Given the construction of a comprehensive, evidence-based database on the victims and perpetrators of the experiments, researchers can now draw on this data, while the data itself can be augmented and refined. The methodology of a comprehensive reconstruction of a victim group can be augmented and expanded to other victim groups: Sabine Hildebrandt is developing this approach for anatomical victims, and other groups such as psychiatric patients abused for research are to be comprehensively reconstructed. The methodology can be expanded to other persecuted Nazi groups such as Sinti and Rome, "asocials" and homosexuals. These are topics that reach deep into the history of Nazi Germany, of occupied territories and of the post-war history of the two Germanies. The implications of science and the Holocaust have yet to be fully taken on board.

Notes

1 Erica Dyck and Larry Stewart (eds), *The Use of Humans in Experiments*, Leiden: Brill, 2016.
2 Howard Brody, Sarah Leonard, Jing-Bao Nie and Paul Weindling, 'United States Responses to Japanese Wartime Inhuman Experimentation after World War II: National Security and Wartime Exigency', *Cambridge Quarterly of Healthcare Ethics*, 23.2 (2014), pp. 220–230.
3 Paul Julian Weindling, *Nazi Medicine and the Nuremberg Trials: From Medical War Crimes to Informed Consent*, Houndmills, Basingstoke: Palgrave Macmillan, 2004.
4 Ibid., pp. 126–132; Volker Roelcke, 'Between Professional Honor and Self-Reflection: The German Medical Association's Reluctance to Address Medical Malpractice during the National Socialist Era, ca. 1985–2012', in idem, Sascha Topp and Etienne Lepicard (eds), *Silence, Scapegoats, Self-Reflection: The Shadow of Nazi Medical Crimes on Medicine and Bioethics*, Göttingen: V&R unipress, 2014, pp. 243–278; Sabine Schleiermacher and Udo Schagen, 'Medizinische Forschung als Pseudowissenschaft; Selbstreinigungsrituale der Medizin nach den Nürnberger Ärzteprozess', in Dirk Rupnow, Veronika Lipphardt, Jens Thiel and Christina Wessely (eds), *Pseudowissenschaft, Konzeptionen von Nichtwissenschaftlichkeit in der Wissenschaftsgeschichte*, Frankfurt am Main: Suhrkamp, 2008.
5 Sabine Hildebrandt, *The Anatomy of Murder. Ethical Transgressions and Anatomical Science during the Third Reich*, New York: Berghahn, 2016.
6 Götz Aly, 'Der saubere und der schmutzige Fortschritt', in idem (ed.), *Reform und Gewissen. "Euthanasie" im Dienst des Fortschritts*, Berlin: Rotbuch Verlag, 1985, pp. 9–78. See also the publications of the neuropathologist Jürgen Peiffer, 'Neuropathology in

the Third Reich. Memorial to victims of National-Socialist atrocities in Germany who were used by medical science', *Brain Pathology*, 1(1991), pp. 125–131; idem, *Hirnforschung im Zwielicht: Beispiele verführbarer Wissenschaft aus der Zeit des Nationalsozialismus. Julius Hallervorden – H.-J. Scherer – Berthold Ostertag*, Husum: Matthiesen, 1997; idem, 'Assessing neuropathological research carried out on victims of the "euthanasia"-programme', *Medizinhistorisches Journal*, 34 (1999), pp. 339–356; idem, 'Neuropathologische Forschung an "Euthanasie"-Opfern in zwei Kaiser-Wilhelm-Instituten', in Doris Kaufmann (ed.), *Die Kaiser-Wilhelm-Gesellschaft im Nationalsozialismus: Bestandsaufnahme und Perspektiven der Forschung*, Göttingen: Wallstein, 2000, pp. 151–173; idem, 'Die Prosektur der brandenburgischen Landesanstalten und ihre Einbindung in die Tötungsaktionen', in Kristina Hübener (ed.), *Brandenburgische Heil- und Pflegeanstalten in der NS-Zeit*, Berlin: Be.bra, 2002, pp. 155–168.

7 Paul Weindling, '"Ressourcen" für medizinische Zwangsforschung, 1933–45', in Rüdiger Hachtmann, Florian Schmaltz and Sören Flachowsky (eds), *Ressourcenmobilisierung. Wissenschaftspolitik und Forschungspraxis im NS-Herrschaftssystem*, Göttingen: Wallstein, 2017, pp. 503–534; Florian Schmaltz, *Kampfstoff-Forschung im Nationalsozialismus. Zur Kooperation von Kaiser-Wilhelm-Instituten, Militär und Industrie*, Göttingen: Wallstein, 2005, pp. 175–177.

8 Paul Weindling, *Victims and Survivors of Nazi Human Experiments: Science and Suffering in the Holocaust*, London: Bloomsbury, 2014.

9 Idem, 'Genetik und Menschenversuche in Deutschland 1940–1960. Hans Nachtsheim, die Kaninchen von Dahlem und die Kinder vom Bullenhuser Damm', in Hans-Walter Schmuhl (ed.), *Rassenforschung an Kaiser-Wilhelm-Instituten vor und nach 1933*, Göttingen: Wallstein, 2003, pp. 245–274.

10 Hermann Langbein, *People in Auschwitz*, Chapel Hill: University of North Carolina Press, 2004, pp. 221–222.

11 Henri Lichtenberger, *L'Allemagne nouvelle*, Paris: Flammarion, 1936.

12 Albert Knoll, 'Humanexperimente im KZ Dachau: Die medizinischen Versuche Dr. Sigmund Raschers', *Beiträge zur Geschichte der nationalsozialistischen Verfolgung in Norddeutschland*, 13(2012), pp. 139–148.

13 Robert Proctor, *Racial Hygiene. Medicine under the Nazis*, Cambridge, MA: Harvard University Press, 1988; Paul Weindling, *Health, Race and German Politics between National Unification and Nazism, 1870–1945*, Cambridge: Cambridge University Press, 1989.

14 Michael Burleigh and Wolfgang Wipperman, *The Racial State. Germany 1933–1945*, Cambridge: Cambridge University Press, 1991.

15 Götz Aly and Susanne Heim, *Vordenker der Vernichtung: Auschwitz und die deutschen Pläne für eine neue europäische Ordnung*, Hamburg: Hoffmann und Campe, 1990; Götz Aly and Karl Heinz Roth, *Die restlose Erfassung. Volkszählen, Identifizieren, Aussondern im Nationalsozialismus*, Berlin: Rotbuch Verlag, 1984, rev. ed., Frankfurt am Main: S. Fischer, 2000.

16 Sören Flachowsky, *Von der Notgemeinschaft zum Reichsforschungsrat*, Stuttgart: Franz Steiner, 2008.

17 Mitchell Ash, 'Wissenschaft und Politik: Eine Beziehungsgeschichte im 20. Jahrhundert', *Archiv für Sozialgeschichte*, 50(2010), pp. 11–46. On the Faustian Pact, see Sheila Weiss, *The Nazi Symbiosis: Human Genetics and Politics During the Third Reich*, Chicago and London: University of Chicago Press, 2010 who echoes Weindling, *Health, Race and German Politics*, p. 538.

18 Volker Roelcke, 'Fortschritt ohne Rücksicht. Menschen als Versuchskaninchen bei den Sulfonamid-Experimenten im Konzentrationslager Ravensbrück', in Insa Eschebach and Astrid Ley (eds), *Geschlecht und Rasse in der NS Medizin*, Berlin: Metropol, 2012, pp. 101–114.

19 Weindling, Health, *Race and German Politics*, p. 574.

20 Idem, Anna von Villiez, Aleksandra Loewenau and Nichola Farron, 'The victims of unethical human experiments and coerced research under National Socialism', *Endeavour*, 40.1(2016), pp. 1–6.

21 Michael H. Kater, Das "Ahnenerbe" der SS 1935–1945. Ein Beitrag zur Kulturpolitik des Dritten Reiches, 4th ed., Munich: Oldenbourg, 2006; Julien Reitzenstein, Himmlers Forscher. Wehrwissenschaft und Medizinverbrechen im "Ahnenerbe" der SS, Paderborn: Verlag Ferdinand Schöningh, 2014.

22 Michael Burleigh, *The Third Reich. A New History*, London: Pan Macmillan, 2000, p. 804.

23 Richard Evans overlooks the importance of Udo Benzenhöfer, *Der Fall Leipzig (alias Fall "Kind Knauer") und die Planung der NS-"Kindereuthanasie"*, Münster: Klemm und Oelschläger, 2008.

24 Tobias Schmidt-Degenhard, Vermessen und Vernichten: der NS-"Zigeunerforscher" Robert Ritter, Stuttgart: Franz Steiner, 2012; Anne Sudrow, *Der Schuh im National-sozialismus. Eine Produktgeschichte im deutsch-britisch-amerikanischen Vergleich*, Göttingen: Wallstein, 2010; Christoph Kopke, Die "politisch denkende Gesundheitsführung". Ernst Günther Schenck (1904–98) und der Nationalsozialismus, PhD thesis, Berlin: Freie Universität, 2008; Weindling, *Victims and Survivors*; idem, von Villiez, Loewenau and Farron, 'Victims of unethical human experiments'; Paul Weindling, 'Consent, Care and Commemoration: the Nuremberg Medical Trial and its Legacies for Victims of Human Experiments", in Volker Roelcke, Sascha Topp and Etienne Lepicard (eds), *Silence, Scapegoats, Self-Reflection. The Shadow of Nazi Medical Crimes on Medicine and Bioethics*, Göttingen: V&R unipress, 2014, pp. 29–46.

25 Annette Hinz-Wessels, *Das Robert Koch-Institut im Nationalsozialismus*, Berlin: Kadmos, 2008.

26 Paul Weindling, Stephan Kolb, Volker Roelcke and Horst Seithe, 'Apologising for Nazi medicine: a constructive starting point', *The Lancet*, 380.9843 (2012), pp. 722–723; Volker Roelcke, 'Zwischen Standesehre und Selbstreflexion: Zur zögerlichen Thematisierung von medizinischem Fehlverhalten im Nationalsozialismus durch die Bundesärztekammer, ca. 1985 – 2012', in Stephan Braese and Dominik Groß (eds), *NS-Medizin und Öffentlichkeit: Formen der Aufarbeitung nach 1945*, Frankfurt am Main: Campus, 2015, pp. 133–176.

27 Ash, 'Wissenschaft und Politik', pp. 11–46.

28 Hildebrandt, *Anatomy of Murder*.

29 Weindling, *Victims and Survivors*, p. 204.

30 www.rki.de/DE/Content/Institut/Geschichte/Dokumente/Erinnerungszeichen_ Broschuere.pdf?__blob=publicationFile (accessed 14 July 2016).

31 Astrid Ley and Annette Hinz-Wessels (eds), *The "Euthanasia Institution" of Brandenburg an der Havel. Murder of the Ill and Handicapped during National Socialism*, Berlin: Metropol, 2012; Henry Friedlander, *The Origins of Nazi Genocide: From Euthanasia To The Final Solution*, Chapel Hill: University of North Carolina Press, 1995.

32 Ernst Klee, *Auschwitz, die NS-Medizin und ihre Opfer*, Frankfurt am Main: S. Fischer, 1997.

33 Arthur Caplan (ed.), *When Medicine Went Mad. Bioethics and the Holocaust*, Totowa: Humana Press, 1992; John J. Michalczyk, *Medicine, Ethics, and the Third Reich: Historical and Contemporary Issues*, Rowman & Littlefield, 1994.

34 Carola Sachse, *Die Verbindung nach Auschwitz: Biowissenschaften und Menschenversuche an Kaiser-Wilhelm-Instituten*. Dokumentation eines Symposiums im Juni 2001, Göttingen: Wallstein, 2003.

35 Volker Roelcke and Simon Duckheim, 'Medizinische Dissertationen aus der Zeit des Nationalsozialismus: Potential eines Quellenbestands und erste Ergebnisse zu "Alltag", Ethik und Mentalität der universitären medizinischen Forschung bis (und ab) 1945', *Medizinhistorisches Journal*, 49(2014), pp. 260–271.

36 Aleksandra Loewenau, *The Impact of Nazi Medical Experiments on Polish Inmates at Dachau, Auschwitz and Ravensbrück*, PhD thesis, Oxford: Oxford Brookes University, 2012.

37 Paul Weindling, *John W. Thompson. Psychiatrist in the Shadow of the Holocaust*, Rochester, NY: Rochester University Press, 2010, pp. 114–126.

38 Idem, *Nazi Medicine*; idem, 'Victims, Witnesses and the Ethical Legacy of the Nuremberg Medical Trial', in Kim Priemel and Alexa Stiller (eds), *Reassessing The Nuremberg Military Tribunals: Transitional Justice, Trial Narratives, and Historiography*, New York: Berghahn, 2014, pp. 74–103.

39 Weindling, *Thompson*, pp. 114–115.

40 Alexander Mitscherlich and Fred Mielke, *Wissenschaft ohne Menschlichkeit*, Heidelberg: Lambert Schneider, 1949; idem, *Doctors of Infamy: the Story of the Nazi Medical Crimes*, New York: Henry Schuman, 1949; idem, *Medizin ohne Menschlichkeit, Dokumente des Nürnberger Ärzteprozesses*, Frankfurt am Main: S. Fischer, 1960.

41 Volker Roelcke, 'Zwischen Standesehre und Selbstreflexion', pp. 133–176.

42 Loewenau, *Impact of Nazi Medical Experiments*.

43 Koblenz, Bundesarchiv Koblenz, Bundesministerium für Finanzen, B 126/121487.

44 Ibid., B 126/121487, Simon Wiesenthal to Bundeskanzler Kohl, 29 Nov 1985; Vienna, Simon Wiesenthal Archive, Mengele files.

45 Günther Schwarberg, *Meine zwanzig Kinder*, Göttingen: Steidl, 1996.

46 Hans-Joachim Lang, *Die Namen der Nummern. Wie es gelang, die 86 Opfer eines NS-Verbrechens zu identifizieren*, Hamburg: Hoffmann und Campe, 2004.

47 Paul Weindling, "Essay Review: 'Deadly Medicine. Creating the Master Race'. Exhibition at the United States Holocaust Memorial Museum, 2004 to October 2005", *Social History of Medicine*, 21.1(2008), pp. 208–212.

48 Thomas Beddies, *Im Gedenken der Kinder: die Kinderärzte und die Verbrechen an Kindern in der NS-Zeit – In memory of the children: Pediatricians and crimes against children in the Nazi period*, Berlin: Deutsche Gesellschaft für Kinder- und Jugendmedizin e.V., 2012.

49 Paul Weindling, ' "Jeder Mensch hat einen Name": Psychiatric Victims of Human Experiments under National Socialism', *Die Psychiatrie*, 7(2010), pp. 255–260; Georg Lilienthal, Elke Martin, Matthias Meissner and Paul Weindling, 'Erfahrungen von Historikern, Gedenkstätten und die Position des Bundesarchivs', in Gerrit Hohendorf, Stefan Raueiser, Michael von Cranach and Sybille von Tiedemann (eds), *Die "Euthanasie"-Opfer zwischen Stigmatisierung und Annerkennung*, Münster: Kontur, 2014, pp. 181–193.

50 www.iaapa.org.il/46024/claim_list_A.

51 Benzenhöfer, *Der Fall Leipzig*. This provides full details of what the author calls "academic piracy". Benzenhöfer accepts the mistaken original identification.

52 See www.pulse-project.org/node/572 (accessed 24 May 2016) for 19 podcasts on the topic at a symposium held in Oxford, 4–7 July 2013 on "Reassessing Nazi Human Experiments and Coerced Research, 1933–1945: New Findings, Interpretations and Problems". For further bibliography on medicine and the Holocaust see: www.medicine aftertheholocaust.org/wp-content/uploads/2014/09/appendices.pdf (accessed 24 May 2016); Sheldon Rubenfeld and Susan Benedict (eds), *Human Subjects Research After the Holocaust*, New York: Springer, 2014.

53 George J. Annas and Michael A. Grodin (eds), *The Nazi Doctors and the Nuremberg Code. Human Rights in Human Experimentation*, New York: Oxford University Press, 1992; Klaus Dörner, Angelika Ebbinghaus and Karsten Linne (eds), in cooperation with Karlheinz Roth and Paul Weindling, on behalf of the Stiftung für Sozialgeschichte des 20. Jahrhunderts, *The Nuremberg Medical Trial 1946/47. Transcripts, Material of the Prosecution and Defense. Related Documents. English Edition*, Microfiche ed., Munich: Saur, 1999.

54 Weindling, *John W. Thompson*, pp. 124–129, 152–156.

Bibliography

Archival sources

Austria

Vienna, Simon Wiesenthal Archive, Mengele files

Germany

Koblenz, Bundesarchiv Koblenz, Bundesministerium für Finanzen, B 126/121487

Literature

Aly, Götz, 'Der saubere und der schmutzige Fortschritt', in Götz Aly (ed.), *Reform und Gewissen. "Euthanasie" im Dienst des Fortschritts*, Berlin: Rotbuch Verlag, 1985, pp. 9–78

—— and Susanne Heim, Vordenker der Vernichtung: Auschwitz und die deutschen Pläne für eine neue europäische Ordnung, Hamburg: Hoffmann und Campe, 1990

—— and Karl Heinz Roth, *Die restlose Erfassung. Volkszählen, Identifizieren, Aussondern im Nationalsozialismus*, Berlin: Rotbuch Verlag, 1984, rev. ed., Frankfurt am Main: S. Fischer, 2000

Annas, George J. and Michael A. Grodin (eds), *The Nazi Doctors and the Nuremberg Code. Human Rights in Human Experimentation*, New York: Oxford University Press, 1992

Ash, Mitchell, 'Wissenschaft und Politik: Eine Beziehungsgeschichte im 20. Jahrhundert', *Archiv für Sozialgeschichte*, 50 (2010), pp. 11–46

Beddies, Thomas, *Im Gedenken der Kinder: die Kinderärzte und die Verbrechen an Kindern in der NS-Zeit – In memory of the children: Pediatricians and crimes against children in the Nazi period*, Berlin: Deutsche Gesellschaft für Kinder- und Jugendmedizin e.V., 2012

Benzenhöfer, Udo, *Der Fall Leipzig (alias Fall "Kind Knauer") und die Planung der NS-"Kindereuthanasie"*, Münster: Klemm und Oelschläger, 2008

Brody, Howard, Sarah Leonard, Jing-Bao Nie and Paul Weindling, 'United States Responses to Japanese Wartime Inhuman Experimentation after World War II: National Security and Wartime Exigency', *Cambridge Quarterly of Healthcare Ethics*, 23.2 (2014), pp. 220–230

Burleigh, Michael, *The Third Reich. A New History*, London: Pan Macmillan, 2000

—— and Wolfgang Wipperman, *The Racial State. Germany 1933–1945*, Cambridge: Cambridge University Press, 1991

Caplan, Arthur (ed.), *When Medicine Went Mad. Bioethics and the Holocaust*, Totowa: Humana Press, 1992

Dörner, Klaus, Angelika Ebbinghaus and Karsten Linne (eds), in cooperation with Karlheinz Roth and Paul Weindling, on behalf of the Stiftung für Sozialgeschichte des 20. Jahrhunderts, *The Nuremberg Medical Trial 1946/47. Transcripts, Material of the Prosecution and Defense. Related Documents. English Edition*, Microfiche ed., Munich: Saur, 1999

Dyck, Erica and Larry Stewart (eds), *The Use of Humans in Experiments*, Leiden: Brill, 2016

Flachowsky, Sören, *Von der Notgemeinschaft zum Reichsforschungsrat*, Stuttgart: Franz Steiner, 2008

Friedlander, Henry, *The Origins of Nazi Genocide: From Euthanasia To The Final Solution*, Chapel Hill: University of North Carolina Press, 1995

Hildebrandt, Sabine, *The Anatomy of Murder. Ethical Transgressions and Anatomical Science during the Third Reich*, New York: Berghahn, 2016

Hinz-Wessels, Annette, *Das Robert Koch-Institut im Nationalsozialismus*, Berlin: Kadmos, 2008

Kater, Michael H., *Das "Ahnenerbe" der SS 1935–1945. Ein Beitrag zur Kulturpolitik des Dritten Reiches*, 4th ed., Munich: Oldenbourg, 2006

Klee, Ernst, *Auschwitz, die NS-Medizin und ihre Opfer*, Frankfurt am Main: S. Fischer, 1997

Knoll, Albert, 'Humanexperimente im KZ Dachau: Die medizinischen Versuche Dr. Sigmund Raschers', *Beiträge zur Geschichte der nationalsozialistischen Verfolgung in Norddeutschland*, 13 (2012), pp. 139–148

Kopke, Christoph, *Die "politisch denkende Gesundheitsführung". Ernst Günther Schenck (1904–1998) und der Nationalsozialismus*, PhD thesis, Berlin: Freie Universität, 2008

Lang, Hans-Joachim, *Die Namen der Nummern. Wie es gelang, die 86 Opfer eines NS-Verbrechens zu identifizieren*, Hamburg: Hoffmann und Campe, 2004

Langbein, Hermann, *People in Auschwitz*, Chapel Hill: University of North Carolina Press, 2004

Ley, Astrid and Annette Hinz-Wessels (eds), *The "Euthanasia Institution" of Brandenburg an der Havel. Murder of the Ill and Handicapped during National Socialism*, Berlin: Metropol, 2012

Lichtenberger, Henri, *L'Allemagne nouvelle*, Paris: Flammarion, 1936

Lilienthal, Georg, Elke Martin, Matthias Meissner and Paul Weindling, 'Erfahrungen von Historikern, Gedenkstätten und die Position des Bundesarchivs', in Gerrit Hohendorf, Stefan Raueiser, Michael von Cranach and Sybille von Tiedemann (eds), *Die "Euthanasie"-Opfer zwischen Stigmatisierung und Annerkennung*, Münster: Kontur, 2014, pp. 181–193

Loewenau, Aleksandra, *The Impact of Nazi Medical Experiments on Polish Inmates at Dachau, Auschwitz and Ravensbrück*, PhD thesis, Oxford: Oxford Brookes University, 2012

Michalczyk, John J. (ed.), *Medicine, Ethics, and the Third Reich: Historical and Contemporary Issues*, Rowman & Littlefield, 1994

Mitscherlich, Alexander and Fred Mielke, *Wissenschaft ohne Menschlichkeit*, Heidelberg: Lambert Schneider, 1949

—— *Doctors of Infamy: the Story of the Nazi Medical Crimes*, New York: Henry Schuman, 1949

—— *Medizin ohne Menschlichkeit, Dokumente des Nürnberger Ärzteprozesses*, Frankfurt am Main: S. Fischer, 1960

Peiffer, Jürgen, 'Neuropathology in the Third Reich. Memorial to victims of National-Socialist atrocities in Germany who were used by medical science', *Brain Pathology*, 1 (1991), pp. 125–131

—— *Hirnforschung im Zwielicht: Beispiele verführbarer Wissenschaft aus der Zeit des Nationalsozialismus. Julius Hallervorden – H.-J. Scherer – Berthold Ostertag*, Husum: Matthiesen, 1997

—— 'Assessing neuropathological research carried out on victims of the "euthanasia"-programme', *Medizinhistorisches Journal*, 34(1999), pp. 339–356

—— 'Neuropathologische Forschung an "Euthanasie"-Opfern in zwei Kaiser-Wilhelm-Instituten', in Doris Kaufmann (ed.), *Die Kaiser-Wilhelm-Gesellschaft im Nationalsozialismus: Bestandsaufnahme und Perspektiven der Forschung*, Göttingen: Wallstein, 2000, pp. 151–173

—— 'Die Prosektur der brandenburgischen Landesanstalten und ihre Einbindung in die Tötungsaktionen', in Kristina Hübener (ed.), *Brandenburgische Heil- und Pflegeanstalten in der NS-Zeit*, Berlin: Be.bra, 2002, pp. 155–168

Proctor, Robert, *Racial Hygiene. Medicine under the Nazis*, Cambridge, MA: Harvard University Press, 1988

Reitzenstein, Julien, *Himmlers Forscher. Wehrwissenschaft und Medizinverbrechen im "Ahnenerbe" der SS*, Paderborn: Verlag Ferdinand Schöningh, 2014

Roelcke, Volker, 'Fortschritt ohne Rücksicht. Menschen als Versuchskaninchen bei den Sulfonamid-Experimenten im Konzentrationslager Ravensbrück', in Insa Eschebach and Astrid Ley (eds), *Geschlecht und Rasse in der NS Medizin*, Berlin: Metropol, 2012, pp. 101–114

—— 'Between professional honor and self-reflection: The German Medical Association's reluctance to address medical malpractice during the National Socialist era, ca. 1985–2012', in Volker Roelcke, Sascha Topp and Etienne Lepicard (eds), *Silence, Scapegoats, Self-Reflection: The Shadow of Nazi Medical Crimes on Medicine and Bioethics*, Göttingen: V&R unipress, 2014, pp. 243–278

—— 'Zwischen Standesehre und Selbstreflexion: Zur zögerlichen Thematisierung von medizinischem Fehlverhalten im Nationalsozialismus durch die Bundesärztekammer, ca. 1985 – 2012', in Stephan Braese and Dominik Groß (eds), *NS-Medizin und Öffentlichkeit: Formen der Aufarbeitung nach 1945*, Frankfurt am Main: Campus, 2015, pp. 133–176

—— and Simon Duckheim, 'Medizinische Dissertationen aus der Zeit des Nationalsozialismus: Potential eines Quellenbestands und erste Ergebnisse zu "Alltag", Ethik und Mentalität der universitären medizinischen Forschung bis (und ab) 1945', *Medizinhistorisches Journal*, 49(2014), pp. 260–271

Rubenfeld, Sheldon and Susan Benedict (eds), *Human Subjects Research After the Holocaust*, New York: Springer, 2014

Sachse, Carola, *Die Verbindung nach Auschwitz: Biowissenschaften und Menschenversuche an Kaiser-Wilhelm-Instituten. Dokumentation eines Symposiums im Juni 2001*, Göttingen: Wallstein, 2003

Schleiermacher, Sabine and Udo Schagen, 'Medizinische Forschung als Pseudowissenschaft; Selbstreinigungsrituale der Medizin nach den Nürnberger Ärzteprozess', in Dirk Rupnow, Veronika Lipphardt, Jens Thiel and Christina Wessely (eds), *Pseudowissenschaft, Konzeptionen von Nichtwissenschaftlichkeit in der Wissenschaftsgeschichte*, Frankfurt am Main: Suhrkamp, 2008

Schmaltz, Florian, *Kampfstoff-Forschung im Nationalsozialismus. Zur Kooperation von Kaiser-Wilhelm-Instituten, Militär und Industrie*, Göttingen: Wallstein, 2005

Schmidt-Degenhard, Tobias, *Vermessen und Vernichten: der NS-"Zigeunerforscher" Robert Ritter*, Stuttgart: Franz Steiner, 2012

Schwarberg, Günther, *Meine zwanzig Kinder*, Göttingen: Steidl, 1996

Sudrow, Anne, *Der Schuh im Nationalsozialismus. Eine Produktgeschichte im deutsch-britisch-amerikanischen Vergleich*, Göttingen: Wallstein, 2010

Weindling, Paul, *Health, Race and German Politics between National Unification and Nazism, 1870–1945*, Cambridge: Cambridge University Press, 1989

—— 'Genetik und Menschenversuche in Deutschland 1940–1960. Hans Nachtsheim, die Kaninchen von Dahlem und die Kinder vom Bullenhuser Damm', in Hans-Walter Schmuhl (ed.), *Rassenforschung an Kaiser-Wilhelm-Instituten vor und nach 1933*, Göttingen: Wallstein, 2003, pp. 245–274

—— *Nazi Medicine and the Nuremberg Trials: From Medical War Crimes to Informed Consent*, Houndmills, Basingstoke: Palgrave Macmillan, 2004

—— 'Essay review: 'Deadly medicine. Creating the master race'. Exhibition at the United States Holocaust Memorial Museum, 2004 to October 2005', *Social History of Medicine*, 21.1 (2008), pp. 208–212

—— ' "Jeder Mensch hat einen Name": Psychiatric Victims of Human Experiments under National Socialism', *Die Psychiatrie*, 7(2010), pp. 255–260

—— John W. Thompson. *Psychiatrist in the Shadow of the Holocaust*, Rochester, NY: Rochester University Press, 2010

—— 'Consent, Care and Commemoration: the Nuremberg Medical Trial and its Legacies for Victims of Human Experiments", in Volker Roelcke, Sascha Topp and Etienne Lepicard (eds), *Silence, Scapegoats, Self-Reflection. The Shadow of Nazi Medical Crimes on Medicine and Bioethics*, Göttingen: V&R unipress, 2014, pp. 29–46

—— *Victims and Survivors of Nazi Human Experiments: Science and Suffering in the Holocaust*, London: Bloomsbury, 2014

—— 'Victims, Witnesses and the Ethical Legacy of the Nuremberg Medical Trial', in Kim Priemel and Alexa Stiller (eds), *Reassessing The Nuremberg Military Tribunals: Transitional Justice, Trial Narratives, and Historiography*, New York: Berghahn, 2014, pp. 74–103

—— ' "Ressourcen" für medizinische Zwangsforschung, 1933–45', in Rüdiger Hachtmann, Florian Schmaltz and Sören Flachowsky (eds), *Ressourcenmobilisierung. Wissenschaftspolitik und Forschungspraxis im NS-Herrschaftssystem*, Göttingen: Wallstein, 2017

—— Stephan Kolb, Volker Roelcke and Horst Seithe, 'Apologising for Nazi medicine: a constructive starting point', *The Lancet*, 380.9843 (2012), pp. 722–723

—— Anna von Villiez, Aleksandra Loewenau and Nichola Farron, 'The victims of unethical human experiments and coerced research under National Socialism', *Endeavour*, 40.1 (2016), pp. 1–6

Weiss, Sheila, *The Nazi Symbiosis: Human Genetics and Politics During the Third Reich*, Chicago and London: University of Chicago Press, 2010

2 The use and abuse of medical research ethics

The German *Richtlinien*/guidelines for human subject research as an instrument for the protection of research subjects – and of medical science, ca. 1931–61/64

Volker Roelcke

Since the Nuremberg Medical Trial in 1946/47, the extent and inhumanity of biomedical research on human subjects during the Nazi period have been the cause of intense debates about the impact of political contexts on medical practice, the specificities of science under Nazism, and the dangers and limits of medical research in general.[1]

A long cherished stereotype about medicine during the Nazi period tried to explain the atrocities that became visible in the immediate post-war period with the claim that they were the result of "pseudoscience", or mere criminal acts of fanatic Nazi physicians under the guise of science.[2] However, the fact that 12 of the 20 physicians who were defendants at the Nuremberg Medical Trial were faculty members of the prestigious Berlin University Medical School may have cast serious doubts about the seemingly quick and easy explanation of the atrocities as "pseudoscience". Indeed, until the 1930s, the Berlin medical school had been a mecca of scientifically ambitious medical students and post-docs from all over the world, including the United States.[3] Johns Hopkins University Medical School, the contemporary model of US academic medicine as judged in the Flexner Report, was itself modelled on German medical schools, in particular the one in Berlin.

Being aware of these circumstances, the Heidelberg neurologist Alexander Mitscherlich, official observer of the West German Chambers of Physicians (*Arbeitsgemeinschaft der Westdeutschen Ärztekammern*) at the Nuremberg Medical Trial, diagnosed that the massive atrocities committed by renowned medical scientists had been the result of an aggressive search for truth, combined with servile obedience to a dictatorship. As a result, the individual suffering human being had become an object. He argued that the Trial was not just one of individual physicians, and murder, but of the dubious ethics of unbridled medical experimentation.[4] Somewhat earlier, in addressing the Nuremberg Trial against the "main war criminals" preceding the Medical Trial, Mitscherlich had posed the even more general question: "How could it happen that a society which perceived itself as a leading nation of culture (*Kulturnation*) lost respect for the dignity of its particularly weak and defenceless members, and made these human beings the object of economic and eugenic programs of optimisation?".[5]

In recent years, medical historiography has to a considerable degree confirmed and substantiated these early evaluations by Mitscherlich. It has been amply documented that many instances of medical research in Nazi concentration camps as well as in psychiatric institutions and hospitals in the German occupied territories, if judged in terms of the standards of the time, had scientific validity, or at least rationality, for the research aims or the applied methodology, while at the same time they ignored the subjectivity and suffering of the research subjects.[6]

These research activities cannot, therefore, be dismissed as having nothing to do with the professionalism of medical scientists. Rather, they point to profound issues about the ethics of human subject research. At the core of these issues is the following question: under what conditions are sane and rational medical scientists, trained in an internationally acclaimed system of academic medicine, prepared to prioritise their aim to produce new medical knowledge to such an extent that they completely disregard the subjectivity, suffering and indeed humanity of their research "objects"?[7] And if this specific value hierarchy of medical researchers was a relevant factor in the configuration of conditions leading to the medical atrocities, why should similar atrocities not occur today, particularly in contexts of legal de-regulation where scientists themselves decide on the limits of their research?

A frequent reply to these questions is the claim that "today, we have strict regulations for human subject research", which supposedly prevent such disregard of humanity, whereas it is assumed that there were no such regulations during the Nazi period. However, as a number of authors have pointed out, there existed state regulations on human experimentation issued by the German Reich's Ministry of the Interior in 1931. As Ruth Faden and Tom Beauchamp claim in their reference work on the history and theory of informed consent, these guidelines are widely considered "the first major document in the history of research ethics to deal with consent in a detailed manner".[8]

The German *Richtlinien*/"Guidelines for new therapies and human experimentation" of 1931

The "Guidelines for new therapies and human experimentation" (*Richtlinien für neuartige Heilbehandlung und für die Vornahme wissenschaftlicher Versuche am Menschen*) were the result of debates in the Reich's parliament and the Reich Health Council (*Reichsgesundheitsrat*) following various research scandals in the 1920s.[9] In these debates, physicians were criticised for their use of human subjects as research objects, their neglect of respect for patients, and their general ignorance regarding issues of medical ethics. The *Richtlinien* were drafted by the Reich Health Council in 1930, and validated by the Reich Ministry of the Interior. The Ministry also published the *Richtlinien* as a circular in the *Reichsgesundheitsblatt* (Bulletin of the Reich Health Office) in February 1931.[10] The *Richtlinien* were never formally invalidated, but in fact they were superseded by the Medicinal Product Act (*Arzneimittelgesetz*) of 1961, specifically by the amendments to § 21 passed in 1964, and by the Declaration of Helsinki of the World Medical Association, agreed in 1964.[11]

The origins of the Guidelines as a consequence of discussions on research scandals and inappropriate care being taken before the introduction of a new vaccine in the late Weimar Republic have been reconstructed in the dissertations of Steinmann (1975) and Reuland (2001).[12] Both authors clearly documented that these regulations had not been initiated by the medical profession or the research community, but were issued after critical public discussion and political debate in which individual physicians, in particular the social hygienist and member of the Reich's parliament Julius Moses had played a key role.[13]

Various authors have argued that the exact legal status of the *Richtlinien* remains unclear. The question of their validity was already an issue at the Nuremberg Trial. Andrew Ivy, one of the expert medical advisors to the Trial, referred to the *Richtlinien* as a contemporary legal regulation for medical researchers. Contradicting this, the defence counsel argued that the Guidelines had no force of law.[14] Along these opposing views, the *Richtlinien* have also been referred to in the historiographical and bioethical research literature. Several authors claimed that the guidelines had constituted a valid, enforceable law up to 1945,[15] whereas others were of the opinion that they had been only recommendations without any legal force. For example, Paul Weindling as well as Vollmann and Winau assume that these directives "were not binding in the legal sense".[16] Beyond the legal status, Ulf Schmidt claimed that the *Richtlinien* "failed to achieve wide circulation", and that "their influence on the profession remained almost negligible".[17] Weindling gives a more cautious, but similar evaluation stating that the guidelines most likely had no impact on research practice.[18] He also pointed to the "mythical status" of the guidelines, since they were used by both the prosecution and the defendants, but with varying interpretations, and for different ends.[19]

The following will address the questions around the legal status of the *Richtlinien*, their public circulation, and the various meanings ascribed to these regulations, as well as their practical impact – as far as this may be reconstructed. The guidelines, apparently, do not simply represent a clearly formulated set of norms addressing medical research on human subjects; rather, the meaning and importance ascribed to them changed in different contexts. A reconstruction and analysis of these changing references and activities related to these regulations may thus be seen as an example of a cultural history of ethical rules in medical research.

The following is divided into three parts. First, after a short summary of the *Richtlinien*'s content and legal status, issues of dissemination and implementation will be addressed for the period between their publication in 1931, and the end of the Nazi regime in 1945. Second, the use of the guidelines in the immediate post-war period will be described, both as a benchmark of research ethics, and an instrument of exculpation. Third, the outlines for a non-public discussion about the *Richtlinien* as an obstacle for efficient clinical research will be reconstructed, which may explain their disappearance from German medical ethics and law in the 1960s, instead of a potential legal enforcement.

Content, legal status, public circulation and implementation, 1931–45

Content and legal status

The *Richtlinien* contained a basic differentiation between innovative interventions and treatments serving a therapeutic purpose (*neuartige Heilbehandlung*) and non-therapeutic experimentation (*wissenschaftliche Versuche*). For these two categories of research, different kinds of informed consent were required:

> Innovative therapy may be carried out only after the subject or his legal representative has unambiguously consented to the procedure in the light of relevant information provided in advance. Where consent is refused, innovative therapy may be initiated only if it constitutes an urgent procedure to preserve life or prevent serious damage to health and previous consent could not be obtained under the circumstances.[20]

Non-therapeutic research ("scientific experimentation") was "prohibited in all cases where consent has not been given".[21] Experimentation involving children or minors under eighteen years of age was prohibited if it implied any risks for the child or minor. The guidelines also included the necessity of previous animal experimentation before any new intervention on human subjects, special protections for vulnerable subjects, the requirement of risk/benefit evaluation and of written documentation, including the purpose of the intervention, its justification and a statement that the subject or, where appropriate, his legal representative was provided with relevant information in advance and had given his consent.

Regarding the legal status of the *Richtlinien*, there were already doubts among contemporary lawyers on the possibility of implementing and enforcing the regulations.[22] In a recent statement (of 2013), the German Ministry of Health claimed that the *Richtlinien* only constituted rules for orientation, or recommendations that did not have the binding force of laws or decrees (*Verordnungen*). Thus, there existed no general obligation for all physicians to follow the guidelines, but only for those who had signed them.[23]

According to the historian of law Peter Collin, the term *Richtlinien* referred to a policy instrument, which originated during the First World War, but became more common during the Weimar Republic.[24] In contrast to a proper law, a decree or a statute, the category of *Richtlinien* was not consistently spelled out in legal theory, with clear and unequivocal implications for the range of validity. Such *Richtlinien* were implemented in very different contexts, they were issued not only by legislative or governmental authorities, but also by semi-state institutions (such as the *Reichskohlerat*/Reich Coal Council). Following this interpretation, the guidelines of 1931 did not constitute direct legal rules for medical research activities, but rather specified existing legal norms regarding physicians' behaviour. They formulated standards for the conduct of human subject research, similar to the formula "the state of science and technology" used in the context of technology law.

Public dissemination and implementation

As previously described by Reuland, the discussions in the Reich Health Council on the ethical issues and necessary limits of human subject research preceding the definite decision on the *Richtlinien* were published in the *Münchener Medizinische Wochenschrift*, one of the most widely circulated medical journals in Germany at the time.[25] Back in the late 1920s, the editor of the journal *Ethik*, physiologist Emil Abderhalden, had initiated a debate in the journal on the nature and limits of human subject research.[26] Immediately after the official decision of the Reich Health Council, the Reich Ministry of the Interior as the super-ordinated political instance published the *Richtlinien* in the official Bulletin of the Reich Health Office (*Reichsgesundheitsblatt*).[27] Within the next few weeks, the regulations were also published in the *Deutsche Medizinische Wochenschrift*, probably the most widely read medical weekly,[28] as well as in the journals *Ärztliche Mitteilungen*, *Deutsches Ärzteblatt* (official journal of the chambers of physicians), *Der Kassenarzt* (journal of the panel doctors of the statutory health insurances), *Die Volkswohlfahrt* (official bulletin of the Ministry of Social Welfare/*Volkswohlfahrt*), the *Zeitschrift für ärztliche Fortbildung*, and *Der Gesundheitslehrer*.[29]

Together, these journals probably reached a large proportion of medical practitioners and functionaries, as well as representatives of public health, and thereby, immediately after their publication, the new regulations quite likely came to the attention of many, if not most German physicians. As periodicals, some of them with a high publication frequency (weekly or monthly), these journals probably had a sharp peak in readership immediately after their publication, followed by a fairly low audience later on.

What is known about the public dissemination of the *Richtlinien* during the Nazi regime? As Thorsten Noack has pointed out, the full text of the guidelines was published in all editions of Carly Seyfarth's *Der Ärzte-Knigge*, a deontological introduction for medical students and young physicians. There, the guidelines were classified under the heading "Laws and Decrees" (*Gesetze und Verordnungen*), together with the Statutes of the Reich Chamber of Physicians (*Reichsärzteordnung*) of December 1935, and the Code of Conduct of the Reich Chamber of Physicians (*Berufsordnung für die deutschen Ärzte*) of November 1937.[30]

In addition to the repeated publication of the guidelines in the *Ärzte-Knigge*, the Professor of Hygiene at the University of Munich, Karl Kisskalt, referred to the preconditions for human subject research in the two editions of his textbook *Theorie und Praxis der medizinischen Forschung* (*Theory and Practice of Medical Research*, 1st ed. 1942, 2nd ed. 1944). He stressed the necessity for the informed consent of research subjects, however, without explicitly naming the *Richtlinien*.[31] Thus, in contrast to Ulf Schmidt's view,[32] the regulations and their core content were repeatedly published in various medical contexts and consecutive editions of widely read reference works, addressing young clinicians, as well as emerging and practicing medical researchers. In contrast, one of the few publications explicitly devoted to ethics in medicine during the Nazi period referred only vaguely to limits of "the scientific urge to research" (*wissenschaftlicher Forscherdrang*).[33]

However, the fact that the *Richtlinien* were readily available through publications does not necessarily imply that they were really known, or applied in the practice of medical research. Indeed, it is difficult to elucidate their practical impact, but there are a number of indicators that give some evidence.

Hans Reiter, from 1933 onwards director of the Reich Health Office (*Reichsgesundheitsamt*) and member of the Expert Committee for Population and Race Policy (*Sachverständigenbeirat für Bevölkerungs- und Rassenpolitik*) in the Reich Ministry of the Interior,[34] insisted on the implementation of the *Richtlinien* in two documented cases. The first was a controversy in 1937 between Reiter and researchers from the prestigious Robert Koch-Institute for Infectious Diseases (RKI) in Berlin.[35] All involved actors were apparently informed about the existence and the content of the *Richtlinien*; Professor Heinrich A. Gins and his assistant Georg Wenckebach, who wanted to organise a clinical trial of a newly developed serum against measles; Eugen Gildemeister, the director of the RKI, who submitted the proposal for the trial to the Reich Health Office, as well as the Berlin Central Health Office (*Hauptgesundheitsamt*), which had already accepted the trial (on convalescent children), and finally Hans Reiter, to whom the proposal was addressed. In his proposal, Gins had explicitly added a remark that the trial would be conducted in accordance with the *Richtlinien*. However, Reiter rejected the trial outright with the following sharp remark: "Trials on healthy children are unacceptable *under all circumstances* [emphasis in the original]! Why no self-experimentation!!".[36] As mentioned above, this qualification regarding trials on children was an integral requirement of the guidelines.

In another case of a request for a clinical trial from Halle University Medical School addressed to Reiter, he made detailed reference to some further preconditions listed in the *Richtlinien*, such as clearly documented approval by the director of the medical institution concerned. After these formal preconditions were fulfilled, Gildemeister – acting as deputy of Reiter – agreed to a revised application for the trial.[37]

These two documented cases illustrate that the *Richtlinien* were not ignored, or even explicitly dismissed by representatives of public institutions in the Nazi context. They rather indicate that a highly ranked Nazi medical functionary, race hygienist and NDSAP member since 1931 (that is, even before the Nazi takeover) was insisting on their implementation – as long as German citizens or children were concerned. This insistence by Reiter is in tune with the repeated reference to the necessity of informed consent of research subjects by Kisskalt, himself not only a professor of hygiene, but also a prominent race hygienist.

However, there is little evidence that the *Richtlinien* were generally followed and implemented in practice. A systematic analysis of the methodologies of clinical trials as documented in the most widely read medical journals during the Nazi period did not report any references to the regulations, nor – more generally – to the informed consent of the research subjects.[38] Further, the *Richtlinien* were not mentioned in any of the medical dissertations conducted at Giessen University Medical School between 1932 and 1951. Of the 771 medical theses completed in this period, 120 involved direct research interventions on human subjects. In no single dissertation was an explicit reference made to the *Richtlinien*, nor do they contain any documentation of informed consent by the research subjects or their legal representatives.[39] Further research is needed to establish whether – and to what extent – informed consent was documented in the records of patients who participated in medical experiments or clinical trials.[40]

1945–47/57: Instrument of exculpation

In the context of the Nuremberg Medical Trial 1946/47, the guidelines assumed a new role.[41] On 22 November 1946, immediately before the beginning of the trial, the Professor of Pharmacology at Heidelberg University Medical School Fritz Eichholtz approached Mitscherlich, the prospective official observer of the Trial delegated by the West German Chambers of Physicians and sent him the regulations. Only a few days later, on 30 November, Eichholtz' colleague, the retired head of the department of pharmacology in the Reich Health Office Eugen Rost,[42] sent a letter to Sir Henry Dale, also a pharmacologist, but in addition a former president of the Royal Society, Nobel laureate, and member of the British Committee on Medical War Crimes.[43] Rost opened the letter with a pathetic statement, saying that at this time when the German medical profession was being attacked in a devastating manner, he was pleased to find an opportunity to inform British colleagues "how the German physician really thought and still thinks about feelings of duty, compassion, and humanity, what is his Magna Charta" (a clumsy allusion to the British tradition of human rights, as Paul Weindling remarked).[44] Rost pointed to the *Richtlinien*, which he also sent as an attachment. His Heidelberg colleague Eichholtz had made the *Richtlinien* a topic during his lectures in the past summer semester, and would repeat this in the winter semester. Rost also mentioned that Wolfgang Heubner, professor of pharmacology in Berlin, shared his views about the regulations and their impact, and that he (Rost) had recently sent the guidelines to Heubner. Together, the three of them (Eichholtz, Heubner and Rost) wanted to let the British colleagues know "how seriously the German health administration took the duties of physicians", and "to document the self-evident ethical standards of German physicians – in contrast to those 23 accused at Nuremberg". Rost concluded with reminiscences of an occasion when he had visited Dale in London in 1934, and of another meeting in Zurich in 1938. In a short additional letter two days later, Rost expressed his wish to clarify that the *Richtlinien* had been binding for German physicians from their publication by authorities of the Reich in 1931 up to the present (1946).[45]

Rost and his two colleagues apparently knew that Dale was a member of the Committee on Medical War Crimes, which had been convened in September 1946 to adjudicate on the scientific value and ethics of the German medical experiments in the war context – but they were also aware that Dale, as Paul Weindling has pointed out, had been an "inveterate Germanophile" since his studies with Paul Ehrlich.[46] Their move to contact Dale on the collegial level of pharmacologists obviously was a very well thought out strategy. In his reply, Dale expressed his understanding for the concerns of the German colleagues, but refrained from formulating any further commitments.[47]

Beyond the immediate response, the initiative of Eichholtz and Rost had a somewhat more lasting effect. In February 1948 Dale drew the attention of Lord Moran, President of the Royal College of Physicians and speaker of the Scientific Committee for Germany to the *Richtlinien*. In his letter, he accepted the assertion of Rost and Eichholtz that all German scientists felt bound by the principle of the consent of the research subject.[48] Instead of imposing more political control and an explicit ethical framework on German medical science, Dale wanted the Western Allies to liberalise the legal structures for greater autonomy in medical research, and set up a German Medical Research Council (MRC) modelled on the British MRC. For that purpose, Dale had visited Germany and also established contacts to Detlev Bronk, chairman of the US National Research Council and previously (until 1946) chief of the Division of Aviation Medicine, Committee of Research of the Office of Scientific Research and Development of the US government.[49]

The strategic use of the guidelines as an instrument of exoneration, or exculpation is also suggested by their otherwise surprising appearance in the textbook of pharmacology (*Lehrbuch der Pharmakologie*) by Eichholtz in the post-war period. Whereas in the 3rd and 4th edition of the textbook published in 1944, there is no reference to the *Richtlinien*, they are mentioned with full title and bibliographical details in all post-war editions from 1947 up to 1957, albeit without any further comment and squeezed in at the very end of the index, at the very bottom of the book's last page.[50]

As the broad availability of the guidelines documents, as well as the insistence on their implementation by the director of the Reich Health Office, the missing reference to the regulations up to the end of the war in Eichholtz's textbook cannot be explained by their repression, or lacking validity during the Nazi period. Rather, the pharmacologist apparently perceived no need to relate any information on the regulations to his potential readers during the Nazi period, but changed his mind after attempting to draw the attention of prominent British physicians to the *Richtlinien* in the context of the Nuremberg Medical Trial. The reference to the regulations at the very end of the book without further details on their content, or explanation of their validity, suggests that the author's primary motivation was not to give a clear and consistent information to his readers on the content of the regulations and related issues, but rather to provide printed proof of his awareness of the guidelines.

At the Nuremberg Medical Trial itself, another voice also expressed the assumption that the *Richtlinien* had been binding legal regulations since 1931. The medical scientist Andrew Ivy, vice-president of the University of Illinois, former president of the American Physiological Association, and expert witness for the prosecution declared this in a statement on the ethics of human experimentation at the court in June 1947. As he explained, in the discussions preceding the trial, he had himself submitted three principles for the proper conduct of human experimentation to the House of Representatives of the American Medical Association (AMA) in December 1946; only afterwards had he received knowledge of the German regulations.[51] In the context of his statement, he referred to the *Richtlinien* to underline his broader claim that the three principles he had formulated and submitted to the AMA had been valid for the "medical profession over the civilized world generally".[52] Asked by defence counsel Fritz Sauter whether these rules had existed in print, as formally published norms in the US, Ivy replied that no such rules had existed for the AMA before 1946, but that "they were understood as a matter of common practice" in medical experimentation.[53]

Ivy had been nominated by the AMA to the "embryonic war crimes commission" (Weindling) in May 1946.[54] Being involved in human subject research himself, and familiar with the concerns of medical scientists, one of his central aims was to prevent publicity of the envisaged trial against German physicians from "stir[ring up] public opinion against the use of humans in any experimental manner whatsoever [so] that a hindrance will therefore result to the progress of science".[55] In a meeting with Judge Telford Taylor who was to become the Chief Counsel for the Medical Trial in early August 1946, Ivy suggested that "caution should be exercised in the release of publicity on the medical trials so that it would not jeopardize ethical experimentation". As Paul Weindling has documented, Taylor consequently introduced Ivy to John Anspacher who was in charge of public relations, to disseminate in public that there was a clear difference between ethical and unethical experimentation. Subsequently, in November 1946, an American press release from Nuremberg denounced the "inhuman experimentation program" that had violated the "ethical rules for human experimentation".[56]

Thus, in late 1946, Ivy was eager to demarcate the limits between ethical and unethical medical research on human subjects in order to avoid a public outcry and distrust in human subject research in general once the atrocities of German medical scientists became known. Being aware that no explicit rules on the relevant issues existed in the AMA, his strategy was to postulate a universal knowledge about such rules among physicians who undertook research. In the context of the trial, he clearly formulated this claim, using the *Richtlinien* to give it some empirical underpinning.

Contradicting Ivy, defence counsel Sauter tried to cast doubt on the supposedly universal acceptance of such rules on human subject research. His first argument consisted in the claim that the *Richtlinien* referred "not to experiments of all sorts, but only to experiments on patients in hospitals". For this differentiation, surprisingly, he did not point to the distinction between experiments and new forms of therapy made in the guidelines themselves, but rather to the fact that the introductory remarks of the regulations stated that the document was directed only to "doctors working in institutions for private or for medical welfare" who had to sign the regulations when they commenced work in such an institution.[57] His second, even stronger claim was that the guidelines had "never become a law", that they were "nothing but a draft, and remained merely a draft".[58]

1949: obstacle for clinical trials

The period immediately following the Nuremberg Trials was marked by attempts to "normalise" medical activities in the realm of clinical services, but also in research. In this context, medical researchers were not only concerned with their public image regarding the ethics of their investigative activities. At the same time, they were eager to safeguard their scope of action with regard to research, and to prevent the state from insisting on – as they perceived it – too narrow limitations on human subject research. Again, the *Richtlinien* were a relevant document, but now they were seen as an obstacle for proper research, rather than a symbol of the German medical scientist's "ethos". This very different perspective is represented in the correspondence between Heinrich Hörlein, representative of the pharmaceutical company IG Farben/ Bayer Leverkusen, and Paul Martini, professor of internal medicine at Bonn University Medical School and the first elected president of the German Association of Internal Medicine (*Deutsche Gesellschaft für Innere Medizin*) in the post-war period.

Hörlein, himself a trained chemist, was not only the director of pharmaceutical research at IG Farben/Bayer Leverkusen, a member of the managing board of the IG Farben concern and member of the Reich Health Council; he had also been one of the defendants at the Nuremberg IG Farben Trial 1947/48 where he was accused of involvement in human experimentation in concentration camps, and of responsibility for the development and production of war chemicals. In 1948, he was acquitted because it could not be proved that he had been aware of the production of Zyklon B, or the atrocious experiments.[59]

Martini had kept some distance from the more active party members on the academic staff at the Bonn medical school during the Nazi period. In the immediate post-war period, he was not only one of the leading figures in the German Association of Internal Medicine and chairman of its first national congress in Karlsruhe 1948. He was also the author of the leading reference work on the methodology of clinical trials (*Methodenlehre der Klinischen Forschung*, 1st ed. 1932, 2nd ed. 1947).

In a letter to Martini, dated 17 May 1949, Hörlein wrote: "... on page 10 of your *Methodenlehre* I read that for a [methodologically sound] trial of new drugs to exclude psychological factors it is essential that the setting include a 'blind' application, that is, an intake by research subjects without their knowledge". This, he argued, was in contrast with paragraph 5 of the *Richtlinien* of 1931 (the paragraph referring to informed consent). Hörlein went on: "This discrepancy played a role in the IG Farben Trial in which I – as director of the pharmaceutical research department of IG Farben – was to be branded [*gestempelt*] a war criminal". The prosecution had systematically translated the German term *(Heil-) Versuch* with the English term "experiment", rather than "test", although in all cases in question, the aim had been to evaluate drugs that had been thoroughly investigated using pharmacological methods.

> It took two expert witnesses (Prof. Butenandt, Tübingen, and Prof. Weese, Elberfeld) to clarify to the Court the difference between an experiment and a clinical trial. Fortunately, the Court did not know the *Richtlinien*, otherwise my situation would have been even more difficult. Resulting from this experience, I see in the *Richtlinien* a certain risk for clinicians involved in trials of new drugs – a risk that should be eliminated.[60]

Indeed, at the IG Farben Trial, the careful separation between *Versuch* and *Experiment* was crucial for the argumentation of the defence.[61] By defining the application of IG Farben drugs as an attempt to improve the condition of the individuals concerned, Hörlein (together with the witnesses supporting him) succeeded in explaining the delivery of the drugs in question to the camps. He claimed that after he had received information about the improper use of these drugs, he had stopped the deliveries – a claim which could not be disproved by the prosecution.

The move by Hörlein and his defence counsel Otto Nelte to invite the testimony of Adolf Butenandt, Nobel laureate and director of the prestigious Kaiser-Wilhelm-Institute for Biochemistry, as an expert witness apparently had the expected effect on the members of the Court.[62] In fact, the defendant and the invited expert witnesses used a core feature of modern medical research ethics – the distinction between experimental (i.e., non-therapeutic) and therapeutic research – for their apologetic purposes. This analytical distinction had been introduced – for the first time internationally – in explicit research regulations by the *Richtlinien*.[63] In his testimony for Hörlein, Butenandt elaborated in detail on this differentiation. He defined "human experiment" as a procedure where "danger for the body and life of the research subject is caused intentionally (e.g. by infection with a disease-causing agent)", whereas "the therapeutic trial is aimed at the avoidance of an already existing danger of life". In the case of an experiment, he argued, "it is self-evident that it is the duty of the experimenter to point out the dangers in all details", whereas in a therapeutic trial, "there might even exist serious reservations for the physician to inform the sick individual about an intended therapy, since in doing so, potential unpleasant, but innocuous side effects might impair the favorable effects of the drug by psychological reactions".[64]

Thus, both Hörlein and Butenandt used the analytical distinction introduced by the *Richtlinien*, but at the same time carefully avoided mentioning them explicitly (as indicated by Hörlein in his letter to Martini) – since that would imply to acknowledge that they made informed consent a requirement for both categories of human subject research. As a matter of fact, in actual research practice, this distinction was not that clear and exclusive as Hörlein and Butenandt suggested. For example, the drug trials carried out in concentration camps using new compounds produced by IG Farben, most notably in the context of research to combat typhoid fever, but also to improve the prognosis of infected war wounds, were certainly intended to test the efficacy and potential side effects of the new substances.[65] But the new knowledge to be gained by this research was clearly not intended to be of benefit for the research subjects themselves, but for German soldiers, or the German population in the context of the war. In quite a number of specific research settings – for example in the context of the Sulfonamide trials in Ravensbrück concentration camp – the conditions which were to be treated experimentally were systematically inflicted on previously healthy prisoners. The research subjects in the drug trials were indeed used like guinea pigs in laboratory experiments (quite consequently, one of the involved physicians used the term *Kaninchen*/rabbits for the victims).[66]

Let us return to the correspondence on the *Richtlinien* in 1949. In his response to Hörlein, Martini wrote:

> You are certainly right that article 5 [of the Guidelines] represents such a trap [*Fussangel*]. It contradicts our present *modus procedendi*, and if one would adhere to this rule, this would imply a severe hindrance for clinical therapeutic research. I have considered what should, and could be done to solve this problem. The present situation is perhaps not yet well suited to attack article 5. Certainly, a step in this direction would not be helpful and would meet with critical resonance in the public. But in general I am aware that something has to be done, and I shall approach the Ministry of Social Affairs which [in this matter] may most likely be seen as the successor to the Reich Ministry of the Interior. . . . Since this is an issue regarding research, I shall put this on the agenda of the German Research Council [*Deutscher Forschungsrat*] of which Herr Butenandt is also a member.[67]

For this kind of activity, Martini was in a privileged position. The new German federal government was established in Bonn in 1949, and as professor of internal medicine and director of the University Department of Internal Medicine, he had both official and private access to members of the new political establishment. Like Heisenberg and Butenandt, Martini was also a member of the newly established *Forschungsrat,* representing clinical medicine.[68]

Hörlein replied a few days later, apparently trying to boost the initiated development. He mentioned that during the Trial and with the help of his advocate, he had written a letter to Privy Council Rost who had been head of the pharmacological department at the Reich Health Office in 1931 when the *Richtlinien* were adopted, and to Professor Eichholtz who was a personal friend of his, and a former colleague at Bayer until his switch to an academic career. In spite of this close relationship, both Eichholtz and Rost were of the opinion that the Guidelines were of "extreme importance" (as they had written in a co-authored letter to Hörlein) in the present situation of German medicine, and therefore should not be questioned. Hörlein concluded his letter by stating that he was prepared to come to Bonn for a discussion of the relevant issues at Martini's convenience.[69]

With some delay, Martini answered:

> . . . considering your last letter, I am even more convinced that it will become necessary to correct the *Richtlinien.* They are really not compatible with clinical research, and for everybody who takes the *Richtlinien* seriously, such research is undermined. However, I am of the opinion that the present time is not suitable for two reasons: on the one hand, as a result of the experiences during the Nazi period, the minds are still so unfavourably sensitised that it would be easy for anybody, be it in government, or the parliament – even with inadequate reasons – to impede a change to the regulations. On the other hand, I am convinced that it will become ever more obvious in the near future in Germany that any unjustified restriction of research will also have most serious economic consequences . . .[70]

There is no evidence that Martini himself took any further initiative on the issue, nor that the German Research Council up to its fusion with the *Notgemeinschaft der Deutschen Wissenschaft* leading to the formation of the German Research Association (*Deutsche Forschungsgemeinschaft, DFG*) in 1951 formulated any recommendations regarding the *Richtlinien.* In fact, the Research Council did establish a "Commission on the Co-Responsibility of Science" (*Kommission zur Mitverantwortung der Wissenschaft*) in response to the "abuse of medical research during the Third Reich" and "the application of the results of research in the natural sciences for purposes of armament". However, neither Martini nor Butenandt were among the members of this commission, and as far as this can be reconstructed, no decision was taken on medical issues.[71]

Conclusion

The German *Richtlinien* of 1931 were an early normative document on the ethical issues of human subject research. They addressed questions of informed consent, documentation, research on minors and exploitation of vulnerable individuals, and introduced the analytical distinction between therapeutic and non-therapeutic research.

From their promulgation onwards, their legal status was vaguely defined, and certainly not that of a binding law. Rather, they represented a reference for the ethical standards of medical research, which was binding only for those physicians who had signed this code of conduct at the commencement of their contract to work in public hospitals. The guidelines were widely disseminated in medical and public health journals with high circulation in the late Weimar Republic. In the Nazi period, the *Richtlinien* were not simply ignored, or even explicitly dismissed by representatives of the regime or medical institutions. In fact, they were regularly reprinted in full in the consecutive editions of a widely read compendium for young physicians and thus easily available, and their core principle of informed consent was also clearly spelled out in two editions of an introductory textbook on medical research. It is also documented that the director of the Reich Health Office, Hans Reiter, insisted on their implementation – in cases where German citizens or children were concerned. There is, however, lacking evidence of their general implementation in "normal" medical research at university medical schools before the Second World War (which may, of course, be due to the lack of historical sources). In contrast to their public dissemination and the documented instances of implementation with regard to "regular" German citizens before the war, the guidelines were clearly disregarded in the contexts of coerced research on vulnerable groups in concentration camps, psychiatric asylums and hospitals in the occupied territories, that is, in spaces of de facto "de-regulated" research where physicians could carry out any kind of research they considered rational to resolve relevant, or even urgent issues, irrespective of the consent, or welfare of the research subjects.

Thus, the historical evidence documents that the *Richtlinien* were not merely a legal fact. Rather, on one level, they represented a set of ethical norms, and rules with limited legal validity. In this respect, they may be considered as a regulative instrument intended to protect research subjects.

On another level, the guidelines may be seen as an instrument to enable the continuation and protection of human subject research in the face of grave public concerns about the motivations and actual behaviour of medical researchers. This function of the *Richtlinien* is already apparent in their origins during the late Weimar Republic. Here, intra-professional, but in particular public debates about scandals of medical research and the implementation of new, non-routine prophylactic interventions were decisive in the formation and promulgation of the guidelines, the very first paragraph of which argues that regulation of medical research is essential to enable the progress of medical science. This progress was not justified any further; it was apparently seen as an end in itself.

This function of the *Richtlinien* – to protect medical science – became even more obvious in the period after the Second World War. At the Nuremberg Medical Trial, highly ranked representatives of German medical science were indicted. The concerns formulated by leading British and US medical researchers such as Nobel-laureate Henry Dale, and the AMA-delegate to the trial Andrew Ivy, document that the trial and public debates that might potentially emerge from it were seen to be not only a problem for German medicine, but to threaten public confidence in the ethics of medical human subject research in general. In various communicative contexts, including the Medical Trial itself, and addressing medical colleagues as well as political instances or the public, Dale and Ivy used the *Richtlinien* to show that explicit German and international standards of human subject research did exist, that these had been binding for German medical scientists as well, and that it had only been a few individual physicians who – reacting to outside political contexts – had violated them. The purpose of this argumentation was to protect the freedom of future medical research from state interference. Similarly, a group of prominent German medical scientists used references to the supposedly legally binding *Richtlinien* to argue that state regulations had existed starting in 1931, and throughout the Nazi period, and that – apart from the 20 medical defendants at Nuremberg – the large majority of German physicians had behaved in an ethical manner.

The common denominator of the remarkable interest of prominent German, British and US-American representatives of medical research in the *Richtlinien* was their aim to safeguard the public image of scientific medicine in Germany and on the international level, and to enable the continuation, and indeed extension of clinical research – not least for economic reasons. The communication between Paul Martini as prominent representative of German medicine, and Heinrich Hörlein as member of the board of directors of IG Farben/Bayer Leverkusen in 1949 underlines this common interest of medical scientists and pharmaceutical industry, but now – ironically – referring to the *Richtlinien* with their strict rules for informed research as a hindrance for the development of drug trials in clinical medicine. Accordingly, both Hörlein and Martini agreed that efforts should be taken on a political level to soften the requirements for informed consent in human subject research.

Notes

1 George Annas and Michael Grodin (eds), *The Nazi Doctors and the Nuremberg Medical Trial: Human Rights in Human Experimentation*, New York and Oxford: Oxford University Press, 1992; Michael Marrus, 'The Nuremberg doctors' trial in historical context', *Bulletin of the History of Medicine*, 73 (1999), pp. 106–123; Christian Bonah, Etienne Lepicard and Volker Roelcke (eds), *La médecine expérimentale au tribunal. Implications éthiques de quelques procès médicaux du XXe siècle européen*, Paris: Éditions des Archives Contemporaines, 2003; Paul J. Weindling, *Nazi Medicine and the Nuremberg Trial*, Houndmills, Basingstoke: Palgrave Macmillan, 2004.

2 See, for example, Nava Cohen, 'Medical experiments', in Israel Gutman (ed.), *Encyclopedia of the Holocaust*, New York: Macmillan, 1990, pp. 957–966; Klaus-D. Henke, 'Einleitung', in idem (ed.), *Tödliche Medizin im Nationalsozialismus. Von der Rassenhygiene zum Massenmord*, Cologne: Böhlau, 2008, p. 9; Winfried Süß, 'Versuche der Wiedergut-machung', in Robert Jütte (ed.) *Medizin und Nationalsozialismus*, Göttingen: Wallstein, 2011, p. 285.

3 Thomas Neville Bonner, *Becoming a Physician. Medical Education in Britain, France, Germany, and the United States, 1750–1945*, Oxford and New York: Oxford University Press, 1995.

4 Alexander Mitscherlich and Fred Mielke (eds), *Medizin ohne Menschlichkeit*, Frankfurt am Main: S. Fischer 1960, Vorwort (Preface).

5 Alexander Mitscherlich, 'Geschichtsschreibung und Psychoanalyse. Gedanken zum Nürnberger Prozess', *Schweizer Annalen*, 11 (1945), pp. 604–613.

6 Compare, for instance, the research in the context of aviation medicine at the Dachau camp in Karl Heinz Roth, 'Tödliche Höhen. Die Unterdruckkammer-Experimente im Konzentrationslager Dachau und ihre Bedeutung für die luftfahrtmedizinische Forschung des "Dritten Reichs" ', in Angelika Ebbinghaus and Klaus Dörner (eds), *Vernichten und Heilen. Der Nürnberger Ärzteprozess und seine Folgen*, Berlin: Aufbau, 2001, pp. 110–151; on the eugenically motivated genetic research of Josef Mengele, see Benoît Massin, 'Mengele, die Zwillingsforschung und die "Auschwitz-Dahlem Connection" ', in Carola Sachse (ed.), *Die Verbindung nach Auschwitz. Biowissenschaften und Menschenversuche an Kaiser-Wilhelm-Institute*, Göttingen: Wallstein, 2003, pp. 201–254; on genetic research in the context of psychiatry, see Volker Roelcke, Gerrit Hohendorf and Maike Rotzoll, 'Psychiatric Research and "Euthanasia". The case of the psychiatric department at the University of Heidelberg, 1941–1945', *History of Psychiatry*, 5(1994), pp. 517–532; and Volker Roelcke, 'Psychiatrische Wissenschaft im Kontext nationalsozialistischer Politik und "Euthanasie": Zur Rolle von Ernst Rüdin und der *Deutschen Forschungsanstalt/Kaiser-Wilhelm-Institut für Psychiatrie*', in Doris Kaufmann (ed.), *Die Kaiser-Wilhelm-Gesellschaft im Nationalsozialismus: Bestandsaufnahme und Perspektiven der Forschung*, Göttingen: Wallstein, 2000, pp. 112–150. For various examples and aspects of bacteriological research, see Paul Julian Weindling. *Epidemics and Genocide in Eastern Europe, 1890–1945*, Oxford: Oxford University Press, 2000; and Wolfgang U. Eckart (ed.), *Man, Medicine, and the State. The Human Body as an Object of Government Sponsored Medical Research in the 20th Century*, Stuttgart: Franz Steiner, 2006; for a recent overview, see Paul Weindling, *Victims and Survivors of Nazi Human Experiments. Science and Suffering in the Holocaust*, London: Bloomsbury, 2015.

7 For an extreme and exemplary case of scientific rationality combined with complete disregard of humanity, see Volker Roelcke, 'Sulfonamide Experiments on Prisoners in Nazi Concentration Camps: Coherent Scientific Rationality Combined with Complete Disregard of Humanity', in Sheldon Rubenfeld and Susan Benedict (eds), *Human Subjects Research after the Holocaust*, Cham: Springer, 2014, pp. 51–66.

8 Ruth Faden and Tom Beauchamp, *A History and Theory of Informed Consent*, New York and Oxford: Oxford University Press, 1986, p. 154.

9 For the debates leading to the *Richtlinien*, see Reinhard Steinmann, *Die Debatte über medizinische Versuche am Menschen in der Weimarer Zeit*, MD thesis, Tübingen: Eberhard Karls University, 1975; Andreas Reuland, *Humanexperimente in der Weimarer Republik und Julius Moses ' "Kampf gegen die Experimentierwut"*, Norderstedt: Books on Demand 2004; Christian Bonah, 'Le drame de Lübeck: La vaccination BCG, le "procès Calmette" et les *Richtlinien* de 1931', in idem, Lepicard and Roelcke, *La médecine expérimentale*, pp. 65–94; and Andreas Frewer, *Medizin und Moral in Weimarer Republik und Nationalsozialismus: Die Zeitschrift "Ethik" unter Emil Abderhalden*, Frankfurt am Main: Campus, 2000, where the debates in the journal *Ethik* preceding the passing of the *Richtlinien* are described.

10 'Richtlinien für neuartige Heilbehandlung und für die Vornahme wissenschaftlicher Versuche am Menschen [Rundschreiben des Reichsministers des Inneren, 28. February 1931]', *Reichsgesundheitsblatt*, 55.6 (1931), pp. 174–175; English translation in Hans-Martin Sass, '*Reichsrundschreiben* 1931: Pre-Nuremberg German Regulation Concerning New Therapy and Experimentation', *Journal of Medicine and Philosophy*, 8(1983), pp. 99–111; as well as Michael Grodin, 'Historical Origins of the Nuremberg Code', in George Annas and Michael Grodin (eds), *The Nazi Doctors and the Nuremberg Medical Trial: Human Rights in Human Experimentation*, New York and Oxford: Oxford University Press, 1992, pp. 121–144.

11 Horst Hasskarl and Hellmuth Kleinsorge, Arzneimittelprüfung, Arzneimittelrecht. Nationale und internationale Bestimmungen und Empfehlungen, Stuttgart: Gustav Fischer, 1974, p. 3.

12 Steinmann, *Debatte*; Reuland, *Humanexperimente*; see also Norman Howard-Jones, 'Human Experimentation in Historical and Ethical Perspective', *Social Science and Medicine*, 16(1982), pp. 1429–1448.

13 See also Jochen Vollmann and Rolf Winau, 'Informed consent in human experimentation before the Nuremberg Code', *British Medical Journal*, 313 (1996), pp. 1445–1449; on the key role of Julius Moses, see Daniel Nadav, 'The "Death Dance" of Lübeck: Julius Moses and the German Guidelines for Human Experimentation', in Volker Roelcke and Giovanni Maio (eds), *Twentieth-Century Ethics of Human Subject Research*, Stuttgart: Franz Steiner, 2004, pp. 129–136.

14 Grodin, 'Historical Origins'.

15 The most prominent example is Faden and Beauchamp, *History and Theory*, p. 154; see also Sass, '*Reichsrundschreiben*'; Sev Fluss, as quoted in Grodin, 'Historical Origins', p. 142n34. Interestingly, all these authors are bioethicists; the homepage of the German Medical Association (*Bundesärztekammer*) until today claims that the *Richtlinien* were binding law: Christoph Fuchs and Thomas Gerst, 'Medizinethik in der Berufsordnung: Entwicklungen der Muster-Berufsordnung', www.bundesaerztekammer.de/recht/ berufsrecht/muster-berufsordnung-aerzte/medizinethik-in-der-berufsordnung/ (accessed 25 April 2016).

16 Vollmann and Winau, 'Informed consent'; similar Weindling, *Victims*, p. 19.

17 Ulf Schmidt, *Justice at Nuremberg: Leo Alexander and the Nazi Doctors' Trial*, Houndmills, Basingstoke: Palgrave Macmillan, 2004, p. 13.

18 Weindling, *Nazi Medicine*, pp. 259–260.

19 Ibid., 260.

20 'Richtlinien', p. 174 (translation according to Grodin, 'Historical Origins', p. 130).

21 Ibid.

22 J[akob] R[ichard] Spinner, 'Wie kann und soll der Laie gegen den üblen Ausgang ärztlicher Experimente geschützt werden', *Der Kassenarzt*, 7 (23 Aug 1930), pp. 5–8.

23 Bundesministerium für Gesundheit to author, 29 Aug 2013.

24 Peter Collin (Max-Planck-Institute for the History of European Law, Frankfurt am Main), e-mails to author, 24 and 28 Sept 2015; I am grateful to Peter Collin for providing this evaluation.

25 See Friedrich Müller, 'Die Zulässigkeit ärztlicher Versuche an gesunden und kranken Menschen: I.', *Münchener Medizinische Wochenschrift* (1931), pp. 104–107; Alfons Stauder, 'Die Zulässigkeit ärztlicher Versuche an gesunden und kranken Menschen: II.', *Münchener Medizinische Wochenschrift* (1931), pp. 107–112; on the *Münchener Medizinische Wochenschrift*, see Christina Rohner, *Medizin und politische Ideologie im Spiegel der MMW und der DMW 1923, 1928, 1933 und 1938*, PhD thesis, Zürich: University of Zürich, 1995; Sigrid Stöckel, 'Veränderungen des Genres "Medizinische Wochenschrift"? Deutsche Medizinische Wochenschrift, Münchener Medizinische Wochenschrift und The Lancet im Vergleich', in eadem, Gerlind Rüve and Wiebke Liesner (eds), *Das Medium Wissenschaftszeitschrift seit dem 19. Jahrhundert*, Stuttgart: Franz Steiner, 2009, pp. 139–162.

26 Frewer, *Medizin und Moral*.

27 'Richtlinien'.

28 On the *Deutsche Medizinische Wochenschrift*, see Rohner, *Medizin und politische Ideologie*, and Stöckel, 'Veränderungen des Genres'.

29 *Deutsche Medizinische Wochenschrift*, 57 (1931), p. 509; *Deutsches Ärzteblatt* (1931), pp. 147–148; *Ärztliche Mitteilungen* (1931), p. 208; *Der Kassenarzt* (28 Mar 1931), pp. 3–4; *Zeitschrift für ärztliche Fortbildung* (1931), p. 300; *Der Gesundheitslehrer*, 34 (1931) A, pp. 110–111; *Die Volkswohlfahrt*, 12 (11 June 1931), 607–609.

30 Carly Seyfarth, *Der Ärzte-Knigge: Über den Umgang mit Kranken und über Pflichten, Kunst und Dienst der Krankenhausärzte*, 1st, 2nd and 4th ed., Leipzig: Thieme 1935, 1938 and 1942, pp. 184–187; for the heading *Gesetze und Verordnungen*, see the table of content of the various editions; see also Thorsten Noack, *Eingriffe in das Selbstbestimmungsrecht des Patienten. Juristische Entscheidungen, Politik und ärztliche Positionen 1890–1960*, Frankfurt am Main: Mabuse-Verlag, 2004), pp. 113–124; Florian Bruns, *Medizinethik im National-sozialismus. Entwicklungen und Protagonisten in Berlin (1939–1945)*, Stuttgart: Franz Steiner, 2009, p. 123n513; also pointed to the fact that the *Richtlinien* were mentioned in the 4th ed. of the *Ärzte-Knigge*. In contrast to the assumption of Wolfgang Eckart, the text of the *Richtlinien* was not reprinted, nor were the guidelines mentioned at all in Werner Catel, Richard Frühwald, Artur Knick *et al.* (eds), *Diagnostisch-Therapeutisches Vademecum für Studierende und Ärzte*, 31st and 32nd ed., Leipzig: Barth 1943 and 1945, nor in the 27th or the 29th editions of 1937 and 1941: see Wolfgang Eckart, *Medizin in der NS-Diktatur: Ideologie, Praxis, Folgen*, Vienna: Böhlau, 2012, pp. 294–295.

31 Karl Kisskalt, *Theorie und Praxis der medizinischen Forschung*, Munich, Lehmanns, 1942, p. 137 (also in the 2nd ed. of 1944, p. 150): experiments on human subjects "are, of course, only permissible with the consent of the subject and after detailed explanation of the potential dangers".

32 Schmidt, *Justice at Nuremberg*, p. 13.

33 Georg B. Gruber, *Von ärztlicher Ethik*, Stuttgart: Hippokrates, 1937, p. 42; similarly, one of the few monographs on medical law of the period does not refer at all to medical research: Rudolf Ramm, *Ärztliche Rechts- und Standeskunde. Der Arzt als Gesundheitser-zieher*, Berlin: de Gruyter, 1942; see Bruns, *Medizinethik im Nationalsozialismus*, p. 123.

34 Robin Maitra, "*. . . wer imstande und gewillt ist, dem Staate mit Höchstleistungen zu dienen!*". *Hans Reiter und der Wandel der Gesundheitskonzeption im Spiegel der Lehr- und Handbücher der Hygiene zwischen 1920 und 1960*, Husum: Matthiesen, 2001.

35 Annette Hinz-Wessels, *Das Robert-Koch Institut im Nationalsozialismus*, Berlin: Kultur-verlag Kadmos, 2008, pp. 128–130.

36 Quotation according to ibid., p. 129.

37 Ibid., p. 130.

38 Christoph Wolkewitz, *Die Methodik klinischer Forschung im frühen 20. Jahrhundert: Untersuchung der methodischen Gestaltung klinisch-therapeutischer Studien in Deutschland zwischen 1933 und 1950*, MD thesis, Lübeck: University of Lübeck, 2009. The author identified 158 publications on clinical trials in the realm of internal medicine for the period between 1933 and 1950: in 13 cases (8 per cent) he found discussions of "ethical problems", in 145 cases (92 per cent), there were no such discussions (92 per cent); however, the author did not further specify his understanding of "ethical problems"; a more in-depth analysis of one specific clinical trial on children at Leipzig University also did not find evidence of any reference to the Richtlinien, or the informed consent of the children's parents: Volker Roelcke and Sascha Topp, 'Friedrich Hartmut Dost (1910–85): Aspekte zu Tätigkeit und Haltung in Nationalsozialismus und Nachkriegszeit', *Monatsschrift Kinderheilkunde*, 164 suppl. 1 (2016), pp. 41–45.

39 Volker Roelcke and Simon Duckheim, 'Medizinische Dissertationen aus der Zeit des Nationalsozialismus: Potential eines Quellenbestandes und erste Ergebnisse zu "Alltag",

Ethik und Mentalität der universitären medizinischen Forschung bis (und ab) 1945',
Medizinhistorisches Journal, 49 (2014), pp. 260–271.

40 One of the few cases where the consent of the patients' parents is documented in the
patient records has been reported by Kamila Uzarczyk for the *Kinderfachabteilung* (special
children's ward) at the psychiatric asylum of Loben; however, as far as it can be reconstructed, this was not an instance of human subject research, but of regular ("routine")
diagnostics in the context of the selection process for the programme of child
"euthanasia"; see the chapter by Kamila Uzarczyk in this volume.

41 For the letters of Eichholtz and Rost referring to the *Richtlinien* in the context of the
Trial, see Weindling, *Nazi Medicine*, p. 260; the letter of Rost is also mentioned in
idem, 'The Origins of Informed Consent. The International Scientific Commission on
War Crimes and the Nuremberg Code', *Bulletin of the History of Medicine*, 75 (2001),
pp. 37–71. In contrast to Paul Weindling's assumption, the move to contact Dale was
not initiated by Heubner, but most likely by Rost who had worked at the
Reichsgesundheitsrat in 1930/31 when the *Richtlinien* were debated; after his retirement,
he had moved to Heidelberg where he was in close contact with his colleague Eichholtz.

42 For an appraisal of Rost on the occasion of his 70th birthday, which also mentioned
his honorary membership in the German Association of Pharmacology, see Wolfgang
Heubner, 'Eugen Rost zum siebzigsten Geburtstage (24. Oktober 1940)', *Klinische
Wochenschrift*, 19 (1940), pp. 1095–1096.

43 London, Royal Society (hereafter RS), Dale Papers, letter of Rost to Dale, 30 Nov
1946; see Weindling, *Nazi Medicine*, p. 260; I am grateful to Paul Weindling for providing
a copy of this letter.

44 Ibid.: ". . .wie der deutsche Arzt über Pflichtbewusstsein, Mitgefühl und Menschlichkeit
gedacht hat und noch denkt. Was seine Magna Charta ist . . .".

45 This statement as a kind of addendum and clarification was sent by Rost two days later:
RS, Dale Papers, letter of Rost to Dale, 2 Dec 1946.

46 Weindling, *Nazi Medicine*, p. 260.

47 Ibid.

48 RS, Dale Papers, Dale to Lord Moran, 6 Feb 1948; quoted according to Weindling,
Nazi Medicine, p. 321.

49 Ibid.

50 Fritz Eichholtz, *Lehrbuch der Pharmakologie*, 3rd and 4th ed., Berlin: Springer, 1944; 5th
ed., Berlin and Heidelberg: Springer, 1947, p. 561; in the 9th ed., Berlin: Springer,
1957, the reference to the *Richtlinien* is to be found the end of the bibliography, at the
end of the book's last p. 581.

51 Klaus Dörner *et al.* (eds), *Der Nürnberger Ärzteprozeß 1946/47. Wortprotokolle, Anklage-
und Verteidigungsmaterial, Quellen zum Umfeld,* Micorfiche ed., Munich: K.G. Saur, 1999,
(MF) 09/9141–9142; for Ivy's three principles and the context, see Weindling, *Nazi
Medicine*, pp. 257–269.

52 Dörner *et al.*, *Der Nürnberger Ärzteprozeß*, (MF) 09/9144.

53 Ibid., (MF) 09/9170.

54 Weindling, *Nazi Medicine*, p. 261.

55 Minutes of Meeting to Discuss War Crimes of Medical Nature Executed in Germany
under the Nazi Regime, 31 July 1946, quoted in ibid., p. 263.

56 Ibid., p. 265.

57 Dörner *et al.*, *Der Nürnberger Ärzteprozeß*, (MF) 09/9170–9171.

58 Ibid.

59 *Trials of War Criminals, Selected and Prepared by the United Nations War Crimes Commission,
vol. X: The IG Farben and Krupp Trials*, London: 1949; see also the somewhat apologetic
passages on Hörlein at the Trial in John E. Lesch, *The First Miracle Drugs. How the Sulfa
Drugs Transformed Medicine*, Oxford: Oxford University Press, 2007, pp. 108–121.

60   Leverkusen, Bayer Unternehmensarchiv (hereafter BUNA), Personalia Heinrich Hörlein (B FA 271), letter Hörlein to Martini, 17 May 1949.
61   For a detailed explanation on the supposed difference between *Versuch* and *Experiment* by the defence witness Karl Koenig at the Trial, see Lesch, *Miracle Drugs*, pp. 116–117.
62   On Butenandt as expert witness in defense of Hörlein, see Paul Weindling, 'Verdacht, Kontrolle, Aussöhnung. Adolf Butenandts Platz in der Aussöhnungspolitik der Westalliierten', in Wolfgang Schieder and Achim Trunk (eds), *Adolf Butenandt und die Kaiser-Wilhelm-Gesellschaft. Wissenschaft, Industrie und Politik im "Dritten Reich"*, Göttingen: Wallstein, 2004, pp. 337–338. Interestingly, Butenandt had past obligations towards Hörlein: In 1935, when Butenandt was still working in a somewhat precarious political situation at the Polytechnic College in Danzig and aspired to a more stable and better funded position in Berlin, Hörlein offered him the directorship of a newly created department of medical-pharmaceutical research – an offer that Butenandt was able to use as a negotiating tool in Berlin; see Wolfgang Schieder, 'Spitzenforschung und Politik. Adolf Butenandt in der Weimarer Republik und im "Dritten Reich"', in ibid., p. 37; Heiko Stoff, 'Adolf Butenandt in der Nachkriegszeit. Reinigung und Assoziierung', in ibid., pp. 379–380.
63   Faden and Beauchamp, *History and Theory*, p. 154.
64   Berlin, Archiv of the Max-Planck-Society, Butenandt papers, testimony of Butenandt for Hörlein, Abt. III, Rep 84/1, Nr. 1159–1160.
65   For trials with IG Farben compounds in the context of research on typhoid, see Weindling, *Nazi Medicine*, passim, as well as idem, *Victims*, passim; for the provision of new IG Farben compounds by Gerhard Domagk to Karl Gebhardt, head of the research to test sulfonamides in the context of gas gangrene infections of war wounds, see BUNA, Wehrmacht 1939–42 (B FA 316 – 002 – 094), letter of Gebhardt to Domagk, 25 July 1942; see also Roelcke, 'Sulfonamide Experiments'.
66   Ibid.
67   BUNA, Personalia Heinrich Hörlein (B FA 271), letter Martini to Hörlein, 28 May 1949.
68   The *Deutscher Forschungsrat* was established in early 1949, as an advisory body for federal research policy, headed by Nobel Laureate Werner Heisenberg; in 1951, it fused with the *Notgemeinschaft der Deutschen Wissenschaft*, resulting in the *Deutsche Forschungsgemeinschaft* (German Research Association), see Cathryn Carson and Michael Gubser, 'Science Advising and Science Policy in Post-War West Germany: The Example of the Deutscher Forschungsrat', *Minerva*, 40 (2002), pp. 147–179.
69   BUNA, Personalia Heinrich Hörlein (B FA 271), letter Hörlein to Martini, 2 June 1949.
70   Ibid., letter Martini to Hörlein, 7 July 1949.
71   H. Eickemeyer, *Abschlussbericht des Deutschen Forschungsrates (DFR). Mit einem Vorwort von Werner Heisenberg*, Munich: Oldenbourg, 1953, pp. 45–46.

Bibliography

Archival sources

Germany

Berlin, Archiv der Max-Planck-Gesellschaft, Butenandt papers
Leverkusen, Bayer Unternehmensarchiv (BUNA):
Personalia Heinrich Hoerlein (B FA 271), Korrespondenz Hörlein – Paul Martini
Wehrmacht 1939–42 (B FA 316 – 002 – 094)

United Kingdom

London, Royal Society (RS), Dale Papers

Literature

Annas, George and Michael Grodin (eds), *The Nazi Doctors and the Nuremberg Medical Trial: Human Rights in Human Experimentation*, New York and Oxford: Oxford University Press, 1992

Bonah, Christian, Etienne Lepicard and Volker Roelcke (eds), *La médecine expérimentale au tribunal. Implications éthiques de quelques procès médicaux du XXe siècle européen*, Paris: Éditions des Archives Contemporaines, 2003

Bonner, Thomas Neville, *Becoming a physician. Medical Education in Britain, France, Germany, and the United States, 1750–1945*, Oxford and New York: Oxford University Press, 1995

Bruns, Florian, *Medizinethik im Nationalsozialismus. Entwicklungen und Protagonisten in Berlin (1939–1945)*, Stuttgart: Franz Steiner, 2009

Carson, Cathryn, and Michael Gubser, 'Science Advising and Science Policy in Post-War West Germany: The Example of the Deutscher Forschungsrat', *Minerva*, 40(2002), pp. 147–179

Cohen, Nava, 'Medical experiments', in Israel Gutman (ed.), *Encyclopedia of the Holocaust*, New York: Macmillan, 1990, pp. 957–966

Dörner, Klaus, Angelika Ebbinghaus and Karsten Linne (eds), in cooperation with Karl Heinz Roth and Paul Weindling, on behalf of the Stiftung für Sozialgeschichte des 20. Jahrhunderts, *Der Nürnberger Ärzteprozeß 1946/47. Wortprotokolle, Anklage- und Verteidigungsmaterial, Quellen zum Umfeld*, Microfiche ed., Munich: K.G. Saur, 1999

Eckart, Wolfgang U. (ed.), *Man, Medicine, and the State. The Human Body as an Object of Government Sponsored Medical Research in the 20th Century*, Stuttgart: Franz Steiner 2006

—— *Medizin in der NS-Diktatur: Ideologie, Praxis, Folgen*, Vienna: Böhlau, 2012

Eichholtz, Fritz, *Lehrbuch der Pharmakologie*, 3rd, 4th, 5th, 7th ed., Berlin: Springer 1944, 1947, 1957

Eickemeyer, H., *Abschlussbericht des Deutschen Forschungsrates (DFR). Mit einem Vorwort von Werner Heisenberg*, Munich, Oldenbourg, 1953

Faden, Ruth, and Tom Beauchamp, *A History and Theory of Informed Consent*, New York and Oxford: Oxford University Press, 1986

Frewer, Andreas, *Medizin und Moral in Weimarer Republik und Nationalsozialismus: Die Zeitschrift "Ethik" unter Emil Abderhalden*, Frankfurt am Main: Campus, 2000

Gruber, Georg B., *Von ärztlicher Ethik*, Stuttgart: Hippokrates, 1937

Hasskarl, Horst and Hellmuth Kleinsorge, *Arzneimittelprüfung, Arzneimittelrecht. Nationale und internationale Bestimmungen und Empfehlungen*, Stuttgart: Gustav Fischer, 1974

Heidler, Mario, 'Die Zeitschriften des J. F. Lehmanns Verlages bis 1945', in Sigrid Stöckel (ed.), *Die "rechte Nation" und ihr Verleger: Politik und Popularisierung im J. F. Lehmanns Verlag 1890–1979*, Berlin: Lehmanns, 2002, pp. 47–102

Henke, Klaus-D., 'Einleitung', in Klaus-D. Henke (ed.), *Tödliche Medizin im Nationalsozialismus. Von der Rassenhygiene zum Massenmord*, Cologne: Böhlau, 2008, pp. 9–29

Heubner, Wolfgang, 'Eugen Rost zum siebzigsten Geburtstage (24. Oktober 1940)', *Klinische Wochenschrift*, 19 (1940), pp. 1095–1096

Hinz-Wessels, Annette, *Das Robert-Koch Institut im Nationalsozialismus*, Berlin: Kultur-verlag Kadmos, 2008

Howard-Jones, Norman, 'Human Experimentation in Historical and Ethical Perspective', *Social Science and Medicine*, 16(1982), pp. 1429–1448

Kisskalt, Karl, *Theorie und Praxis der medizinischen Forschung*, Munich: Lehmanns, 1942

Laukötter, Anja, 'Wie aus den Pocken Karies wurde – Die Forschung von Heinrich A. Gins am Robert Koch-Institut', in Marion Hulverscheidt and Anja Laukötter (eds), *Infektion und Institution: Zur Wissenschaftsgeschichte des Robert Koch-Instituts im Nationalsozialismus*, Göttingen: Wallstein, 2009, pp. 128–146

Lesch, John E., The First Miracle Drugs. How the Sulfa Drugs Transformed Medicine, Oxford: Oxford University Press, 2007

Maitra, Robin, "... *wer imstande und gewillt ist, dem Staate mit Höchstleistungen zu dienen!*". *Hans Reiter und der Wandel der Gesundheitskonzeption im Spiegel der Lehr- und Handbücher der Hygiene zwischen 1920 und 1960*, Husum: Matthiesen, 2001

Marrus, Michael, 'The Nuremberg doctors' trial in historical context', *Bulletin of the History of Medicine*, 73(1999), pp. 106–123

Massin, Benoît, 'Mengele, die Zwillingsforschung und die "Auschwitz-Dahlem Connection"', in Carola Sachse (ed.), *Die Verbindung nach Auschwitz. Biowissenschaften und Menschenversuche an Kaiser-Wilhelm-Institute*, Göttingen: Wallstein, 2003, pp. 201–254

Mitscherlich, Alexander, 'Geschichtsschreibung und Psychoanalyse. Gedanken zum Nürnberger Prozess', *Schweizer Annalen*, 11(1945), pp. 604–613

——— and Fred Mielke (eds), *Medizin ohne Menschlichkeit. Dokumente des Nürnberger Ärzteprozesses*, Frankfurt: S. Fischer, 1978

Müller, Friedrich, 'Die Zulässigkeit ärztlicher Versuche an gesunden und kranken Menschen: I.', *Münchener Medizinische Wochenschrift* (1931), pp. 104–107

Nadav, Daniel, 'The "Death Dance" of Lübeck: Julius Moses and the German Guidelines for Human Experimentation', in Volker Roelcke and Giovanni Maio (eds), *Twentieth-Century Ethics of Human Subject Research*, Stuttgart: Franz Steiner, 2004, pp. 129–136

Noack, Thorsten, *Eingriffe in das Selbstbestimmungsrecht des Patienten. Juristische Entscheidungen, Politik und ärztliche Positionen 1890–1960*, Frankfurt am Main, Mabuse-Verlag 2004, pp. 113–124

Ramm, Rudolf, *Ärztliche Rechts- und Standeskunde. Der Arzt als Gesundheitserzieher*, Berlin: de Gruyter, 1942

Reuland, Andreas, *Humanexperimente in der Weimarer Republik und Julius Moses' "Kampf gegen die Experimentierwut"*, Norderstedt: Books on Demand 2004

'Richtlinien für neuartige Heilbehandlung und für die Vornahme wissenschaftlicher Versuche am Menschen [Rundschreiben des Reichsministers des Inneren, 28. February1931]', *Reichsgesundheitsblatt*, 55.6 (1931), pp. 174–175

Roelcke, Volker, Gerrit Hohendorf and Maike Rotzoll, 'Psychiatric Research and "Euthanasia". The case of the psychiatric department at the University of Heidelberg, 1941–1945', *History of Psychiatry*, 5(1994), pp. 517–532

Roelcke, Volker, 'Psychiatrische Wissenschaft im Kontext nationalsozialistischer Politik und "Euthanasie": Zur Rolle von Ernst Rüdin und der *Deutschen Forschungsanstalt/ Kaiser-Wilhelm-Institut für Psychiatrie*', in Doris Kaufmann (ed.), *Die Kaiser-Wilhelm-Gesellschaft im Nationalsozialismus: Bestandsaufnahme und Perspektiven der Forschung*, Göttingen: Wallstein, 2000, pp. 112–150

——— 'Repräsentation – Reduktion – Standardisierung: Zur Formierung des "Tiermodells" menschlicher Krankheit in der experimentellen Medizin des 19.

Jahrhunderts', in Roland Borgards and Nicolas Pethes (eds), *Tier – Experiment – Literatur, 1880–2010*, Würzburg: Königshausen & Neumann, 2013, pp. 15–36

—— 'Sulfonamide Experiments on Prisoners in Nazi Concentration Camps: Coherent Scientific Rationality Combined with Complete Disregard of Humanity', in Sheldon Rubenfeld and Susan Benedict (eds), *Human Subjects Research after the Holocaust*, Cham: Springer, 2014, pp. 51–66

—— and Simon Duckheim, 'Medizinische Dissertationen aus der Zeit des Nationalsozialismus: Potential eines Quellenbestandes und erste Ergebnisse zu "Alltag", Ethik und Mentalität der universitären medizinischen Forschung bis (und ab) 1945', *Medizinhistorisches Journal*, 49 (2014), pp. 260–271

—— and Sascha Topp, 'Friedrich Hartmut Dost (1910–1985): Aspekte zu Tätigkeit und Haltung in Nationalsozialismus und Nachkriegszeit', *Monatsschrift Kinderheilkunde*, 164 suppl. 1 (2016), pp. 41–45

Rohner, Christina, *Medizin und politische Ideologie im Spiegel der MMW und der DMW 1923, 1928, 1933 und 1938*, PhD thesis, Zürich: University of Zürich, 1995

Roth, Karl Heinz, 'Tödliche Höhen. Die Unterdruckkammer-Experimente im Konzentrationslager Dachau und ihre Bedeutung für die luftfahrtmedizinische Forschung des "Dritten Reichs"', in Angelika Ebbinghaus and Klaus Dörner (eds), *Vernichten und Heilen. Der Nürnberger Ärzteprozess und seine Folgen*, Berlin: Aufbau, 2001, pp. 110–151

Saretzki, Thomas, *Reichsgesundheitsrat und Preußischer Landesgesundheitsrat in der Weimarer Republik*, Berlin: Weißensee, 2000

Sass, Hans-Martin, '*Reichsrundschreiben* 1931: Pre-Nuremberg German Regulation Concerning New Therapy and Experimentation', *Journal of Medicine and Philosophy*, 8 (1983), pp. 99–111

Schieder, Wolfgang, 'Spitzenforschung und Politik. Adolf Butenandt in der Weimarer Republik und im "Dritten Reich"', in Wolfgang Schieder and Achim Trunk (eds), *Adolf Butenandt und die Kaiser-Wilhelm-Gesellschaft. Wissenschaft, Industrie und Politik im "Dritten Reich"*, Göttingen: Wallstein, 2004, pp. 23–77

Schmidt, Ulf, *Justice at Nuremberg: Leo Alexander and the Nazi Doctors' Trial*, Houndmills, Basingstoke: Palgrave Macmillan, 2004

Seyfarth, Carly, *Der Ärzte-Knigge*, 1st, 2nd and 4th ed., Leipzig: Thieme 1935, 1938 and 1942

Stauder, Alfons, 'Die Zulässigkeit ärztlicher Versuche an gesunden und kranken Menschen: II.', *Münchener Medizinische Wochenschrift* (1931), pp. 107–112

Steinmann, Reinhard, *Die Debatte über medizinische Versuche am Menschen in der Weimarer Zeit*, MD thesis, Tübingen: Eberhard Karls University, 1975

Stöckel, Sigrid, 'Veränderungen des Genres "Medizinische Wochenschrift"? Deutsche Medizinische Wochenschrift, Münchener Medizinische Wochenschrift und The Lancet im Vergleich', in Sigrid Stöckel, Gerlind Rüve and Wiebke Liesner (eds), *Das Medium Wissenschaftszeitschrift seit dem 19. Jahrhundert*, Stuttgart: Franz Steiner, 2009, pp. 139–162

Süß, Winfried, 'Versuche der Wiedergutmachung', in Robert Jütte (ed.), *Medizin und Nationalsozialismus*, Göttingen: Wallstein, 2011, pp. 283–294

Vollmann, Jochen and Rolf Winau, 'Informed consent in human experimentation before the Nuremberg Code', *British Medical Journal*, 313 (1996), pp. 1445–1449

Weindling, Paul Julian, *Epidemics and Genocide in Eastern Europe, 1890–1945*, Oxford: Oxford University Press, 2000

—— 'The Origins of Informed Consent. The International Scientific Commission on War Crimes and the Nuremberg Code', *Bulletin of the History of Medicine*, 75 (2001), pp. 37–71

—- *Nazi Medicine and the Nuremberg Trials*, Houndmills, Basingstoke: Palgrave Macmillan, 2004

—— *Victims and Survivors of Nazi Human Experiments. Science and Suffering in the Holocaust*, London: Bloomsbury, 2015

Wolkewitz, Christoph, *Die Methodik klinischer Forschung im frühen 20. Jahrhundert: Untersuchung der methodischen Gestaltung klinisch-therapeutischer Studien in Deutschland zwischen 1933 und 1950*, MD thesis, Lübeck: University of Lübeck, 2009

3 The Society of German Neurologists and Psychiatrists and research in the context of eugenics and "euthanasia"[1]

Hans-Walter Schmuhl

The mass murder of mentally disabled and psychiatric patients in National Socialist Germany, which claimed around 300,000 fatalities, opened up entirely new possibilities for psychiatric research. Humans who were sorted out in the screening process and released for extermination, but who had attracted the attention of researchers as "interesting cases", were initially subjected to psychiatric, neurological and internal examination, and then underwent clinical observation and psychological tests, medical experiments and anthropometric measurements before they were murdered, after which their brains were dissected and examined pathologically. At the beginning of 1941 – probably on 23 January – a conference with the *Reichsdozentenführer* (Reich Leader of University Teachers) took place, at which a large-scale research plan was drafted in connection with the Nazi "euthanasia" campaign. Fourteen of the 30 anatomical institutes of the German Reich were to be included in the plans for mass examinations.[2] While the course of the war prevented the realisation of this ambitious plan, the "euthanasia" headquarters of 1942 maintained two research departments of its own, one at the Brandenburg-Görden Psychiatric Hospital, directed by Hans Heinze, and the other at the Psychiatric Hospital in Wiesloch, Baden under the direction of Carl Schneider, which was later moved to Heidelberg University Psychiatric Clinic.

The history of these two research departments has since been researched in great detail.[3] In the following chapter, the role of the psychiatric-neurological professional association will be clarified in this context. Did the leadership of the Society of German Neurologists and Psychiatrists (GDNP) know about the research on "euthanasia" victims? What position did it take on this subject? Did it perhaps even support such research? The account centres around a key document: the "Recommendations for psychiatric-neurological research in war" (*Empfehlungen zur psychiatrisch-neurologischen Forschung im Krieg*), which Ernst Rüdin, as chairman of the GDNP, submitted to the *Reichsgesundheitsführung* (Reich Health Leadership) in October 1942. However, I will first outline the role of the professional association of scientists at the interface between science and politics.

I Institutional background

The Society of German Neurologists and Psychiatrists was created in 1935, when the German Association for Psychiatry (*Deutscher Verein für Psychiatrie*) merged with the German Association for Mental Hygiene (*Deutscher Verband für psychische Hygiene*) and the Association of German Neurologists (*Gesellschaft Deutscher Nervenärzte*). A quick study of the sources reveals that the long-established conception that three independent scientific professional societies had been consolidated from above, and turned into an extension of National Socialist eugenics policy against their will, does not correspond with reality. On the contrary, it is much more accurate to say that psychiatry and neurology on the one hand, and the biopolicy of National Socialism on the other, functioned as "resources for each other" (Mitchell Ash).[4] Political actors sought an alliance with the merged scientific professional society in order to integrate psychiatry and neurology into the practical implementation of the sterilisation law and other eugenic measures; for its part, the society attempted to bring psychiatrists and neurologists into line in order to strengthen the two disciplines' social-policy function of asserting professional interests and offsetting any undesired secondary effects of eugenic policy.

Pulling the strings in the background was a tightly knit network centred on Ernst Rüdin, who was director of the German Institute for Psychiatric Research (*Deutsche Forschungsanstalt für Psychiatrie*) in Munich since 1931; he was considered the leading scientist in the field of psychiatric genetics in Germany. Up to May 1933 Rüdin did not hold *any* central position within the system of scientific professional societies. However, within just two years he succeeded in ascending to *Reichsleiter* of the newly founded GDNP and thus bringing under his control the professional societies for psychiatry, mental hygiene and neurology. His success was certainly assisted by his alliance with Dr Arthur Gütt in the Reich Ministry of the Interior, who up until 1938 was indisputably the strong man in the state's "health leadership" (*Gesundheitsführung*). His position was never completely uncontested, however, as he was constantly confronted with conflicts about the respective authority of the health leadership of the Nazi Party under Chief Physician of the Reich (*Reichsärzteführer*) Gerhard Wagner. Wagner died in 1939. His successor was Leonardo Conti, who up to that time had been the highest-ranking medical official in Berlin. He managed to oust Arthur Gütt, who had been seriously injured in a hunting accident. Shortly before the outbreak of the Second World War, on 27 August 1939, Conti was appointed state secretary in the Reich Ministry of the Interior. From that day on he thus became the Reich Health Leader (*Reichsgesund-heitsführer*), at the head the both the state's and the Party's health leadership.[5] With Gütt ousted, Ernst Rüdin also lost his direct connection to power – Leonardo Conti was closely allied with one of Rüdin's nemeses, Eugen Fischer and his Kaiser Wilhelm Institute for Anthropology, Human Genetics and Eugenics in Berlin.[6] As part of the "euthanasia" programme, however, Rüdin gained new access to the centre of the regime. With the appointment of Paul

Nitsche, managing director of the GDNP until 1939 and one of Rüdin's closest confidants within the professional society, to medical director of *Aktion T4*, Rüdin had a direct line to the Führer's Chancellery.

II Rüdin's research manifesto

The third year of the war was well under way before any opportunity arose to renew the connection to the health leadership of the Reich. On 7 October 1942 Walter Schütz, personal advisor to the Reich Health Leader, contacted the managing director of the GDNP – since 1939 this position had been held by a medical officer to the provincial administration of the Rhineland, Walter Creutz. Schütz inquired as to the opinion of the Psychiatric-Neurological Society about which research issues should be pursued most urgently during the war.[7] Creutz forwarded the inquiry to Rüdin on 13 October 1942. At the same time he sent a copy of the inquiry to the deputy chairman and director of the neurological department of the GDNP, Heinrich Pette in Hamburg. As far as the "direct motive"[8] of the inquiry was concerned, Creutz presumed that Conti wanted to deliver recommendations to the Reich Research Council.

Creutz offered to answer the inquiry himself if Rüdin were to give him "instructions". In case Rüdin preferred to take on the task of responding to the inquiry himself, Creutz made his own suggestions. In addition to "genetic research", which had to be continued even under conditions of war, one would want to point to the primary importance of "neuropathology research in connection with war injuries to the brain and the rest of the nervous system and with neurosurgical experiences". Furthermore, Creutz believed it "appropriate . . . to draw attention to the fact that research in the area of psychoses, and currently especially those in the areas of electro-shock therapy, [must] not come to a standstill". To this end it was necessary, he continued, to maintain the manufacture of the apparatus this therapy required. In this context Creutz referred to an initiative by the Reich officer responsible for psychiatric hospitals, Herbert Linden, to supply the German psychiatric hospitals with electro-convulsators manufactured by the Siemens-Reiniger company. In fact, after initial hesitation, the GDNP was eager to anchor the new somatic therapies in psychiatric practice.[9]

Heinrich Pette also hastened to write to Rüdin. His letter to Munich was dispatched on 16 October 1942. In the "foreground"[10] of neurological research at times of war, Pette confirmed, were 'of course the traumatic injuries of the central and peripheral nervous systems'. Moreover, increased research efforts should be directed "to the area of infectious diseases of the nervous system"; the longer the war lasted, the more "the great importance of these diseases for their effect on the armed forces" would be recognised.

The proposals from Walter Creutz and Heinrich Pette corresponded with the emphases of the first two days of the 6th Annual Meeting of the GDNP, which was supposed to have taken place exactly one year before in Würzburg from 5 to 7 October 1941, before it had to be cancelled at short notice because of the wartime situation.[11] The main topic of the first day of the meeting, 5 October 1941, was supposed to be "War Experiences of Brain Injuries". The agenda of the second day, 6 October 1941, was headed up with "The Therapy of Psychoses", whereby no less than 11 of the 17 lectures planned on this day were to deal with shock therapies, especially the newly developed electroconvulsive therapy. However, the meeting in Würzburg was supposed to follow a dramaturgy to which Creutz and Pette were oblivious. In the run-up to the meeting, Paul Nitsche had written a memo for Viktor Brack from the Führer's Chancellery, who headed up the administration of the on-going "euthanasia" campaign. In this memo Nitsche had demanded that German psychiatrists be officially notified about the "euthanasia" campaign, in order to make clear to them that the psychiatry of the future was not to be content merely with the custodianship of incurable patients – clinical operations would constitute its new focus. The annual meeting of the GDNP was to serve as the occasion for this change of course.[12] Apparently, Viktor Brack a high ranking official of the Führer's Chancellery had been convinced: the Führer's Chancellery sponsored the upcoming annual meeting with a subsidy of 10,000 Reichsmarks.[13] The main lecture on the "Therapy of Psychoses" was to be held by Carl Schneider, professor of psychiatry at the University of Heidelberg – and, as can be gleaned from Schneider's surviving "concluding remarks", in this address he intended to treat the mass murder of psychiatric patients as an open secret.[14] Schneider's lecture was to be framed on one side by the section on the treatment of brain injuries, which was to show the high level of neurosurgery and its military importance in a positive light, and on the other by the presentations on electroconvulsive therapy, which were to illuminate the tremendous progress achieved in therapy for psychoses. Both sets of issues were thus intended to contribute indirectly to legitimising "euthanasia".

Incidentally, an exchange of letters between Ernst Rüdin and Paul Nitsche in June 1941 showed that these psychiatrists, both of whom were deeply implicated in the "euthanasia" campaign, encountered Walter Creutz with some suspicion – delaying tactics in his area of responsibility suggested that Creutz would offer some resistance for a policy of mass murder.[15] Rüdin and Nitsche therefore agreed that all abstracts for the planned annual meeting in Würzburg should be routed over Rüdin's desk. With this decision Creutz's function as secretary of the GDNP was subject to scrutiny. Indeed, Nitsche left no doubt as to the purpose of this step: "Just as the new state cannot allow its work in developing racial hygiene to be disturbed by any kind of obstructionism by scientific antagonists, neither can it tolerate such disturbance . . . in light of the imminent euth.[anasia] law".[16]

This may well be the reason why Rüdin responded to the query from the Reich Health Leadership, rather leaving this task to his managing director. Within a few days he had worked out a brief 17-point plan, which he sent to Schütz on 23 October 1942. Accordingly, the entire process took only two weeks – although the query went from Berlin to Düsseldorf, from Düsseldorf to Munich and Hamburg, and from Munich to Berlin, suggesting that Rüdin saw this as an opportunity to use the political influence of the Reich Health Leader to promote psychiatric and neurological research. Yet his prospects of success were unclear. As he confessed to Creutz, he did not know "whether [the matter was] a mere formality"[17] or whether "anything significant for research [was] to be expected". All the same, he had used the opportunity to draft a research design according to his own ideas. In so doing he had picked up on the impulses supplied by Creutz and Pette, but placed them in a general context oriented above all on psychiatric genetics, racial hygiene, and "euthanasia". In my opinion this was a key document that throws a spotlight on the ideas of the doctors and scientists involved in the "euthanasia" program.[18]

III Eugenic parameters

The point of departure of the research plan designed by Rüdin was the by then classical question of eugenics after the damaging effects of counter-selection caused by the war. Rüdin was particularly adamant about the need for studies on the development of fertility in the so-called "selection profes-sion[s]";[19] conditions of war at the front and on the home front should be studied, as should the effects of war conditions on the rate of suicide.[20]

In addition, the "biological status" of those women who had borne illegitimate children during the war should be researched. This final point referred to a discussion that had been triggered in 1940 by an article in the *Schwarzes Korps*, which had spoken out decisively *against* social discrimination against single mothers and *for* state incentives for single, working mothers to have children out of wedlock. Fritz Lenz, director of the Department for Eugenics at the Kaiser Wilhelm Institute for Anthropology, Human Genetics and Eugenics, had expressed his strong opposition – under the aspects of racial hygiene the state should concentrate on promoting *legitimate* births.[21] Rüdin now demanded an unprejudiced examination of the eugenic importance of illegitimate births – this was also a barb against the institute in Berlin. That he himself tended toward the position advocated by Fritz Lenz was apparent in the fact that an article appeared in 1942 in the *Archiv für Rassen- und Gesellschaftsbiologie* (Archive for the Biology of Race and Society) under his editorship, entitled "Die unehelich Geborenen, ein empfindlicher Wertmesser für die sittliche Kraft unseres Volkes" (The Illegitimately Born, a Sensitive Gauge of Values for the Moral Strength of our Nation),[22] which took a decided position on this issue. As a consequence Rüdin had to accept sharp critique from both Walter Groß on the part of NSDAP Race Policy office and from Herbert Linden from the Reich Ministry of the Interior. The Press Department of the Reich government in the Reich Ministry of Popular Enlightenment and Propaganda even saw 'subversive aspirations' at work and demanded from Rüdin a "rectification".[23] Rüdin hastened to fulfil this demand. He not only reprinted a critical text entitled "Unehelichkeit und Rassenpflege" (Illegitimacy and Racial Care) by Karl Valentin Müller, director of the Institute for Social Anthropology and Biology of the Nation at the German University in Prague, in the *Archiv für Rassen- und Gesellschaftsbiologie*;[24] in an editorial at the turn of the year 1942/43 he further emphasised his political orthodoxy under the headline "Zehn Jahre nationalsozialistischer Staat" (Ten Years of the National Socialist State).[25]

Yet Rüdin remained on secure political terrain when, in his catalogue of research questions important for the war effort, he advocated in favour of a "genetic characterisation" of German women who had been impregnated by prisoners of war and foreign forced labourers – this was a highly dangerous demand, considering the draconian punishments for "racial defilement". In such cases there was general assent for at least compulsory sterilisation, and possibly also for abortion for reasons of racial policy. Rüdin's demand to press ahead with research on early detection and segregation of those genetically predisposed to become "socially incompetent" from those "who are primarily victims of environment" found similar support. This demand was quite clearly related to considerations about a *Gemeinschaftsfremdengesetz* (Community Aliens Act), which was to stipulate the internment and sterilisation of hereditary "anti-socials" and "psychopaths".[26]

To consolidate such eugenic research by providing direct relation to practice, Rüdin further advocated the promotion of theoretical research on genetics, to the extent that such research was possible under conditions of war. In this context Rüdin pointed to two research projects in progress at his own institute. The first concerned the heritability of serious physical defects – that was being conducted in opposition to the Kaiser Wilhelm Institute for Anthropology, Human Genetics and Eugenics in Berlin, which had a research focus in this field.[27] The second project Rüdin mentioned was on the psychiatric genetic evaluation of schizophrenias with short, non-recurring, attacks and longer periods of complete remission.[28] Both projects – but above all the latter project on schizophrenia – again, picked up directly on the practical problems of implementing the *Gesetz zur Verhütung erbkranken Nachwuchses* (Law for the Prevention of Genetically Diseased Offspring). As the jurisdiction of the Genetic Health Courts was inconsistent and contradictory on these points, race hygienists and psychiatrists in Munich, Berlin and elsewhere were working vigorously at this time to clarify the legislation and provide the courts with precise guidelines.

IV Euthanasia targets

A central aspect of Rüdin's plan – item 10 of his 17-point plan – elaborated on the "euthanasia" measures still under way. In his words:

> Of outstanding importance for racial hygiene, due to its significance as the foundation for a humane and secure response against counter-selective processes of every kind in the body of our German nation, would be the exploration of the question as to *which children* (infants and toddlers) *can, even as early as childhood, be clinically and genetically* (in terms of family ancestry)

classified to the parents and/or their legal representatives as inferior and thus worthy of elimination, with complete conviction and evidentiary power and so irreproachably that, both in their own interest and in the interest of the German nation, they can be recommended for euthanasia?

In this Rüdin quite openly alluded to the work of the "Research Department" of the Brandenburg-Görden Psychiatric Hospital under the direction of Hans Heinze, set up by the "T4" headquarters in January 1942. In September 1941 Paul Nitsche had suggested making the institution useful for research by "simply transferring the cases of congenital imbecility and epilepsy from the institutions located relatively nearby to Görden as an intermediate station, in order to pass them on to one of our other institutions after performing the necessary examinations".[29] A series of preliminary talks between Nitsche and Heinze took place between November 1941 and January 1942. On the basis of an agreement between the *Reichsarbeitsgemeinschaft Heil- und Pflegeanstalten* (Reich Working Group for Psychiatric Hospitals and Homes) and the association of the Mark Brandenburg province, from 26 January 1942 on, the research department had 80 beds at Görden at its disposal. On 6 July 1942 half of the research department's beds were transferred to the *Wehrmacht*, so that research had to be restricted to relatively few cases. By September 1942, a total of 97 patients had been examined in the research department at Görden; one year later, in September 1943, this number had climbed to 135. So far 98 children aged between 3 and 19 have been identified, 48 of whom died in the institution, many after spending several years there, including 30 before 31 March 1945.[30]

In a research report submitted to the "euthanasia" headquarters by Heinze on 9 September 1942 – and thus nearly two months before Rüdin delivered his recommendations, two research emphases stand out. First, Heinze was concerned with the nosology of forms of imbecility. This also involved the investigation of the "dressage capability of the profoundly imbecile". Even before the war, Heinze had set up a "school of living" at the Brandenburg-Görden Hospital, in which "feeble-minded" children, whose theoretical intelligence was too low to learn skills like reading and writing, but whose practical intelligence was sufficient to perform manual work, were trained as unskilled workers. Heinze's second research emphasis was on the diagnostic differentiation between various forms of "imbecility" and between mental disabilities and neurodegenerative diseases. The research department was officially dissolved as of 31 March 1943, yet on the part of the institution the work continued until 1945 with the support of the Reich Working Group for Psychiatric Hospitals and Homes.

The second research department of the "T4" headquarters, which launched operations under the direction of Carl Schneider in late 1942, initially at the Psychiatric Hospital in Wiesloch, Baden, and then later moved to the University Psychiatric Hospital in Heidelberg, was still in planning at the time Rüdin drafted his programme. Here Rüdin emphasised how important it would be to use the opportunity the "euthanasia" programme opened up for research on genetic psychiatry and racial hygiene – the background of this was the terrible possibility of expanding the clinical and psychological findings to include the anatomical and histological investigation of the brains of the murdered children. At the same time, with a nod to the Reich Health Leadership, Rüdin accentuated the importance of research in the context of the "euthanasia" programme with regard to the public acceptance of mass murder: if one could convince the parents of the murdered children that their "worthiness of elimination" had been proven scientifically, according to Rüdin's implicit thesis, one could give "euthanasia" an established basis of legitimacy. As Volker Roelcke documented, in late autumn 1943 Rüdin seconded a member of the German Institute for Psychiatric Research staff, Dr Julius Deussen, to Heidelberg in order to co-ordinate the psychological research on children at the "research station" located there.[31] Thus Rüdin was also personally involved in the research programme in the context of "euthanasia".

V Neurological advances

The passage about research in the context of the "euthanasia" programme was followed by remarks about the field of neurology. In these Rüdin adhered for the most part to the recommendations by Heinrich Pette and Walter Creutz. Picking up on Creutz's proposal, Rüdin warned that even in war, research on therapy for psychoses, especially with regard to electroconvulsive therapy, must not come to a standstill. Further, Rüdin, as suggested by Creutz, advocated maintaining the production of the equipment required for electroconvulsive therapy. However, Rüdin felt it necessary to explain to the Reich Health Leadership that:

> We may not have any interest in preserving the lives of incurable, ruined victims of heredity, nor in the reproduction of those humans who are carriers of the genes required for the development of serious genetic diseases. But in the case of the latter group of patients, we do have an interest in intervening in [the] course of the disease early enough to save at least those individuals who can be saved, in order to preserve at least their utility for society.

In the penultimate point of his plan Rüdin discussed malaria therapy for general paralysis. Here, too, it is worth analysing the wording precisely:

> It is desirable to treat paralytics
>
> 1   by attempting to treat their paralysis
> 2   with large-scale tests of remedies for malaria, in order to utilise the results for members of the army who suffer from an early stage of syphilis or from malaria.

This illustrates a fluid transition from a psychiatric "attempt to heal" all the way to a tropical medicine experiment on human subjects. Rüdin referred to a common practice. After the loss of the colonies, German research on malaria had found a new field of research in the psychiatric hospitals, where the malaria therapy for general paralysis proposed by Julius Wagner-Jauregg became established in the 1920s. It seemed harmless to use patients who were already infected with malaria to test malaria remedies. Yet in this way, as Marion Hulverscheidt showed using the example of the Robert Koch Institute, psychiatric patients increasingly became guinea pigs for tropical medicine. And that is not all: staff began infecting psychiatric patients with malaria merely to keep the pathogens alive. On the quiet, the "attempted healing" had transformed into the reduction of helpless humans to "host animals" in order to keep alive pathogens for research.[32] With his position paper of 1942 Ernst Rüdin, chairman of the professional association for psychiatry and neurology, legitimated this practice.

VI A militant programme

Let us summarise briefly. The 17-point plan of October 1942 shows that Ernst Rüdin regarded psychiatric research, individual therapy, eugenics, sterilisation and "euthanasia" as complementary elements in a comprehensive scientific-political complex; and that he used the channels of the professional scientific society in the midst of war in order to submit his ideas to political decision-makers while indicating the support of the professional society for psychiatry and neurology. The plan bears Ernst Rüdin's signature. The documents offer no support for the claim that he was privately opposed to "euthanasia", as has long been contended.[33] On the contrary: the plan of 1942 proves that he actively supported the "euthanasia" programme, that he had no interest at all in preserving the lives of presumably incurably ill, socially useless persons. His proposal did not have any recognisable practical consequences. Yet this did not prevent Rüdin and his closest colleagues from working out a comprehensive expose in 1943 and sending it to the Reich Health Leader, laying out their ideas for reforming the field of psychiatry in Germany on the basis of murdering patients.[34] The psychiatric hospital of the future was to be organised as a clinical operation focusing on newly developed forms of therapy. The safekeeping of mentally disabled and chronically ill patients was to be its purpose no longer.

Notes

1 This chapter pools findings from a research group on the history of the Society of German Neurologists and Psychiatrists in the National Socialist era, which was initiated and financed by the German Association for Psychiatry, Psychotherapy and Psychosomatics (DGPPN). Cf. Hans-Walter Schmuhl, *Die Gesellschaft Deutscher Neurologen und Psychiater im Nationalsozialismus*, Berlin and Heidelberg: Springer, 2016. I thank the German Association for Psychiatry, Psychotherapy and Psychosomatics for covering the expenses for translating this chapter.

2 Berlin, Bundesarchiv Berlin (hereafter BAB), R 96 I/5, Memorandum by Nitsche of 18 Sept 1941; BAB, R 96 I/4, Carl Schneider's report 'über Stand, Möglichkeiten und Ziele der Forschung an Epileptikern im Rahmen der Aktion' for Paul Nitsche, 24 Jan 1944. Dating based on a document entitled 'Anatomischer Forschungsplan gemäß Besprechung vom 23. January 1941' in BAB, All. Proz. 7, Roll 12, Fr. 220.

3 On Brandenburg-Görden, see for example: Thomas Beddies, 'Kinder und Jugendliche in der brandenburgischen Heil- und Pflegeanstalt Görden als Opfer der NS-Medizinverbrechen', in Kristina Hübener (ed.), *Brandenburgische Heil- und Pflegeanstalten in der NS-Zeit*, Berlin: Be.bra, 2002, pp. 129–154; idem, 'Die Forschungsabteilung in der Landesanstalt Brandenburg-Görden', in idem and Kristina Hübener (eds), *Dokumente zur Psychiatrie im Nationalsozialismus*, Berlin: Be.bra, 2003, pp. 261–270; Beatrice Falk and Friedrich Hauer, *Brandenburg-Görden. Geschichte eines psychiatrischen Krankenhauses*, Berlin: Be.bra, 2007; Schmuhl, *Gesellschaft*, pp. 293–298. On Wiesloch/Heidelberg, see: Volker Roelcke, Gerrit Hohendorf and Maike Rotzoll, 'Psychiatric Research and "Euthanasia": The Case of the Psychiatric Department at the University of Heidelberg, 1941–1945', *History of Psychiatry*, 5 (1994), pp. 517–532; Gerrit Hohendorf and Maike Rotzoll, 'Medical Research and National Socialist Euthanasia: Carl Schneider and the Heidelberg Research Children from 1942 until 1945', in Sheldon Rubenfeld and Susan Benedict (eds), *Human Subjects Research after the Holocaust*, Heidelberg: Springer, 2014, pp. 127–138; Götz Aly, *Die Belasteten. "Euthanasie" 1939–1945. Eine Gesellschaftsgeschichte*, Frankfurt am Main: S. Fischer, 2013, pp. 199–212; Schmuhl, *Gesellschaft*, pp. 298–303.

4 Mitchell G. Ash, 'Wissenschaft und Politik als Ressourcen für einander', in Rüdiger vom Bruch and Brigitte Kaderas (eds), *Wissenschaften und Wissenschaftspolitik. Bestandsaufnahmen zu Formationen, Brüchen und Kontinuitäten im Deutschland des 20. Jahrhunderts*, Stuttgart: Franz Steiner, 2002, pp. 32–51.

5 Ernst-Alfred Leyh, "Gesundheitsführung", "Volksschicksal", "Wehrkraft". Leonardo Conti (1900–45) und die Ideologisierung der Medizin in der NS-Diktatur, MD thesis, Heidelberg: Heidelberg University, 2002; Hans-Walter Schmuhl, 'Die biopolitische Entwicklungsdiktatur des Nationalsozialismus und der "Reichsgesundheitsführer" Dr. Leonardo Conti', in Klaus-Dietmar Henke (ed.), Tödliche Medizin im Nationalsozialismus. Von der Rassenhygiene zum Massenmord, Cologne: Böhlau, 2008, pp. 101–117.

6 On this at length: Hans-Walter Schmuhl, The Kaiser Wilhelm Institute for Anthropology, Human Heredity and Eugenics, 1927–45. Crossing Boundaries, Dordrecht: Springer, 2008, pp. 254–262.

7 Munich, Max-Planck-Institut für Psychiatrie, Historisches Archiv (hereafter MPIP-HA), GDA 128, Reichsgesundheitsführer/Doz. Dr. Schütz, to Creutz, 7 Oct 1942.

8 MPIP-HA, GDA 128, Creutz to Rüdin, 13 Oct 1942. Subsequent citations also from this source.

9 Sascha Lang, 'Psychiatrie, technische Innovation und Industrie. Die Siemens-Reiniger-Werke und die Entwicklung des Elektrokrampftherapiegerätes "Konvulsator" im Zweiten Weltkrieg', in Hans-Walter Schmuhl and Volker Roelcke (eds), *"Heroische Therapien". Die deutsche Psychiatrie im internationalen Vergleich 1918–1945*, Göttingen: Wallstein, 2013, pp. 216–232.

10 MPIP-HA, GDA 129, Pette to Rüdin, 16 Oct 1942. Subsequent citations also from this source. Pette's suggestions appear in Rüdin's programme as items 12 and 13.

11 Ibid.

12 BAB, All. Proz. 7, Roll 12, Frame 220, Memorandum by Paul Nitsche of 9 Apr 1941. Subsequent citations also from this source.

13 Washington, DC, National Archives Washington (hereafter NAW), Record Group 549, box 1, folder 5, Bl. 124914, Nitsche to Brack, 23 May 1941; NAW, Record Group 549, Stack 290, Row 59, Comp. 17, Fol. 125819, Rüdin to Buhler [sic], 19 July 1941.

14 BAB, R 96 I/9, Carl Schneider, 'Schlussbemerkungen. Wissenschaftliche, wirtschaftliche und soziale Bedeutung und Zukunft der psychiatrischen Therapien'. All subsequent citations also from this source. Also discussed in Aly, *Die Belasteten*, pp. 201–203; Schmuhl, *Gesellschaft*, pp. 365–369.

15 Creutz's role in this research is disputed. Cf. Hans-Walter Schmuhl, 'Walter Creutz und die "Euthanasie" in der Rheinprovinz. Zwischen Resistenz und Kollaboration', *Der Nervenarzt*, 84 (2013), pp. 1069–1074; idem, *Gesellschaft*, pp. 310–315.

16 BAB, R 96 I/11, Nitsche to Rüdin, 17 June 1941.

17 MPIP-HA, GDA 128, Rüdin to Creutz, 26 Oct 1942. Subsequent citation also from this source.

18 This document is addressed frequently in research and sections of it have been cited. Cf. Matthias M. Weber, *Ernst Rüdin. Eine kritische Biographie*, Berlin: Springer, 1993, p. 279; Volker Roelcke, Gerrit Hohendorf and Maike Rotzoll, 'Psychiatrische Genetik und "Erbgesundheitspolitik" im Nationalsozialismus. Zur Zusammenarbeit zwischen Ernst Rüdin, Carl Schneider und Paul Nitsche', *Schriftenreihe der Deutschen Gesellschaft für Geschichte der Nervenheilkunde*, 6 (2000), p. 67; Volker Roelcke, 'Psychiatrische Wissenschaft im Kontext nationalsozialistischer Politik und "Euthanasie": Zur Rolle von Ernst Rüdin und der Deutschen Forschungsanstalt/Kaiser-Wilhelm-Institut für Psychiatrie', in Doris Kaufmann (ed.), *Die Kaiser-Wilhelm-Gesellschaft im Nationalsozialismus, Bd. 1*, Göttingen: Wallstein, 2000, pp. 130 f. and 135 f.; Volker Roelcke, Gerrit Hohendorf and Maike Rotzoll, 'Psychiatrische Forschung, "Euthanasie" und der "Neue Mensch". Zur Debatte um Menschenbild und Wertsetzungen im Nationalsozialismus', in Andreas Frewer and Clemens Eickhoff (eds), *"Euthanasie" und die aktuelle Sterbehilfe-Debatte*, Frankfurt am Main and New York: Campus, 2000, p. 201; Volker Roelcke, 'Ernst Rüdin – renommierter Wissenschaftler, radikaler Rassenhygieniker', *Der Nervenarzt*, 83 (2012), pp. 303–310. In order to elaborate the overall conception of this research program in more detail, the document will be discussed comprehensively below.

19 MPIP-HA, GDA 129, Rüdin to Reichsgesundheitsführer, z. Hd. Doz. Dr. Schütz, 23 Oct 1942. Subsequent citations also from this source (emphases in the original).

20 During his leave from military service from October 1942 to March 1943, Bruno Schulz investigated the frequency of suicide in manic-depressive men, see 'XXII. Bericht über die Deutsche Forschungsanstalt für Psychiatrie, Kaiser-Wilhelm-Institut in München', *Zschr. ges. Neurol. Psychiatr.*, 175 (1942), pp. 483–484.

21 On this at length: Schmuhl, *Kaiser Wilhelm Institute*, pp. 316–318.

22 Siegfried Tzschucke, 'Die unehelich Geborenen, ein empfindlicher Wertmesser für die sittliche Kraft unseres Volkes', *Archiv für Rassen- und Gesellschaftsbiologie*, 36 (1942), pp. 83–148. On the following: Weber, *Ernst Rüdin*, pp. 265 f.

23 Cited in ibid., p. 266.

24 Karl Valentin Müller, 'Unehelichkeit und Rassenpflege. Eine Stellungnahme zu dem Aufsatz von S. Tzschucke', *Archiv für Rassen- und Gesellschaftsbiologie*, 36 (1942), pp. 346–357. At the *Deutsche Forschungsanstalt für Psychiatrie*, on 1 Oct 1940 Dr Erwin Schröter had begun studying the files of the family division of the Munich circuit court for a project on 'the hereditary biological worth of the illegitimate child'. However, he was drafted into the *Waffen-SS* temporarily in Nov 1940, and permanently in Feb 1941. According to Rüdin's statements, as a physician with the *Waffen-SS* he continued to work on evaluating the collected material, see 'XXI. Bericht über die Deutsche Forschungsanstalt für Psychiatrie, Kaiser-Wilhelm-Institut in München', *Zschr. ges. Neurol. Psychiatr.*, 173 (1941), p. 795; 'XXII. Bericht über die Deutsche Forschungsanstalt für Psychiatrie', pp. 482 f.; 'XXIII. Bericht über die Deutsche Forschungsanstalt für Psychiatrie, Kaiser-Wilhelm-Institut in München', *Zschr. ges. Neurol. Psychiatr.*, 177 (1943), p. 319.

25　Ernst Rüdin, 'Zehn Jahre nationalsozialistischer Staat', *Archiv für Rassen- und Gesellschaftsbiologie*, 36 (1942), p. 321 f. Cf. also Sheila Faith Weiss, *The Nazi Symbiosis: Human Genetics and Politics in the Third Reich*, Chicago and London: University of Chicago Press, 2010, pp. 170 f.

26　Until 1944 Rüdin attempted to exert influence on a future *Gemeinschaftsfremdengesetz* (Community Aliens Act). Cf. Weber, *Ernst Rüdin*, p. 280.

27　This refers to the research by Karlheinz Idelberger on the heritability of the clubfoot, of congenital hip displaysia and lip, jaw and palate clefts, see Weber, *Ernst Rüdin*, p. 246; Weiss, *Nazi Symbiosis*, p. 158 f.

28　Here Rüdin was apparently referring to the research Bruno Schulz had been performing for so long, who, on leave from the *Wehrmacht* from Oct 1942 to Mar 1943, had resumed working at his Institute in Munich, as well as on two research projects on "the hereditary predisposition of patients who [suffer] from short, non-recurring, attacks and longer periods of complete remission". Cf. 'XXII. Bericht über die Deutsche Forschungsanstalt für Psychiatrie', p. 484 and 'XXIII. Bericht über die Deutsche Forschungsanstalt für Psychiatrie', p. 319.

29　BAB, R 96 I/5, Memorandum by Nitsche of 20 Sept 1941. Cf. Falk and Hauer, *Brandenburg-Görden*, pp. 112–118.

30　Beddies, 'Forschungsabteilung'; idem, 'Kinder', pp. 146 ff.

31　Volker Roelcke, Gerrit Hohendorf, Maike Rotzoll, 'Erbpsychologische Forschung im Kontext der "Euthanasie". Neue Dokumente zu Carl Schneider, Julius Deussen und Ernst Rüdin', *Fortschritte der Neurologie – Psychiatrie*, 66 (1998), pp. 331–336; Volker Roelcke, 'Kontinuierliche Umdeutungen: Biographische Repräsentationen am Beispiel der Curricula vitae des Psychiaters Julius Deussen (1906–1974)', in Kornelia Grundmann and Irmtraut Sahmland (eds), *Concertino. Ensemble aus Kultur- und Medizingeschichte. Festschrift zum 65. Geburtstag von Prof. Dr. Gerhard Aumüller*, Marburg: Univ.-Bibliothek, 2008, pp. 221–232.

32　Marion Hulverscheidt, 'Die Beteiligung von Mitarbeitern des Robert-Koch-Instituts an Verbrechen gegen die Menschlichkeit – tropenmedizinische Menschenversuche im Nationalsozialismus', in eadem and Anja Laukötter (eds), *Infektion und Institution. Zur Wissenschaftsgeschichte des Robert Koch-Instituts im Nationalsozialismus*, Göttingen: Wallstein, 2009, pp. 147–168.

33　Weber, *Ernst Rüdin*, p. 279 f. Also see: Roelcke, 'Ernst Rüdin'; Weiss, *Nazi Symbiosis*, pp. 174–180.

34　On this at length: Schmuhl, *Gesellschaft*, pp. 384–390.

Bibliography

Archival sources

Germany

Berlin, Bundesarchiv Berlin (BAB):
All. Proz. 7, Roll 12, Fr. 220
R 96 I/4–5, 9 and 11
Munich, Max-Planck-Institut für Psychiatrie, Historisches Archiv (MPIP-HA), GDA 128–129

USA

Washington, DC, National Archives Washington (NAW), Record Group 549

Literature

'XXI. Bericht über die Deutsche Forschungsanstalt für Psychiatrie, Kaiser-Wilhelm-Institut in München', *Zschr. ges. Neurol. Psychiatr.*, 173 (1941), pp. 783–796

'XXII. Bericht über die Deutsche Forschungsanstalt für Psychiatrie, Kaiser-Wilhelm-Institut in München', *Zschr. ges. Neurol. Psychiatr.*, 175 (1942), pp. 476–484

'XXIII. Bericht über die Deutsche Forschungsanstalt für Psychiatrie, Kaiser-Wilhelm-Institut in München', *Zschr. ges. Neurol. Psychiatr.*, 177(1943), pp. 311–320

Aly, Götz, *Die Belasteten. "Euthanasie" 1939–1945. Eine Gesellschaftsgeschichte*, Frankfurt am Main: S. Fischer, 2013

Ash, Mitchel G., 'Wissenschaft und Politik als Ressourcen für einander', in Rüdiger vom Bruch and Brigitte Kaderas (eds), *Wissenschaften und Wissenschaftspolitik. Bestandsaufnahmen zu Formationen, Brüchen und Kontinuitäten im Deutschland des 20. Jahrhunderts*, Stuttgart: Franz Steiner, 2002, pp. 32–51

Beddies, Thomas 'Kinder und Jugendliche in der brandenburgischen Heil- und Pflegeanstalt Görden als Opfer der NS-Medizinverbrechen', in Kristina Hübener (ed.), *Brandenburgische Heil- und Pflegeanstalten in der NS-Zeit*, Berlin: Be.bra, 2002, pp. 129–154

—— 'Die Forschungsabteilung in der Landesanstalt Brandenburg-Görden', in idem and Kristina Hübener (eds), *Dokumente zur Psychiatrie im Nationalsozialismus*, Berlin: Be.bra, 2003, pp. 261–270

Falk, Beatrice and Friedrich Hauer, *Brandenburg-Görden. Geschichte eines psychiatrischen Krankenhauses*, Berlin: Be.bra, 2007

Hohendorf, Gerrit, and Maike Rotzoll, 'Medical Research and National Socialist Euthanasia: Carl Schneider and the Heidelberg Research Children from 1942 until 1945', in Sheldon Rubenfeld and Susan Benedict (eds), *Human Subjects Research after the Holocaust*, Heidelberg: Springer, 2014, pp. 127–138

Hulverscheidt, Marion, 'Die Beteiligung von Mitarbeitern des Robert-Koch-Instituts an Verbrechen gegen die Menschlichkeit – tropenmedizinische Menschenversuche im Nationalsozialismus', in eadem and Anja Laukötter (eds), *Infektion und Institution. Zur Wissenschaftsgeschichte des Robert Koch-Instituts im Nationalsozialismus*, Göttingen: Wallstein, 2009, pp. 147–168

Lang, Sascha, 'Psychiatrie, technische Innovation und Industrie. Die Siemens-Reiniger-Werke und die Entwicklung des Elektrokrampftherapiegerätes "Konvulsator" im Zweiten Weltkrieg', in Hans-Walter Schmuhl and Volker Roelcke (eds), *"Heroische Therapien". Die deutsche Psychiatrie im internationalen Vergleich 1918–1945*, Göttingen: Wallstein, 2013, pp. 216–232

Leyh, Ernst-Alfred, *"Gesundheitsführung", "Volksschicksal", "Wehrkraft". Leonardo Conti (1900–1945) und die Ideologisierung der Medizin in der NS-Diktatur*, MD thesis, Heidelberg: Heidelberg University, 2002

Müller, Karl Valentin, 'Unehelichkeit und Rassenpflege. Eine Stellungnahme zu dem Aufsatz von S. Tzschucke', *Archiv für Rassen- und Gesellschaftsbiologie*, 36(1942), pp. 346–357

Roelcke, Volker, 'Psychiatrische Wissenschaft im Kontext nationalsozialistischer Politik und "Euthanasie": Zur Rolle von Ernst Rüdin und der Deutschen Forschungs-anstalt/Kaiser-Wilhelm-Institut für Psychiatrie', in Doris Kaufmann (ed.), *Die Kaiser-Wilhelm-Gesellschaft im Nationalsozialismus, Bd. 1*, Göttingen: Wallstein, 2000, pp. 112–150

—— 'Kontinuierliche Umdeutungen: Biographische Repräsentationen am Beispiel der Curricula vitae des Psychiaters Julius Deussen (1906–74)', in Kornelia Grundmann and Irmtraut Sahmland (eds), *Concertino. Ensemble aus Kultur- und Medizingeschichte. Festschrift zum 65. Geburtstag von Prof. Dr. Gerhard Aumüller*, Marburg: Univ.-Bibliothek, 2008, pp. 221–232

—— 'Ernst Rüdin – renommierter Wissenschaftler, radikaler Rassenhygieniker', *Der Nervenarzt*, 83 (2012), pp. 303–310

Roelcke, Volker, Gerrit Hohendorf and Maike Rotzoll, 'Psychiatric Research and "Euthanasia": The Case of the Psychiatric Department at the University of Heidelberg, 1941–1945', *History of Psychiatry*, 5(1994), pp. 517–532

—— 'Erbpsychologische Forschung im Kontext der "Euthanasie". Neue Dokumente zu Carl Schneider, Julius Deussen und Ernst Rüdin', *Fortschritte der Neurologie – Psychiatrie*, 66 (1998), pp. 331–336

—— 'Psychiatrische Forschung, "Euthanasie" und der "Neue Mensch". Zur Debatte um Menschenbild und Wertsetzungen im Nationalsozialismus', in Andreas Frewer and Clemens Eickhoff (eds), *"Euthanasie" und die aktuelle Sterbehilfe-Debatte*, Frankfurt am Main and New York: Campus, 2000, pp. 193–217

—— 'Psychiatrische Genetik und "Erbgesundheitspolitik" im Nationalsozialismus. Zur Zusammenarbeit zwischen Ernst Rüdin, Carl Schneider und Paul Nitsche', *Schriftenreihe der Deutschen Gesellschaft für Geschichte der Nervenheilkunde*, 6(2000), pp. 59–73

Rüdin, Ernst, 'Zehn Jahre nationalsozialistischer Staat', *Archiv für Rassen- und Gesellschaftsbiologie*, 36 (1942), pp. 321–322

Schmuhl, Hans-Walter, 'Die biopolitische Entwicklungsdiktatur des Nationalsozialismus und der "Reichsgesundheitsführer" Dr. Leonardo Conti', in Klaus-Dietmar Henke (ed.), *Tödliche Medizin im Nationalsozialismus. Von der Rassenhygiene zum Massenmord*, Cologne: Böhlau, 2008, pp. 101–117

—— The Kaiser Wilhelm Institute for Anthropology, Human Heredity and Eugenics, 1927–1945. Crossing Boundaries, Dordrecht: Springer, 2008

—— 'Walter Creutz und die "Euthanasie" in der Rheinprovinz. Zwischen Resistenz und Kollaboration', *Der Nervenarzt*, 84(2013), pp. 1069–1074

—— Die Gesellschaft Deutscher Neurologen und Psychiater im Nationalsozialismus, Berlin and Heidelberg: Springer, 2016

Tzschucke, Siegfried, 'Die unehelich Geborenen, ein empfindlicher Wertmesser für die sittliche Kraft unseres Volkes', *Archiv für Rassen- und Gesellschaftsbiologie*, 36(1942), pp. 83–148

Weber, Matthias M., *Ernst Rüdin. Eine kritische Biographie*, Berlin: Springer, 1993

Weiss, Sheila Faith, *The Nazi Symbiosis: Human Genetics and Politics in the Third Reich*, Chicago and London: University of Chicago Press, 2010

Part Two

Clinics and the sciences

4   Research on the boundary between life and death

Coercive experiments on pregnant women and their foetuses during National Socialism

Gabriele Czarnowski and Sabine Hildebrandt

Victims of National Socialism became subjects of coercive medical experiments not only in life but also in death, when their bodies were used for further research. Some investigations were even situated at the boundary between life and death, such as the collaborative studies by Karl Ehrhardt, Chairman of Gynaecology, and Alfred Pischinger, Chairman of Embryology and Histology, at the University of Graz. In 1941 these scientists published results on experiments performed on pregnant women and their foetuses surgically removed from the uterus while undergoing abortions and sterilisations for medical and eugenic reasons.

The following study will explore the historical and personal background that led to this cooperation, including the researchers' scientific and political biographies and the situation at the Women's Hospital of the University of Graz during National Socialism (NS, Nazi). Whereas for Pischinger the research on a human foetus was an exception from his usual investigative efforts in histochemistry, for Ehrhardt this human experiment was one of several coercive studies performed on women during the Second World War. In this collaboration Pischinger and Ehrhardt made the planned death of their study subjects part of their experimental design. The clinician Ehrhardt, whose traditional work was with the living, crossed the boundary towards work with the dead, while the anatomist and embryologist Pischinger, whose traditional work was with the dead, crossed this boundary towards work with the living. Other anatomists moved even further by starting to work with the "future dead", meaning living persons who were used for research purposes with the knowledge of their certain death at the hands of the NS regime.[1]

The experiments

In January 1941, the *Zentralblatt für Gynäkologie*,[2] a prominent weekly journal for gynaecologists and obstetricians, published two articles that reveal a local interdisciplinary network of scientists at the University of Graz that focused on the "biology of intra-uterine life". The initiator of this research was Karl Ehrhardt, who had been appointed as the new Chairman of Gynaecology at the University of Graz after the annexation of Austria by NS Germany in 1938. His article on "Further insights into my method of intraamnial Thorium injections (foetal organography)"[3] was the third in a series of six publications with results from his foetographic experiments on pregnant women and their foetuses, performed between 1937 and 1945. Ehrhardt had little interest in foetography as a diagnostic tool, although he did comment on the potential clinical use of the method in his publications. Instead, his chief objective was to understand the physiology of intrauterine life. He claimed to have been the first to demonstrate radiographically the physiological drinking and breathing movements of the intrauterine foetus, after having studied these questions in experiments on pregnant women and their foetuses during terminations of pregnancies for medical and eugenic reasons. Between 1943 and 1945 he experimented on a large number of forced labourers.

Instead of performing the abortion procedure in one session as was standard of care at the time, Ehrhardt started his experiments by removing a defined volume of amniotic fluid with a syringe inserted through the abdominal wall of the woman, and injecting the same volume of the radiographic contrast media Thorotrast or Umbrathor into the womb. In early pregnancies he performed the procedure vaginally via the cervical canal. He described his method as a "small procedure, easily performed under local anaesthesia and done within a few minutes".[4] The abortion itself was delayed for several hours or days (up to three days and more), during which Ehrhardt used X-rays to monitor the extent to which the foetal gastrointestinal tract and lungs filled with the contrast medium. Finally he removed the foetus from the womb via *sectio parva*,[5] which allowed him to "extract" the foetus ("egg", "fruit" in the nomenclature of the time) "unharmed"[6] and still alive in its embryonic sac. He then observed the movements of the dying foetus through the translucent membranes for five minutes, taking three radiographs during that time: one each of the foetus within and outside the membranes, and one of the isolated dissected intestines. The time of death of the foetus is not mentioned. The mother was able to leave the hospital after 14 days. There is no indication that any of the women in Ehrhardt's studies were cognisant of the nature of the experiments or that the abortion procedure was delayed and more extensive than a normal one. Ehrhardt concluded from his investigations that foetuses were capable of drinking, and he proceeded to study the topic of foetal breathing in the following years.[7]

The second member of the local research network was Alfred Pischinger, Chairman of the Institute for Histology and Embryology at the University of Graz. His study "On the nature of the child's breathing before birth" was published alongside Ehrhardt's in 1941. Pischinger wanted to investigate "the question raised of late if breathing is a physiological, normal function of the foetus".[8] This investigation remained unique among Pischinger's published research. Never before, and never after, did he report on the exploration of the physiology of the intrauterine human foetus. Pischinger explained the origins of this collaboration with Ehrhardt in the opening paragraph of the paper:

> On the occasion of a discussion of the nature of the respiration of the intrauterine foetus, which was first definitively described by Ehrhardt, Ehrhardt invited me to study several foetuses in which after the intraamnial injection of a contrast medium its accumulation in the foetal lungs could be shown by radiography.[9]

In his histological investigation Pischinger came to a conclusion that did not support Ehrhardt's hypothesis of a physiological breathing function in the foetus. While confirming the drinking movements, Pischinger found no clear evidence for foetal breathing. He argued that the respiratory foetal actions described by Ehrhardt were of an artificial nature, induced by the termination of the pregnancy by Caesarean section and the irritation of the foetal intestines and breathing centre by the radiographic contrast media. Thus breathing movements were not part of the normal foetal physiology in an undisturbed pregnancy and subsequent spontaneous delivery. In order to demonstrate the stimulating effect of Umbrathor, Pischinger suggested additional experiments with a less irritant contrast medium such as India ink. Studies of foetuses with intraamnial injection of India ink had previously only been performed on animals.[10] Thus Pischinger initiated a new set of human experiments, which were performed by Ehrhardt in four further cases. However, the results were the same, and in Pischinger's opinion did not support Ehrhardt's hypothesis of foetal breathing.

Collaborations between the Women's Hospital and the Institute of Embryology and Histology existed already, as in 1940 Richard Bayer, an assistant at the Women's Hospital and Lecturer in Physiology, published a paper under the auspices of both institutions.[11] He became another member of the Graz research network and reached conclusions similar to Pischinger's. Bayer performed experiments on two so-called 'non-viable' neonates born prematurely in the 7th month of gestation. He administered an Umbrathor-water solution via gastric tube and discovered significant changes in the child's breathing pattern compared to reactions following normal tube feeding.[12] There is no explanation why the children were considered "non-viable" when they were apparently capable of spontaneous breathing. Pischinger further involved Georg Gorbach (1901–70), Chairman of Biochemistry and Microbiology at the Technical University of Graz, in this teamwork, as he asked him for help in measuring the Thorium absorption by various tissues with ultraviolet light spectral analysis. Gorbach studied samples of cardiac blood, liver and myocardium from one of the preterm babies and one of the foetuses, but Pischinger considered the results to be inconclusive.[13] Another local supporter of this research effort was Anton Leb (1891–1965), Director of the Central-Radiology-Institute, whom Ehrhardt acknowledged for assistance with the radiographies.[14]

The work with Pischinger was not Ehrhardt's first collaboration with an anatomist. During his time in Frankfurt, Ehrhardt connected with Wilhelm Pfuhl (1889–1956), Chairman of Anatomy at the University of Frankfurt. In 1938 Pfuhl presented results from Ehrhardt's experiments on swallowing and breathing actions in 5–6-month-old foetuses in Ehrhardt's name at the annual meeting of the *Anatomische Gesellschaft*.[15] This conference report stated that the women received a "necessary abortion", and Ehrhardt emphasised that the intra-amniotic Thorotrast injections for foetography were tolerated well by "mother and child" without the induction of a miscarriage. It seems that Ehrhardt did not realise the deep cynicism of his comment: the method was perfect because it did not induce a miscarriage. However, the subsequent surgical removal of the foetus and its death were part of the original research design. Pischinger, on the other hand, was also experienced in collaborations between basic scientist and clinician through a study on a malformed foetus with the gynae-cologist Erich Engelhart from the Women's Hospital in Graz.[16] The result of that investigation was to caution against the detrimental effect of radiation on human foetuses, while in the collaborative study with Ehrhardt he used radiation as an investigative method.

Thorotrast and Umbrathor had been on the market since 1929 and contained the radioactive element Thorium as their active ingredient. Intravenously administered Thorium is permanently stored in the human body, which made the contrast media controversial in the US and Europe as early as the 1930s. Ehrhardt was as much aware of the discussion concerning a possible stem cell effect of Thorium as his colleagues. However, the substances were used until their ban 20 years later because of their carcinogenic potential. Ehrhardt was the first to use these contrast media on pregnant women in Germany.[17]

In 1945 Ehrhardt took up the question of foetal breathing again after additional experiments on pregnant women and their foetuses, including two cases in late pregnancy.[18] While admitting that the breathing actions of the foetus still needed further elucidation, he did not agree with Pischinger's interpretation. He saw his own observations supported by W. Reifferscheid and R. Schmiemann from the University of Würzburg. These gynaecologists were apparently the only other German research group working on the question, and competed with Ehrhardt for precedence in the radiographic confirmation of this phenomenon in the human foetus.[19] Stöhr's FIAT review of German embryology from 1939 to 1945, which does not include Austrian embryologists, reveals that most researchers worked in animal systems or, like Erich Blechschmidt, on the earliest stages of human development in the embryo, and not on foetal physiology.[20] The question of foetal breathing was an active area of research internationally at the time, but in Canada and the US similar experiments were performed exclusively on small mammals, such as rabbits, guinea-pigs, cats and rats, and not on human foetuses.[21] Indeed, Ehrhardt was not the first or only "foetographer". Approximately 20 scientists and groups worldwide had been experimenting on animals and pregnant women with different contrast media and with various scientific and therapeutic aims since the late 1920.[22] They included six researchers or research groups in Italy alone, three in the United States, two each in Japan and Britain, and individual scientists in Mexico, Turkey and Hungary. The German gynaecologist Joachim Erbslöh conducted research at the Women's Hospital in Bydgoszcz (Bromberg) in occupied Poland. The US-American gynaecologists Menees, Miller and Holly published the first paper on amniography in 1930.[23]

The research subjects

Evidence from Ehrhardt and Pischinger 1941

Who were the women used by these researchers as "research material" for their experiments? Ehrhardt and Pischinger differ somewhat in their description of the patients. In his 1941 article, the gynaecologist mentioned "women, for whom an abortion was planned for medical or eugenic reasons",[24] and spoke about "numerous radiographs, which I was able to obtain with my method of intraamnial Thorium injection over the last two years".[25] The radiographs in the paper show five foetal torsos "in actual size" from the 3rd to the 6th month of gestation. According to the figure legends, these are images of four foetuses whose mothers had been injected intraamnially with Thorotrast, and one more with Umbrathor. Four of the radiographs had been produced in Graz, and Figure 2 originated from an earlier study performed during Ehrhardt's time in Frankfurt am Main.[26] He had included it here with the purpose of strengthening his claim on the first proof of foetal breathing by radiography. Ehrhardt did not elaborate which of the women had had an abortion on medical or eugenic grounds, but had described the patient in the 1937 study as a 21-year-old single woman undergoing abortion and sterilisation because of a diagnosis of "congenital feeblemindedness".[27] Pischinger on the other hand wrote: "Similar to previous investigations, Ehrhardt injected women, for whom an abortion and sterilisation for eugenic reasons was planned . . . After the termination of the pregnancy I received the foetuses . . . for anatomical and histological investigations".[28] Whereas Ehrhardt did not mention the sterilisations in connection with the eugenic abortions, Pischinger omitted to reference abortions for medical reasons as sources of the foetuses.

Abortions on medical grounds

In any discussion of the potential abuse of pregnant women for medical experiments it is important to consider the specific dates, places and reasons for the abortions and sterilisations in their political context. In the first three decades of the twentieth century in Germany and Austria, the termination of a pregnancy existed in a grey zone, overshadowed by the criminalisation of abortion in criminal law.[29] An abortion on medical grounds was practised by physicians if the mother's health or life were endangered by the pregnancy or the delivery due to a medical condition. Some physicians recognised social-medical grounds for performing an abortion as well. Neither in NS Germany nor under Austro-Fascist rule (1934–38) were choices concerning abortions left to the private relationship between patient and physician, as these decisions were governed by restrictive legislation. In Austria a new law for the "Protection of unborn life" had been introduced on 30 June 1937,[30] which laid the assessments into the hands of "evaluation committees". These groups were associated with hospitals and medical consultants, and headed by a public health officer. In NS Germany, special "evaluation committees for abortions on medical grounds" within the Reich Physicians' Chamber were created and regulated by guidelines decreed in 1935.[31] From 1940 on Austria also saw the introduction of "evaluation committees" within the Reich Physicians' Chamber. Documents from Graz hospital reflect decisions from both types of committees, the original Austrian and the later NS German ones. Both stipulated the abortion and sterilisation procedure to be performed in a hospital setting.

Abortions on eugenic grounds

In Nazi Germany, legal abortions for eugenic reasons were only performed in conjunction with the forced sterilisation of the woman concerned. The "Law for the Prevention of Hereditary Diseased Offspring" (*Gesetz zur Verhütung erbkranken Nachwuchses*, GzVeN) regulated all aspects of this intervention, including the proceedings at the specially created Genetic Health Courts (*Erbgesundheitsgerichte*); the verdict of *Minderwertigkeit* (literally: status of lesser worth, based on the diagnoses of the "hereditary" diseases explicated in the law); the role of the public health authorities in the determination and enforcement of the verdict; and the regulations for hospitals and physicians performing the surgical and radiological procedures.[32] A defined set of diagnoses required sterilisation under NS law: congenital feeblemindedness, schizophrenia, manic depression, epilepsy, Chorea Huntington, congenital blindness, congenital deafness, severe physical malformation, and chronic alcoholism. Appeals against the verdicts were decided by the Genetic Health High Courts (*Erbgesundheitsobergerichte*). The law came into effect in Germany in January 1934, and in annexed Austria on 1 January 1940.[33] In spring 1934, the first forced sterilisations were performed in Germany, and in Austria in the spring and summer of 1940. In Styria, 16 physicians were authorised as sterilisation specialists at 13 hospitals, which included two University hospitals in Graz, the Women's Hospital for women and the I. Hospital of Surgery for men.[34] From 1940 on Alfred Pischinger served as a judge on the Genetic Health High Court Graz, first as a substitute and from 1942 on as a full member.[35]

The patients

As the information in the 1941 articles on the patients was incomplete and somewhat contradictory, and the Women's Hospital files do not exist any longer, some of the relevant data can be reconstructed from the *Standesprotokolle* (status records). These are tabulated account books kept by the administration of the State Hospital, which included notes on costs and diagnoses of the patients of all University hospitals.[36] While forced sterilisations based on the GzVeN were not specifically listed for gynaecological patients, a eugenic sterilisation can be safely assumed when a patient in the gynaecological hospital is recorded with one of the diagnoses of the sterilisation law. This is verified by corresponding entries from the out-patient-clinic books. Looking at the timeframe for Pischinger's and Ehrhardt's experiments and publications in January 1941, there were five forced sterilisations until late 1940, and only one of them was in combination with a termination of pregnancy. Rosa S., a "single" and "unemployed" woman, was admitted on 13 August 1940, five days before her 22nd birthday. The abortion was performed on 16 August 1940, and Rosa was discharged on 29 August. Under the rubric "diagnosis, result" it was noted that her "epilepsy [had] improved".[37] As epilepsy could be the cause for either a medical or a eugenic sterilisation, it remains undetermined which indication applied to Rosa. If Pischinger was working with foetuses from Graz, it is not quite clear why he chose the term "eugenic" as an indication for the abortions without including the more frequent medical ones.

Thus it is important to look at the other abortions performed at the Women's Hospital after Ehrhardt's arrival in Graz on 15 April 1939. The clinical term "abortus" included many different conditions at the time; among them were spontaneous miscarriages and premature births, also "criminal" and "artificial" abortions, and finally medical and eugenic ones. The number of women admitted to the Women's Hospital in Graz with the diagnosis "abortus" ranged from 36 to 64 cases per month in 1940, altogether 558.[38] Additional information comes from the *Sterbeprotokolle* (death records) of the city of Graz, which not only list neonates, children and adults, but also miscarriages with the names of their mothers. The death records reflected Austrian legislation concerning external post-mortem exams, which differed from Germany in that foetuses had to be examined and buried.[39] All patients who died at one of the university hospitals underwent an external post-mortem exam at the Institute of Pathology, which registered the deaths with the public health authority. In 1940, 11 to 36 miscarried or aborted foetuses were recorded monthly by the state hospital, a total of 271. Seventeen of these entries plus two stillborn children were marked with the note "scientific use", as evidenced by their obvious signs of previous dissection; three of them in January and seven in February. From May to December 1939, three miscarried or aborted foetuses were marked as "scientific use" in September, eight and one stillborn in October, five plus one prematurely born child in November, and one more in December, altogether 19 bodies. A comparison with the *Direktionsbuch* (department records)[40] of the Women's Hospital confirms that all but two of these bodies from 1939 hailed from there (two from the Medical Hospital). This is also highly likely for 1940, even though the relevant books do not exist any longer.

It remains unclear which of these foetuses were the ones used by Ehrhardt and Pischinger. There were at least 13 patients mentioned in their 1941 papers;

only one abortion was potentially performed for eugenic reasons by Ehrhardt in Graz during that period, and one stemmed from an earlier eugenic abortion in Frankfurt. There was a multitude of foetuses available in the Women's Hospital, including those from medical abortions. However, both authors mentioned the use of foetuses from eugenic abortions as a matter of fact and apparently considered these as a legitimate "material" that needed no further justification.

Coercive abortions on forced labourers[41]

Whereas for Pischinger the research on foetal physiology was completed with the publication of the 1941 paper, this was not the case for Ehrhardt. From the spring of 1943 until the end of the war he had control over and access to a new group of patients: pregnant women and girls from Poland and the countries of the former Soviet Union, which were forced to undergo an abortion. After the occupation of these countries in 1940 and 1941/42 respectively, millions of mostly young women and men had been deported to Germany and forced to do labour in industries such as mining, farming, manufacturing, and several hundred girls also in private households.[42] In the National Socialist racist state, "Eastern labourers" and Poles ranged on the lowest hierarchical rank of the civilian work force. They were subject to repressive restrictions in their daily lives, and decisively harsher working conditions than foreign labourers from Western and Northern Europe, and certainly than any individuals of the German and Austrian "Master-Race". Pregnant Polish women and "Eastern labourers" were sent back to their home countries until late 1942, but then the increasing shortage of workers led to a change in policy. Instead of repatriation, *Reichsgesundheitsführer* (Reich Leader of Health) Dr Leonardo Conti together with *Reichskommissar zur Festigung des deutschen Volkstums* (Reich Commissioner for the Strengthening of the German People) Heinrich Himmler organised mass abortions for "racial" reasons.[43] These terminations of pregnancies mostly took place in labour camps, but also in hospitals. About 500 of these involuntary patients could be identified at the Women's Hospital in Graz. They increased the number of potential and actual research subjects for Ehrhardt and his colleagues many times over.

One surviving original research protocol designed by Ehrhardt documents his unscrupulous use and abuse of these women. It describes experiments on 85 pregnant women and girls from the Ukraine, Russia and Poland, and reveals how Ehrhardt performed two sets of studies simultaneously on these patients, who had agreed to the abortion only under pressure and – moreover – had not been informed about the exact procedures or their consequences. One series of pharmacological investigations concerned new approaches to non-surgical abortions in middle and late pregnancies with intraamnial injections, most frequently and effectively with formalin. He presented his results to members of the Medical Society of Styria in March 1944.[44] In another set of studies Ehrhardt continued his foetographic endeavours, as he injected 67 women not only with pharmaceuticals that killed the foetus, but also with radiographic contrast media. He recorded detailed statistical data on the foetuses: length, weight and sex. Ehrhardt killed the child of 22-year-old Anna H. from Kiev shortly before the delivery with a formalin-injection. The child was 51 cm long and weighed 3,000 g.

The researchers

Karl Ehrhardt – life, work and political affiliations[45]

Karl Ehrhardt was born as a teacher's son on 24 February 1895 in Weyer/Hessen and died on 27 May 1993 in Frankfurt am Main. After a teacher training he served as an officer in the First World War from 1915 to 1918, and finished high school in 1919. He started his medical studies in 1919, became a member of the *Germania* fraternity, and as such joined the *Marburger Studentencorps*, a right-wing militia, which fought the labour unrest in Thuringia.[46] After receiving his medical degree in 1922, Ehrhardt worked first as an assistant at the Municipal Hospital in Offenbach, and from 1925 on at the Gynaecological Hospital at the University of Frankfurt, under its Chairman Ludwig Seitz. In 1931 he received his *Venia Legendi*[47] and became attending physician in gynaecology and obstetrics. His early research was focused on endocrinology, an active area of research in Germany at the time.[48] He published numerous studies in this field and founded the hormone lab at the Women's Hospital of Frankfurt University.

Ehrhardt joined the NSDAP in April 1933, and six weeks later the Cavalry Corps of the SS.[49] He was actively involved in representing the group in sports contests and in political functions, as well as in the organisation and education of the health squadron of the 10th SS Cavalry Corps.

In the early 1930s Ehrhardt had begun animal studies in placentography, whereby the placentae were visualised radiographically after intravenous application of contrast media to pregnant animals.[50] From this he developed his new methodology of foetography by intraamnial contrast injection.[51] His preferred contrast media were the radioactive Thorotrast and Umbrathor. He considered the method as safe for the mother, as he had observed the retention of Thorotrast in the placenta without spill-over effect into the mother's other tissues. Thus he started experimenting on pregnant woman slated for abortions at his hospital. The new NS laws on forced sterilisations came "timely" for his purposes, as they made great numbers of such patients available which he would consider "suitable" for his experiments. Among all the physicians at the Women's Hospital of the University of Frankfurt, he was the one who most frequently performed forced sterilisations, often in combination with abortions.[52] Ehrhardt and his colleague Doerr also performed forced sterilisations of girls aged 11 to 16 years, who were the children of German mothers and French Occupational Forces soldiers of South-East Asian and Moroccan descent. Not within the purview of the GzVeN, but on the basis of the secret decree "*Geheime Reichssache- R[heinland]-B[astarde]*" and with support from the Gestapo, these girls were rendered infertile by surgical means, with the goal of the *Reinhaltung des deutschen Blutes* (maintenance of the purity of the German blood).[53]

Ehrhardt married Elisabeth Hoffman in 1935. In 1937 he was promoted to associate professor in Frankfurt, and became a full professor through his recruitment to Graz in 1939. This appointment was a political one and would never have occurred outside the conditions of the NS regime. It was prepared by the NSDDB (the NS lecturers union), enforced by the NS Reich Ministry of Education (REM) in Berlin and purportedly supported by the SS. With his recruitment, Ehrhardt was promoted from *SS-Unterstumführer* to *SS-Sturmbannführer*, skipping two ranks of the promotion ladder from 2nd Lieutenant to Major. Ehrhardt was trained in the surgically conservative, radiology focused school of gynaecology of Ludwig Seitz, and in Graz he encountered the Viennese tradition of active surgical intervention founded by Ernst Wertheim and Friedrich Schauta. The Austrian attending physicians and assistants were superior surgeons compared to their German chief, not only in cancer surgery, but also in obstetrical procedures such as forceps deliveries. Despite the colleagues' shared memberships in NSDAP or SS, severe personal and professional conflicts erupted after a while, which became known outside the hospital. Two committees, one from the university and another from the Berlin REM, investigated circulating rumours and charges, which accused Ehrhardt of mistakes and malpractice in the fields of gynaecology and obstetrics, leading to deaths in some cases. Both committees, with support from the faculty, declared him innocent of the allegations. In particular, the second committee report noted that Ehrhardt had recognised his "surgical insufficiency" and had "acquired new expertise . . . by studious surgical practice on dead bodies, and by journeys to recognised surgeons, especially of the Viennese school".[54] Thus the chairman emerged victoriously from these investigations, and his subordinates who had criticised him, including Dr Bayer, were reprimanded. However, these events resulted in a dynamic that ultimately led to Ehrhardt's move beyond "surgery on dead bodies" to criminal surgical practices on living human beings, who had been declared "sub-human" by NS politics. Ehrhardt performed invasive vaginal surgery on young women from Poland, Russia and the Ukraine who were slated for racial abortions. In at least nine cases, the gynaecologist used a Schuchardt-incision, which was only indicated in hysterectomies for cancer, in combination with a vaginal *sectio parva*, to terminate the 2nd to 4th month pregnancies of these involuntary patients. In effect, he made a wide incision through the skin and muscles of the woman's perineum into the vaginal wall to access and cut into the uterus and then to remove the foetus and placenta, thereby extensively traumatising the women's pelvic floor.[55] The connection with the foetographic experiments is evident.

Ehrhardt left Austria shortly before the end of the war and returned to Germany. In 1945/46 preliminary criminal proceedings were launched against him in Austria, but were cancelled in 1952, because the German justice system did not extradite German suspects to foreign judicial authorities. The Frankfurt prosecutor's office pursued further investigations, but dropped them when the statute of limitations was reached. Ehrhardt never returned to an academic career. He opened a private practice and hospital in Frankfurt and continued to attend meetings of his peers. Ehrhardt was a prolific writer and published a great number of scientific papers in a relatively short time. All of them appeared in traditional and renowned scientific journals. Some of his work, including his first studies in foetography, was funded by the *Deutsche Forschungs-gemeinschaft*.[56]

Alfred Pischinger – life, work and political affiliations

Alfred Pischinger was born on 15 July 1899 in Urfahr near Linz and died in Vienna on 7 July 1983. After serving in a medical corps in the First World War from 10 March 1917 to 29 September 1918, he decided on a career in medicine. During his medical studies in Graz, Pischinger started work for Hans Rabl, Chairman of Embryology and Histology, and ultimately became his successor in 1936.[57] Apart from histology and embryology, Pischinger's teaching activities included lectures on topics of heredity and racial hygiene.[58] Pischinger was married and had several children. His son Klaus died as a child.[59]

Pischinger joined the NSDAP on 20 April 1933.[60] The party was banned in Austria in June 1933, and he acted in the underground as an *Illegaler* (illegal party member). From 1938 on he was also a member of the SA, the NSDDB (National Socialist German lecturers union), the NSV (NS welfare organisation) and a supporting member of the SS. Within the NS political system he held various leadership positions, among others as *SA-Sanitätsobersturmführer* (medical lieutenant in the SA), president of the *Gauehrengericht* of the NSDDB (regional court of honour) from 1940 to 1941, and leader of the section for science within the NSDDB from 1942 to 1944. Pischinger served as consultant on questions of racial politics for the SA,[61] and he was a member of the *Grazer Gesellschaft für Eugenik*, the local eugenics society founded in 1924. The organisation was integrated into the *Deutsche Gesellschaft für Rassenhygiene*, the German Society for Racial Hygiene, after the annexation of Austria in 1938.[62] According to one of his students, during a lecture Pischinger had prided himself on having killed his own "brain-damaged" child.[63] There is no official documentation of Pischinger's son Klaus health problems or that Pischinger was involved in his son's death. The death certificate for the two-year-old,[64] who was born on 6 October 1937, and died on 21 May 1940, stated his cause of death as "double-sided focal pneumonia". Somewhat unusual is the fact that the original diagnosis of "bronchopneumonia, developmental delay" was crossed out, and that no attending physician or midwife was listed. The diagnosis "developmental delay" could indicate that Klaus had a neurological problem. After the war a neighbour remembered that Pischinger's wife and first child had been very sick for months in early 1938, and that the child never recovered.[65] There is no evidence that Klaus was hospitalised in the *Heil- und*

Pflegeanstalt Feldhof,[66] the local mental care facility where a so-called *Kinderfachabteilung* (hospital unit specialised on "euthanasia") existed from 1941 on. In these "special departments" disabled children and youth of "foreign race" were murdered during the Nazi *Kindereuthanasie*.[67]

After the war Pischinger was dismissed from his position and incarcerated by the British Military from 9 June 1945 to 20 December 1946. All former members of the NSDAP and its organisations had to register at their place of residence within a certain time period. Illegal Austrian members (1933–38), party functionaries and NS military leaders from the rank of second lieutenant up were considered as *belastet* (incriminated) or *minderbelastet* (less incriminated) and were subject to "atonement consequences and charges", as well as permanent or temporary dismissal and ban from their profession (*Verbotsgesetz 1945*; *Nationalsozialistengesetz 1947*). In addition, preliminary proceedings for high treason were initiated against these persons. Pischinger was investigated because of his activities in the illegal NSDAP and as an SA-officer.[68] Interestingly, his work for the Genetic Health High Court was not mentioned at all. During a court hearing in February 1947, Pischinger explained the membership in the NSDAP with his initial enthusiasm for National Socialism, and the one in the SA as a manoeuvre to evade accusations by the SS for his support of a Jewish friend, Nobel laureate Otto Loewi. He claimed to have become disenchanted with the regime during the war.[69] Many of his acquaintances were willing to testify for him, none more so than his former colleague and friend, the forensic pathologist Walter Schwarzacher, who had been dismissed for political reasons by the National Socialists as chairman in Graz in 1938.[70] Schwarzacher echoed Pischinger's excuses, but also added: "I know that he has completely distanced himself from this time, and I hope and wish that he, in awareness of his tragically caused guilt, feels remorse about his error".[71] There is no explanation as to what Schwarzacher meant by "tragically caused guilt". Many witness statements were in his favour, and the preliminary investigation was terminated in January 1948. His registration as an "incriminated" person persisted, however, his plea for clemency was granted on 11 August 1948.[72] With this, the professional ban was lifted and he received the status of emeritus professor on 19 January 1949.[73]

Between 1948 and 1958 Pischinger worked in private practice, and pursued his research activity as a guest at various institutes. Throughout his life, his research focus lay on histochemistry with a view to exploring the difference of tissues in life and death. After visits to the laboratories of the anatomist Wilhelm von Moellendorff in Kiel and the physiologist Albrecht Bethe in Frankfurt in the 1920s, Pischinger pursued systematic experiments in histochemistry, which were supported by the Rockefeller Foundation.[74] Three embryological investigations dealt with the development of the head and neck in animals, and were published between 1933 and 1937.[75] Not listed in the obituary[76] is a 1939 study on a human foetus with a malformation due to accidental irradiation of the mother in early pregnancy. In this investigation, performed in collaboration with the gynaecologist Erich Engelhart from the Graz University Women's Hospital, the authors determined that radiation exposure should be avoided at all stages of pregnancy due to the risk of foetal malformations.[77] Their conclusion that after accidental exposure to deep radiation in early pregnancy "in all circumstances an abortion has to be demanded"[78] reflected the political situation of 1939, which prioritised negative selection for eugenic reasons.

While Pischinger's published research until 1945 was entirely in the basic sciences, from 1949 on he started to include explorations of problems in alternative medicine with the scientific tools available to him. He studied the cells of the reticuloendothelial system and other "soft" connective tissue,[79] and evaluated their potential for holistic therapeutic approaches in medicine. Through a special contract with the Austrian Federal Ministry for Education, Pischinger was allowed to perform his research at the Institute for Histology and Embryology in Vienna, with additional funding from the *Österreichische Gesellschaft für Erforschung und Bekämpfung der Krebskrankheit* (Austrian Cancer Society) and the *Deutsche Forschungsgemeinschaft*.[80] In 1958 he was recruited as Chairman of Histology and Embryology at the University of Vienna,[81] a position he held until his retirement in 1969.[82] His studies on "soft" connective tissue were the topic of his inaugural address on 8 October 1958.[83] Several years later Pischinger believed to have found evidence for the regulation of connective tissue by the autonomic nervous and endocrine systems, and recommended the application of this concept within the context of cancer treatment.[84] This work culminated in the publication of his book *Das System der Grundregulation* in 1975, which has been re-published since in German and English.[85] Practitioners of alternative medicine saw in Pischinger's "system of ground regulation" the scientific basis for such therapeutic approaches as regulation-therapy, electro-acupuncture and bioresonance therapy.[86] He was awarded the *Hufeland-Medaille* by the *Zentralverband der Ärzte für Naturheilverfahren*, the Association of Physicians for Complementary Medicine.[87] For several years the *Österreichische Gesellschaft für Akupunktur*, the Austrian Society for Acupuncture, presented an award in his name for outstanding contributions to the field of alternative medicine; however, the prize has been renamed since.[88]

Schwarzacher's bibliography of Pischinger's publications is incomplete.[89] It fails to mention not only Pischinger's 1941 study on the foetal breathing function, but also the collaborative study on a human foetus with Engelhart in 1939, and several papers dealing with holistic aspects of medicine.[90] The latter omission is possibly due to Schwarzacher's own reservations concerning Pischinger's hypotheses on the "soft" connective tissue. He carefully alluded to this when he formulated: "Not all of his works in this area met full acceptance, even though some of our newer insights . . . confirm the basic truth of Pischinger's approach".[91]

Richard Bayer – life, work and political affiliations

Richard Bayer was born in Graz on 4 April 1907, and died on 31 August 1989.[92] He started his medical studies in Graz in 1925 and joined the national-conservative fraternity *Corps Teutonia Graz*.[93] After receiving his medical degree in 1930, Bayer became an assistant at the Institute of Physiology. From 1932 to1938 he worked in private practice for family reasons, but continued his research during these years and joined the Graz Women's Hospital in 1938. After acceptance of his senior thesis (*Habilitation*) and receiving the *Venia Legendi* (permission to teach) for physiology Bayer became a Lecturer in Physiology in 1939/1940. While he was promoted to attending physician at the Women's Hospital in 1941, his application to extend his *Venia Legendi* to gynaecology was rejected thrice for non-scientific reasons, in 1941/43, 1949/50 and 1956. He was only successful after a complaint with the Minister of Education in 1958.[94]

He married Erika Pillwitzer in 1939 and they had four children.[95] As a young student, from 1926 to 1933, Bayer was a member of the *Steirische Heimatschutz*, an Austrian right wing paramilitary organisation,[96] and joined the NSDAP and the SS on 11 January 1933.[97] He held various positions in these formations and worked for the SD, the security service of the SS. His highest rank in the non-military branch of the SS was *Sanitäts-SS-Obersturmführer* (medical lieutenant), the same as Pischinger held in the SA. After the dispute with Ehrhardt, with whom he had been previously on good terms, Bayer tried to withdraw from his positions in the SS.[98] He then volunteered for military service at the front.[99] After the war Bayer was dismissed from his academic position, spent nine months in detention and went through denazification in 1947. He then worked in private practice, resumed his research and publishing activities, and promoted cancer prevention strategies.[100]

One of Bayer's research areas at the Graz University Women's Hospital had been in the area of premature births.[101] Much of this work was of a statistical nature, but his expertise in physiology and gynaecology made him an ideal candidate for the investigation of Pischinger's questions concerning the irritant nature of Umbrathor/Thorotrast. Another research area of Bayer was the physiology of the uterus. Since 1940/41 he experimented on women "of varying uterine statuses" by inserting a small rubber bladder into the uterine cavity, injecting different pharmaceuticals and documenting the uterine contractions via so-called "internal uterine mechanograms". His wartime substitute Franz Hoff continued this research by abusing a large number of pregnant forced labourers as experimental subjects. In their 1956 monograph, Bayer and Hoff reported data from experiments on more than 600 women investigated between 1940 and 1945, of whom 300 had been pregnant.[102] A systematic analysis of Bayer's extensive research oeuvre is still missing, thus it is not known if he performed experiments with foetuses at other times.

Conclusion: research on the boundary between life and death

National Socialist ideology and politics made it abundantly clear that certain groups of the population were not worthy of living and should be eliminated from German society. Physicians played an important role in the ensuing process of selection and killing.[103] Along the way they made coercive use of the living and dead victims of the NS regime for research purposes. Prisoners became the research subjects of SS physicians in human experiments in concentration camps, and the same happened to diverse groups of patients routinely admitted to university hospitals.[104] The bodies of dead NS victims were used by all those scientists whose knowledge gain traditionally depended on bodies of the dead, among them anatomists, neuropathologists, pathologists and forensic scientists.[105]

However, the experimental activities went further, and into new areas of scientific inquiry. The clinicians, who usually worked with the living, began making the death of the patient part of their research design, e.g. the paediatrician Elmar Türk in Vienna,[106] and the psychiatrist Carl Schneider in Heidelberg.[107] And those normally working with the dead now started work with the "future dead" in human experimentation. Among them were the anatomists Max Clara, Johann Paul Kremer and August Hirt,[108] the forensic pathologists Siegfried Krefft and Gerhart Panning,[109] the pathologist Robert Neumann[110] and the neuropathologist Julius Hallervorden.[111] The gynaecologist Ehrhardt and the embryologist/histologist Pischinger performed research right at the boundary between life and death, on dying foetuses. For Ehrhardt this human experiment was one among many other coercive studies performed on women during the Second World War.[112] For Pischinger it remained the only publication of its kind.

In all discussions on coercive human experiments in the first half of the twentieth century, it is important to note that there was no clearly delineated border between the abuse of NS victims and that of other patients. The transitions from one group to the other were fluent, and none of these people were ever informed about the planned experimental procedures or asked for their consent. While guidelines for informed consent had existed for Prussia and Germany since 1931, their legal status was ambiguous and their application rare.[113] Among the most vulnerable human beings were women admitted for abortions, whereby it did not matter whether the planned termination of pregnancy was based on medical grounds, or was forced for racist and eugenic reasons. Relevant for the scientists was that the women undergoing abortions for political reasons greatly increased the number of potential "research subjects".

Ehrhardt's and his colleagues' abortion treatment of the forced labourers even in the latest stages of pregnancy made them complicit with the NS genocidal system, which intended the annihilation and selective incorporation of the *Ostvölker*.[114] However, the abuse of women for scientific experiments in general followed an older tradition, which treated poor and disenfranchised patients as "material" for research and medical education. In National Socialism it was not only the economic and social, but also the "racial" difference that led to an unprecedented increase of "patient material".[115] The discriminatory approach to patients as "material" persisted at least until the 1960s and can still be found sporadically.

The collaboration of Ehrhardt and Pischinger is an example of scientific networking under the conditions of the Third Reich. Ehrhardt gained Pischinger's scientific interest in an area originally outside Pischinger's research focus, but at the time made easily accessible for scientific inquiry through Ehrhardt's activities. Once Pischinger was involved, the histologist developed his own conclusions and devised new experiments on the foetuses, for which he recruited assistance from Bayer, who performed studies that were also outside his own primary field of research. The ethical transgressions committed by Ehrhardt, Pischinger and Bayer lay less in their observations of the dying and dead foetuses or preterm babies, as the "method" of experimenting with freshly aborted foetuses was actually an accepted practice at the time, pursued in the US and published in such popular media as *Time Magazine* in 1938.[116] Even if this approach seems unconscionable from a modern point of view following the changes in ethical thinking concerning foetal research and social perceptions of foetuses,[117] the true iniquity committed by the scientists in Graz lay in their willingness to join in the officially sanctioned abuse of vulnerable women and their foetuses, patients who were forced into abortion, against their will and without a real understanding of the consequences of the surgeries performed on them, including the potential long-term damage to their health. Even if Pischinger may not have worked on foetuses from eugenic abortions, he apparently had no reservations about doing so and assumed that they hailed indeed from eugenic abortions. He also assisted the regime as a consultant on questions of racial hygiene and member of the Genetic Health High Courts, which were responsible for verdicts on eugenic measures. Ehrhardt performed eugenic abortions, which generated the "opportunity" for scientific studies on the resulting "material". The scientists established a local network of abusive research that drew in their colleagues Bayer and others. Under the conditions created by the National Socialist regime, all manner of transgressions were committed by those scientists who were prepared to cross the traditional boundaries of research ethics.

Notes

1   Sabine Hildebrandt, 'Stages of Transgression: Anatomical Research in National Socialism', in Sheldon Rubenfeld and Susan Benedict (eds), *Human Subjects Research after the Holocaust*, New York: Springer, 2014, pp. 68–85.

2   The editor of the *Zentralblatt für Gynäkologie* was the Berlin Chairman of Gynaecology Walter Stoeckel (1871–1961).

3   Karl Ehrhardt, 'Weitere Erfahrungen mit meiner Methode der intraamnialen Thorium-injektion (Fetale Organographie)', *Zentralblatt für Gynäkologie*, 65(1941), pp. 114–120. All translations by author S.H.

4   Ibid., p. 115.

5   Literally: small Caesearian section; a Caesarian section that was employed for the termination of pregnancies after the 3rd month and could be performed transvaginally or via an abdominal incision. In 1936 the gynaecologist Mikulicz-Radecki recommended the transabdominal route for pregnancies from the 3rd month on; see: Karl Heinrich Bauer and Felix von Mikulicz-Radecki, *Die Praxis der Sterilisierungsoperationen*, Leipzig: Verlag von Johann Ambrosius Barth, 1936, p. 148.

6 Here and in the following: Karl Ehrhardt, 'Der trinkende Fötus: Eine röntgenologische Studie', *Münchener Medizinische Wochenschrift*, 84 (1937), p. 1699.

7 Idem, 'Atmet das Kind im Mutterleib? Eine röntgenologische Studie', *Münchner Medizinische Wochenschrift*, 86(1939), pp. 915–918; idem, 'Weitere Erfahrungen'; idem, 'Atmet das Kind im Mutterleib? Ein weiterer Beitrag zur intrauterinen Biologie des Kindes', *Medizinische Zeitschrift*, 5 (1945), pp.182–183.

8 Alfred Pischinger, 'Über das Wesen kindlicher Atembewegungen vor der Geburt', *Zentralblatt für Gynäkologie*, 65(1941), p. 124.

9 Ibid., p. 120.

10 Ibid., p. 122.

11 Richard Bayer, 'Die Molenbildung als Abortusursache', *Zeitschrift für Geburtshilfe und Frauenheilkunde*, 2(1940), pp. 641–650.

12 Pischinger, 'Über das Wesen', p. 123.

13 Ibid.

14 Ehrhardt, 'Weitere Erfahrungen', p. 120.

15 Idem, 'Der trinkende und atmende Fetus. (vorgezeigt und mitgeteilt von W. Pfuhl, Frankfurt a. M.)', *Verhandlungen der Anatomischen Gesellschaft (Suppl.)*, 87(1938), pp. 420–422.

16 Erich Engelhart and Alfred Pischinger, 'Über eine durch Röntgenstrahlen verursachte menschliche Missbildung', *Münchener Medizinsche Wochenschrift*, 34(1939), pp. 1315–1316.

17 Gabriele Czarnowski, 'Involuntary Abortion and Coercive Research on Pregnant Forced Laborers in National Socialism', in Rubenfeld and Benedict, *Human Subjects Research*, pp. 99–108.

18 Ehrhardt, 'Atmet das Kind' (1945).

19 W. Reifferscheid and R. Schmiemann, 'Röntgenographischer Nachweis der intrauterinen Atembewegung des Fetus', *Zentralblatt für Gynäkologie*, 3(1939), pp. 146–153. Ehrhardt, 'Weitere Erfahrungen', p. 119.

20 Philipp Stöhr, *FIAT Review of German Science 1939–1945. Anatomy, Histology and Embryology*, Wiesbaden: Dieterich'sche Verlagsbuchhandlung, 1947, pp. 144–148.

21 Franklin F. Snyder and Morris Rosenfeld, 'Intrauterine Respiratory Movements of the Human Fetus', *Journal of the American Medical Association*, 108(1937), pp. 1946–1948, idem, 'Fetal Respiration and its Relation to Abnormalities of the Newborn', *The Canadian Medical Association Journal*, 38.4 (1938), pp. 338–339; W.H. Whitehead, W.F. Windle and R.F. Becker, 'Changes in Lung Structure during Aspiration of Amniotic Fluid and During Air-Breathing at Birth', *Anatomical Record*, 83 (1942), pp. 255–265.

22 Gabriele Czarnowski, 'Fetography: A National Socialist Crime on Pregnant Forced Laborers and the International Research context', paper presented at the International Symposium "Reassessing Nazi Human Experiments and Coerced Research, 1933–1945: New Findings, Interpretations and Problems", Wadham College, Oxford, 4–7 July, 2013.

23 T.O. Menees, J.D. Miller and L.E. Holly, 'Amniography: Preliminary report', *American Journal of Roentgenology and Radiation*, 24(1930), pp. 363–366.

24 Erhardt, 'Weitere Erfahrungen', p. 114.

25 Ibid., p. 119.

26 Idem, 'Der trinkende und atmende Fetus', p. 421.

27 Idem, 'Der trinkende Fötus', p. 1699.

28 Idem, 'Weitere Erfahrungen', p. 121.

29 For Austria, see Maria Mesner, Geburten/Kontrolle. Reproduktionspolitik im 20. Jahrhundert, Vienna: Böhlau 2010. For Germany, see Atina Grossmann, *Reforming Sex. The Movement for Birth Control and Abortion Reform, 1920–1950*, New York and Oxford: Oxford University Press. 1995; Cornelie Usborne, *The Politics of the Body in Weimar Germany: Women's Rights and Women's Duty*, London: Palgrave Macmillan,

1992; Gabriele Czarnowski, 'Women's crimes, state crimes: abortion in Nazi Germany', in Margaret L. Arnot and Cornelie Usborne (eds), *Gender and Crime in Modern Europe*, London: UCL Press, 1999, pp. 238–256.

30 *Bundesgesetz zum Schutz des keimenden Lebens*, Bundesgesetzblatt für den Bundesstaat Österreich 1937, [30.6.1937] Stück 57, Nr. 203, pp. 885–888.

31 Reichsärztekammer (ed.), Richtlinien für Schwangerschaftsunterbrechung und Unfruchtbarmachung aus gesundheitlichen Gründen, Munich: J.F. Lehmanns Verlag, 1936.

32 Arthur Gütt, Ernst Rüdin and Falk Ruttke, Gesetz zur Verhütung erbkranken Nachwuchses vom 14. Juli 1933 nebst Ausführungsverordnungen, 2nd rev. ed., Munich and Berlin, J.F. Lehmanns Verlag, 1936; Gisela Bock, Zwangssterilisation im Nationalsozialismus. Studien zur Rassenpolitik und Geschlechterpolitik, repr. 1st ed., Münster: Monsenstein und Vannedat, 2010.

33 Kundmachung des Reichskommissars für die Wiedervereinigung Österreichs mit dem deutschen Reich, wodurch die Verordnung über die Einführung des Gesetzes zur Verhütung erbkranken Nachwuchses und des Gesetzes zum Schutze der Erbgesundheit des deutschen Volkes in der Ostmark vom 14. November 1939 bekanntgemacht wird, Gesetzblatt für das Land Österreich 1939, Nr. 1438, pp. 4953–4990.

34 Birgit Poier, ' "Erbbiologisch unerwünscht". Die Umsetzung rassenhygienisch motivierter Gesundheits- und Sozialpolitik in der Steiermark', in Wolfgang Freidl and Werner Sauer (eds), *NS-Wissenschaft als Vernichtungsinstrument. Rassenhygiene, Zwangssterilisation, Menschenversuche und NS-Euthanasie in der Steiermark*, Vienna: Facultas, 2004, p. 214.

35 Ibid., p. 211. A register concerning the Genetic Health High Court reveals that in late 1940, at the time of Pischinger's writing of the paper on foetal breathing, the Court dealt with complaints from men, and not with any case connected to the foetographic experiments, see Graz, Steiermärkisches Landesarchiv (hereafter StLA), OLG Graz, Beschwerderegister des Erbgesundheitsobergerichts.

36 All hospitals and institutes of the medical faculty of Graz University were institutions of the State Hospital (Landeskrankenhaus, LKH) Graz.

37 StLA, LKH Standesprotokolle 502, 17051.

38 StLA, Frauenklinik Gebärhaus K. 66.

39 Since the reign of Empress Maria Theresia of Austria, *Totenbeschau* (external non-invasive post-mortem exam to ascertain the fact and cause of death and to decide on the necessity of a further invasive autopsy, *Obduktion*) and subsequent burial were mandatory for all deceased, including miscarriages, see Georg Bauer, *Gerichtsmedizin. Repetitorium für Studierende, Ärzte u Juristen*, Vienna: Verlag Wilhem Maudrich, 1991, pp. 9–10; Fritz Reuter, 'Forensische Medizin', in Josef Halban and Ludwig Seitz (eds), *Biologie und Pathologie des Weibes. Ein Handbuch der Frauenheilkunde und Geburtshilfe*, VIII. Band, 3. Teil, Berlin and Vienna: Urban und Schwarzenberg, 1929, p. 1129.

40 StLA, Frauenklinik Gebärhaus 1936–1940 K. 65.

41 See Czarnowski, 'Involuntary Abortion', pp. 102–104; eadem, 'Russenfeten. Abtreibung und Forschung an schwangeren Zwangsarbeiterinnen in der Universitätsfrauenklinik Graz 1943–1945', *VIRUS. Beiträge zur Sozialgeschichte der Medizin*, 7 (2008), pp. 53–67.

42 Prisoners of war, Hungarian Jews in *Judenlager* (camps for Jews), and prisoners from concentration camps also served as forced labourers, see Florian Freund, Bertrand Perz and Mark Spoerer, *Zwangsarbeiter und Zwangsarbeiterinnen auf dem Gebiet der Republik Österreich 1939–1945. Veröffentlichungen der Österreichischen Historikerkommission 26*, Vienna and Munich: Oldenbourg, 2004; Ulrich Herbert, *Hitler's Foreign Workers: Enforced Foreign Labor in Germany under the Third Reich*, Cambridge: Cambridge University Press, 1997 (translation of *Fremdarbeiter. Politik und Praxis des "Ausländer-Einsatzes" in der Kriegswirtschaft des Dritten Reiches*, Bonn: Dietz, 1985).

43 Children born despite these policies were separated from their mothers sometime after birth and either left to die or "Germanised" in institutions or adoptive families, see Gabriella Hauch, 'Ostarbeiterinnen. Vergessene Frauen und ihre Kinder', in Fritz Mayrhofer and Walter Schuster (eds), *Nationalsozialismus in Linz (Band 2)*, Linz: Archiv der Stadt Linz, 2001, pp. 1271–1310; Gisela Schwarze, *Kinder, die nicht zählten. Ostarbeiterinnen und ihre Kinder im Zweiten Weltkrieg*, Essen: Klartext, 1997.

44 Karl Ehrhardt, 'Schwangerschaftsunterbrechung jenseits des IV. bis V. Monats durch intraamniale Injektion von Wirkstoffen', *Medizinische Klinik*, 40 (1944), p. 507.

45 This biography is based on the following sources: Berlin, Bundesarchiv Berlin, ehem. Berlin Document Center, SSO Ehrhardt, Dr. Karl 24.2.1895; Frankfurt am Main, Dekanatsarchiv des Fachbereichs Medizin der Johann Wolfgang Goethe Universität Frankfurt am Main im Senckenbergischen Institut für Geschichte der Medizin, Habilitationsakte 91 Karl Ehrhardt; Graz, Universitätsarchiv Graz (hereafter UAG), Personalakt Karl Ehrhardt. See also: Petra Scheiblechner, *". . .Politisch ist er einwandfrei. . .". Kurzbiographien der an der Medizinischen Fakultät der Universität Graz in der Zeit von 1938 bis 1945 tätigen Wissenschaftlerinnen*, Graz: Akademische Druck-u. Verlagsanstalt, 2002, pp. 33–35; Gabriele Czarnowski, 'Österreichs "Anschluss" an Nazi-Deutschland und die österreichische Gynäkologie', in C. Anthuber, M.W. Beckmann, J. Dietl, F. Dross and W. Frobenius (eds), *Herausforderungen. 100 Jahre Bayerische Gesellschaft für Geburtshilfe und Frauenheilkunde*, Stuttgart and New York: Thieme, 2012, pp. 138–148.

46 James J. Weingartner, 'Massacre at Mechterstedt: The Case of the *Marburger Studentencorps*, 1920', *The Historian*, 37.4 (1975), pp. 598–618.

47 Licence to teach at an academic institution.

48 Compare: Carl Clauberg, *Die weiblichen Sexualhormone in ihren Beziehungen zum Genitalzyklus und zum Hypophysenvorderlappen*, Berlin: Verlag von Julius Springer, 1933. Clauberg also started his career in endocrinology and proceeded to perform coercive sterilisation experiments on women at Auschwitz concentration camp.

49 Paul J. Wilson, *The Equestrian SS: Organization, Function and Leadership*, PhD thesis, Mississippi State University, 1997.

50 Karl Ehrhardt, 'Zur Biologie der intravenösen Plazentographie. IV. Mitteilung', *Fortschritte auf dem Gebiet der Röntgenstrahlen*, 48 (1933), pp. 405–418.

51 Idem, 'Weitere Erfahrungen', p. 117.

52 Seventy-nine of 509 sterilisations, including 148 in conjunction with abortions, see H.D. Taubert, 'Zwangssterilisierungen 1933–1945: Ein Versuch der Vergangenheitsbewältigung', *Zentralblatt für Gynäkologie*, 120 (1998), p. 22.

53 Rainer Pommerin, *Sterilisierung der Rheinlandbastarde. Das Schicksal einer farbigen deutschen Minderheit 1918–1937*, Düsseldorf: Droste, 1979; Frankfurt am Main, Archiv der Klinik für Frauenheilkunde und Geburtshilfe an der Johann Wolfgang Goethe Universität Frankfurt am Main, Operationsbücher, 1933–1939.

54 UAG, Personalakt Prof. Dr. Karl Ehrhardt, Bericht Prof. Dr. Wagner v.12.6.1942.

55 Czarnowski, 'Russenfeten'.

56 German Research Association; see Gabriele Czarnowski, 'Vom "reichen Material . . . einer wissenschaftlichen Arbeitsstätte". Zum Problem missbräuchlicher medizinischer Praktiken an der Grazer Universitäts-Frauenklinik in der Zeit des Nationalsozialismus', in Freidl and Sauer, *NS-Wissenschaft als Vernichtungsinstrumen*, p. 254.

57 Scheiblechner, *Kurzbiographien*; Hans-Georg Schwarzacher, 'In memoriam Prof. Dr. A. Pischinger', *Wiener Klinische Wochenschrift*, 96.2 (1984), p. 79; idem, 'Nachruf auf Alfred Pischinger', *Zeitschrift für Mikroskopisch- Anatomische Forschung*, 98.6 (1984), pp. 801–804.

58 Gerald Lichtenegger, 'Vorgeschichte, Geschichte und Nachgeschichte des Nationalsozialismus an der Universität Graz', in Freidl and Sauer, *NS-Wissenschaft als Vernichtungsinstrument*, pp. 61–85.

59 UAG, Med Fak Exhibitenprotokoll 1940/41–578, 29 May 1940.

60 Pischinger's party number was 1602320.

61 All political information from: Scheiblechner, *Kurzbiographien*.

62 Maria Ladinig, 'Das Gesundheitswesen, das Erb- und Blutschutzgesetz, die Vorgaben der NS-Rassenpolitik und ihre Umsetzung im Gau Steiermark', in Wolfgang Freidl, Alois Kernbauer, Richard H. Noack and Werner Sauer (eds), *Medizin und Nationalsozialismus in der Steiermark*, Innsbruck: StudienVerlag, 2001, pp. 78–82.

63 ÖCV, 'Fritz Mankowski' (2012), *www.oecv.at/Biolex/Detail/11400472* (accessed 9 Oct 2014); Friedrich Mankowski, *Herz, steig in den Morgen. Gedichte und Briefe eines großen Liebenden. Erläutert u herausgegeben von Irene Mertens und Georg Schaller*, Graz: Verlag Styria, 1985.

64 Graz, Stadtarchiv Graz, Sterbeprotokoll Mai 1940, Journal-Nr. 307.

65 StLA, LG f Strafsachen Graz Vr 7223/46, Maria Abel, 25 Nov 1947.

66 The authors would like to thank Norbert Weiß for this information.

67 Sandra Kristöfl, NS-"Euthanasie": Ihre Struktur und Systematik in Österreich. Der Grazer "Feldhof", seine Nebenanstalten und Vernetzungen mit Niedernhart und Hartheim, Diplomarbeit History, Graz: Karl Franzens University, 2012.

68 StLA, LG f Strafsachen Graz Vr 7223/46, Polizeidirektion Graz an das Landesgericht, 10 Feb 1947.

69 Ibid., Vernehmung des Beschuldigten, 4 Feb 1947.

70 Scheiblechner, *Kurzbiographien*, pp. 235–236.

71 StLA, LG f Strafsachen Graz Vr 7223/46, Erklärung Walter Schwarzacher, 28 Nov 1945.

72 StLA, Ärztekammer Steiermark K. 186 H. 3053 (Alfred Pischinger), Republik Österreich an Pischinger, 11 Aug 1948.

73 Scheiblechner, *Kurzbiographien*, p. 193.

74 Alfred Pischinger, 'Die Lage des isolelektrischen Punktes histologischer Elemente als Ursache ihrer verschiedenen Färbbarkeit', *Zeitschrift für Zellforschung und mikroskopische Anatomie*, 3 (1926), p. 197; idem, 'Diffusibilität und Dispersität von Farbstoffen und ihre Beziehung zur Färbung bei verschiedenen H-Ionenkonzentrationen', *Zeitschrift für Zellforschung und mikroskopische Anatomie*, 5 (1927), p. 385.

75 Idem, 'Über die Anlage der vierten und fünften Schlundtasche bei der weissen Ratte', *Zeitschrift für Anatomie und Entwicklungsgeschichte*, 99 (1933), pp. 113–116; idem, 'Über die Entwicklung und das Wesen des Carotislabyrinthes bei Anuren', *Zeitschrift für Anatomie und Entwicklungsgeschichte*, 103 (1934), pp. 45–52; idem, 'Kiemenanlagen und ihre Schicksale bei den Amnioten. Schilddrüse und epitheliale Organe der Pharynxwand bei Tetrapoden', *Handbuch der vergleichenden Anatomie*, 3(1937), pp. 1–70.

76 Schwarzacher, 'Nachruf'.

77 Engelhart and Pischinger, 'Missbildung', p. 1316.

78 Ibid., p. 1315.

79 Alfred Pischinger, 'Über die rote Pulpa der Milz, nebst Bemerkungen über das unspezifische Bindegewebe im allgemeinen', *Zeitschrift für Mikroskopisch-Anatomische Forschung*, 59(1953), pp. 286–299.

80 Idem, 'Über die Zellen des weichen Bindegewebes', *Wiener Klinische Wochenschrift*, 71.5 (1959), p. 73.

81 BiographiA, 'Boerner-Patzelt, Dora, geb. Dorothea Sophie Boerner, Histologin', www.univie.ac.at/biografiA/daten/text/bio/boerner-patzelt.htm (accessed 3 Oct 2014).

82 Schwarzacher, 'Nachruf', p. 802.

83 See note 57.

84 Alfred Pischinger, 'Krebs und Abwehreinrichtungen des Organismus', *Der Krebsarzt*, 21.5 (1966), pp. 297–311.

85 Idem, Das System der Grundregulation, Heidelberg: K.F.Haug-Verlag, 1975; idem and Hartmut Heine, *The Extracellular Matrix and Ground Regulation: Basis for a Holistic Biological Medicine*, Berkeley: North Atlantic Books, 2007.

86 Uwe Heyll, Wasser, Fasten, Luft und Licht. Die Geschichte der Naturheilkunde in Deutschland, Frankfurt am Main: Campus Verlag, 2006, pp. 281–282.

87 Ernst Klee, *Das Personenlexikon zum Dritten Reich. Wer war was vor und nach 1945?*, Frankfurt am Main: S. Fischer, 2003; N.N., 'Ankündigung', *Physikalische Medizin und Rehabilitation*, 8.7 (1967), www.zaen.gruen.net/archiv/pdf/1967/1967–07 (accessed 6 Oct 2014).

88 ÖGA, 'Johannes Bischko Preis', hwww.akupunktur.at/index.php?id=91 (accessed 7 Oct 2014).

89 Schwarzacher, 'Nachruf', pp. 803–804.

90 Lebenswecker, 'Die Baunscheidtmethode. Literaturverzeichnis', hwww.lebenswecker.de/baunscheidtmethode/45.htm (accessed 3 Oct 2014).

91 Schwarzacher, 'In memoriam', p. 79.

92 Scheiblechner, *Kurzbiographien*, pp. 6–8.

93 Czarnowski, 'Politische und soziale Netze der Ärzte an der Universitäts-Frauenklinik/ LKH Graz (1934/38 – 1945/48)', paper presented at the annual meeting of the Verein für Sozialgeschichte der Medizin, Vienna, 2006.

94 UAG, Habilitationsakt Dr. Richard Bayer.

95 Scheiblechner, *Kurzbiographien*, p. 7.

96 Bruce F. Pauley, Hahnenschwanz and swastika. The Styrian Heimatschutz and Austrian National Socialism, 1918–1934, PhD thesis, Rochester, NY: University of Rochester, 1966; idem, Hahnenschwanz und Hakenkreuz. Der Steirische Heimatschutz und der österreichische Nationalsozialismus 1918–1934, Vienna: Europaverlag, 1972.

97 Scheiblechner, *Kurzbiographien*, pp. 6–8.

98 Czarnowski, 'Politische und soziale Netze'.

99 Scheiblechner, *Kurzbiographien*, p. 7.

100 H. Pickel, 'Richard Bayer (1907–89), ein Pionier der Früherfassung des Zervixkarzinoms', *Der Gynäkologe*, 48 (2015), pp. 483–486.

101 Richard Bayer, 'Zur Frage der Übergeburtlichkeit männlicher Früchte in verschiedenen Fetalmonaten', *Archiv für Gynäkologie*, 169.4 (1939), pp. 619–624; idem, 'Molenbildung'; idem, 'Zur Ätiologie der Frühgeburt', *Geburtshilfe und Frauenheilkunde*, 12 (1941), pp. 198–249.

102 Franz Hoff and Richard Bayer, *Ovarialhormone und Uterusmotilität. Beilageheft der Zeitschrift für Geburtshilfe und Gynäkologie 144*, Stuttgart: Enke, 1956; Czarnowski, 'Vom reichen Material', pp. 263–273.

103 Michael H Kater, *Doctors under Hitler*, Chapel Hill: The University of North Carolina Press, 1989.

104 Paul Weindling, *Victims and Survivors of Nazi Human Experiments: Science and Suffering in the Holocaust*, London: Bloomsbury, 2015.

105 Sabine Hildebrandt, 'Current Status of Identification of Victims of the National Socialist Regime whose Bodies were used for Anatomical Purposes', *Clinical Anatomy*, 27 (2013), pp. 514–536; Jürgen Peiffer, 'Neuropathology in the Third Reich: Memorial to those Victims of National-Socialist Atrocities in Germany who were used by Medical Science', *Brain Pathology*, 1 (1991), pp. 125–131; Cay-Rüdiger Prüll, *Medizin am Toten oder am Lebenden. Pathologie in Berlin und in London, 1900–1945*, Basel: Schwabe & Co AG Verlag, 2003; Friedrich Herber, *Gerichtsmedizin unterm Hakenkreuz*, Leipzig: Militzke Verlag, 2002.

106 Matthias Dahl, 'Die Tötung behinderter Kinder in der Anstalt am Spiegelgrund 1940–1945', in Eberhard Gabriel and Wolfgang Neugebauer (eds), *NS-Euthanasie in Wien*, Vienna: Böhlau, 2000, pp. 75–92.

107 Gerrit Hohendorf and Maike Rotzoll, 'Medical Research and National Socialist Euthanasia: Carl Schneider and the Heidelberg Research Children from 1942 until 1945', in Rubenfeld and Benedict, *Human Subjects Research*, pp. 127–138.

108 Hildebrandt, 'Stages of Transgression', pp. 68–85.

109 Herber, *Gerichtsmedizin*; Johanna Preuss and Burkhard Madea, 'Gerhard Panning (1900–1944): a German Forensic Pathologist and his Involvement in Nazi Crimes during Second World War', *The American Journal of Forensic Medicine and Pathology*, 30 (2009), pp. 14–17.
110 Astrid Freyeisen, *Shanghai und die Politik des Dritten Reiches*, Würzburg: Königshausen & Neumann, 2000; Prüll, *Medizin am Toten*.
111 Benno Müller-Hill, *Tödliche Wissenschaft*, Reinbek bei Hamburg: Rowohlt Taschenbuch Verlag, 1984.
112 Czarnowski, 'Vom reichen Material'.
113 Volker Roelcke, 'The Use and Abuse of Medical Research Ethics: The German *Richtlinien*/Guidelines for Human Subject Research as an Instrument for the Protection of Research Subjects- and of Medical Science, ca. 1931–1961/64', chapter in this volume.
114 Literally: "people of the East", NS term for Eastern European nations.
115 For a review of the history of discriminatory anatomical body procurement, see Sabine Hildebrandt, 'The Anatomy of Murder: Ethical Transgressions and Anatomical Science during the Third Reich', New York: Berghahn, 2016, pp. 29–43.
116 Emily K. Wilson, 'Ex Utero: Live Human Fetal Research and the Films of Davenport Hooker', *Bulletin of the History of Medicine*, 88 (2014), pp. 132–160.
117 Ibid.

Bibliography

Archival sources

Austria

Graz, Stadtarchiv Graz: Sterbeprotokolle Mai 1939 bis Dezember 1940
Graz, Steiermärkisches Landesarchiv (StLA):
Ärztekammer Steiermark K.186 H. 3053 (Alfred Pischinger)
Frauenklinik Gebärhaus 1936–40 K. 65; 1937–41 K. 66
Landesgericht (LG) für (f) Strafsachen Graz Vr 7223/46
Oberlandesgericht (OLG) Graz: Beschwerderegister des Erbgesundheitsobergerichts Graz
Standesprotokolle LKH 1939 und 1940
Graz, Universitätsarchiv Graz (UAG):
Medizinische Fakultät Graz, Exhibitenprotokoll1940/41 Zl. 578
Habilitationsakt Dr. Richard Bayer
Personalakt Prof. Dr. Karl Ehrhardt

Germany

Berlin, Bundesarchiv Berlin, ehem. Berlin Document Center: SSO (SS-Führer-Personalakten) Ehrhardt, Dr. Karl 24.2.1895
Frankfurt am Main, Archiv der Klinik für Frauenheilkunde und Geburtshilfe an der Johann Wolfgang Goethe Universität Frankfurt am Main: Operationsbücher, 1933–39
Frankfurt am Main, Dekanatsarchiv des Fachbereichs Medizin der Johann Wolfgang Goethe Universität Frankfurt am Main im Senckenbergischen Institut für Geschichte der Medizin: Habilitationsakte 91 Karl Ehrhardt

Literature

Bauer, Georg, *Gerichtsmedizin*. *Repetitorium für Studierende, Ärzte u Juristen*, Vienna: Verlag Wilhelm Maudrich, 1991

Bauer, Karl Heinrich, and Felix von Mikulicz-Radecki, *Die Praxis der Sterilisierungs-operationen*, Leipzig: Verlag von Johann Ambrosius Barth, 1936

Bayer, Richard, 'Zur Frage der Übergeburtlichkeit männlicher Früchte in verschiedenen Fetalmonaten', *Archiv für Gynäkologie*, 169.4 (1939), pp. 619–624

—— 'Die Molenbildung als Abortusursache', *Geburtshilfe und Frauenheilkunde*, 2 (1940), pp. 641–650

—— 'Zur Ätiologie der Frühgeburt', *Geburtshilfe und Frauenheilkunde*, 12 (1941), pp. 198–249

BiographiA,'Boerner-Patzelt, Dora, geb. Dorothea Sophie Boerner, Histologin', *www.univie.ac.at/biografiA/daten/text/bio/boerner-patzelt.htm* (accessed 3 Oct 2014)

Bock, Gisela, *Zwangssterilisation im Nationalsozialismus. Studien zur Rassenpolitik und Geschlechterpolitik*, repr. 1st ed., Münster: Monsenstein und Vannedat, 2010

Clauberg, Carl, *Die weiblichen Sexualhormone in ihren Beziehungen zum Genitalzyklus und zum Hypophysenvorderlappen*, Berlin: Verlag von Julius Springer, 1933

Czarnowski, Gabriele, 'Women's crimes, state crimes: abortion in Nazi Germany', in Margaret L. Arnot and Cornelie Usborne (eds), *Gender and Crime in Modern Europe*, London: UCL Press, 1999, pp. 238–256

—— 'Vom "reichen Material. . . einer wissenschaftlichen Arbeitsstätte". Zum Problem missbräuchlicher medizinischer Praktiken an der Grazer Universitäts-Frauenklinik in der Zeit des Nationalsozialismus', in Wolfgang Freidl and Werner Sauer (eds), *NS-Wissenschaft als Vernichtungsinstrument. Rassenhygiene, Zwangssterilisation, Menschen-versuche und NS-Euthanasie in der Steiermark*, Vienna: Facultas, 2004, pp. 225–273.

—— 'Politische und soziale Netze der Ärzte an der Universitäts-Frauenklinik/LKH Graz (1934/38 – 1945/48)', paper presented at the annual meeting of the Verein für Sozialgeschichte der Medizin, Vienna, 2006

—— '*Russenfeten*. Abtreibung und Forschung an schwangeren Zwangsarbeiterinnen in der Universitätsfrauenklinik Graz 1943–1945', *VIRUS. Beiträge zur Sozialgeschichte der Medizin*, 7 (2008), pp. 53–67

—— 'Österreichs "Anschluss" an Nazi-Deutschland und die österreichische Gynäkologie', in C. Anthuber, M.W. Beckmann, J. Dietl, F. Dross and W. Frobenius (eds), *Herausforderungen. 100 Jahre Bayerische Gesellschaft für Geburtshilfe und Frauenheilkunde*, Stuttgart New York: Thieme, 2012, pp. 138–148

—— 'Fetography: A National Socialist Crime on Pregnant Forced Laborers and the International Research context', paper presented at the International Symposium "Reassessing Nazi Human Experiments and Coerced Research, 1933–1945: New Findings, Interpretations and Problems", Wadham College, Oxford, 4–7 July, 2013

—— 'Involuntary Abortion and Coercive Research on Pregnant Forced Laborers in National Socialism', in Sheldon Rubenfeld and Susan Benedict (eds), *Human Subjects Research after the Holocaust*, New York: Springer, 2014, pp. 99–108

Dahl, Matthias, 'Die Tötung behinderter Kinder in der Anstalt am Spiegelgrund 1940–1945', in Eberhard Gabriel and Wolfgang Neugebauer (eds), *NS-Euthanasie in Wien*, Vienna: Böhlau, 2000, pp. 75–92

Ehrhardt, Karl, 'Zur Biologie der intravenösen Plazentographie. IV. Mitteilung', *Fortschritte auf dem Gebiet der Röntgenstrahlen*, 48 (1933), pp. 405–418

—— 'Der trinkende Fötus: Eine röntgenologische Studie', *Münchner Medizinische Wochenschrift*, 84 (1937), pp. 1699–1670

—— 'Der trinkende und atmende Fetus (vorgezeigt und mitgeteilt von W. Pfuhl, Frankfurt a. M.)', *Verhandlungen der Anatomischen Gesellschaft (Suppl.)*, 87 (1938), pp. 420–422

—— 'Atmet das Kind im Mutterleib? Eine röntgenologische Studie', *Münchner Medizinische Wochenschrift*, 86 (1939), pp. 915–918

—— 'Weitere Erfahrungen mit meiner Methode der intraamnialen Thoriuminjektion (Fetale Organographie)', *Zentralblatt für Gynäkologie*, 65 (1941), pp. 114–120

—— 'Schwangerschaftsunterbrechung jenseits des IV. bis V. Monats durch intraamniale Injektion von Wirkstoffen', *Medizinische Klinik*, 40 (1944), p. 507

—— 'Atmet das Kind im Mutterleib? Ein weiterer Beitrag zur intrauterinen Biologie des Kindes', *Medizinische Zeitschrift*, 5 (1945), pp. 182–183

Engelhart, Erich, and Alfred Pischinger, 'Über eine durch Röntgenstrahlen verursachte menschliche Missbildung', *Münchener Medizinische Wochenschrift*, 34 (1939), pp. 1315–1316

Freund, Florian, Bertrand Perz and Mark Spoerer, *Zwangsarbeiter und Zwangsarbeiterinnen auf dem Gebiet der Republik Österreich 1939–1945. Veröffentlichungen der Österreichischen Historikerkommission 26*, Vienna and Munich: Oldenbourg, 2004

Freyeisen, Astrid, *Shanghai und die Politik des Dritten Reiches*, Würzburg: Königshausen & Neumann, 2000

Grossmann, Atina, *Reforming sex*, New York: Oxford University Press, 1995.

Gütt, Arthur, Ernst Rüdin and Falk Ruttke, *Gesetz zur Verhütung erbkranken Nachwuchses vom 14. Juli 1933 nebst Ausführungsverordnungen*, 2nd rev. ed., Munich and Berlin: J.F. Lehmanns Verlag, 1936

Hauch, Gabriella, 'Ostarbeiterinnen. Vergessene Frauen und ihre Kinder', in Fritz Mayrhofer and Walter Schuster (eds), *Nationalsozialismus in Linz (Band 2)*, Linz: Archiv der Stadt Linz, 2001, pp. 1271–1310

Herber, Friedrich, *Gerichtsmedizin unterm Hakenkreuz*, Leipzig: Militzke, 2002

Herbert, Ulrich, *Fremdarbeiter. Politik und Praxis des "Ausländer-Einsatzes" in der Kriegswirtschaft des Dritten Reiches*, Bonn: Dietz, 1985

—— *Hitler's Foreign Workers: Enforced Foreign Labor in Germany under the Third Reich*, Cambridge: Cambridge University Press, 1997

Heyll, Uwe, *Wasser, Fasten, Luft und Licht. Die Geschichte der Naturheilkunde in Deutschland*, Frankfurt am Main: Campus Verlag, 2006

Hildebrandt, Sabine, 'Current Status of Identification of Victims of the National Socialist Regime whose Bodies were used for Anatomical Purposes', *Clinical Anatomy*, 27 (2013), pp. 514–536

—— 'Stages of Transgression: Anatomical Research in National Socialism', in Sheldon Rubenfeld and Susan Benedict (eds), *Human Subjects Research after the Holocaust*, New York: Springer, 2014, pp. 68–85

—— *The Anatomy of Murder: Ethical Transgressions and Anatomical Science during the Third Reich*, New York: Berghahn, 2016

Hoff, Franz and Richard Bayer, *Ovarialhormone und Uterusmotilität. Beilageheft der Zeitschrift für Geburtshilfe und Gynäkologie 144*, Stuttgart: Enke, 1956

Hohendorf, Gerrit and Maike Rotzoll, 'Medical Research and National Socialist Euthanasia: Carl Schneider and the Heidelberg Research Children from 1942 until 1945', in Sheldon Rubenfeld and Susan Benedict (eds), *Human Subjects Research after the Holocaust*, New York: Springer, 2014, pp. 127–138.

Kater, Michael H., *Doctors under Hitler*, Chapel Hill: The University of North Carolina Press, 1989

Klee, Ernst, *Das Personenlexikon zum Dritten Reich. Wer war was vor und nach 1945?*, Frankfurt am Main: S. Fischer, 2003

Kristöfl, Sandra, *NS-"Euthanasie": Ihre Struktur und Systematik in Österreich. Der Grazer "Feldhof", seine Nebenanstalten und Vernetzungen mit Niedernhart und Hartheim*, Diplomarbeit History, Graz: Karl Franzens University, 2012

Ladinig, Maria, 'Das Gesundheitswesen, das Erb- und Blutschutzgesetz, die Vorgaben der NS-Rassenpolitik und ihre Umsetzung im Gau Steiermark', in Wolfgang Freidl, Alois Kernbauer, Richard H. Noack and Werner Sauer (eds), *Medizin und Nationalsozialismus in der Steiermark*, Innsbruck: StudienVerlag, 2001, pp. 58–85

Lebenswecker, *Die Baunscheidtmethode. Literaturverzeichnis*, www.lebenswecker.de/baunscheidtmethode/45.htm (accessed 3 Oct 2014)

Lichtenegger, Gerald, 'Vorgeschichte, Geschichte und Nachgeschichte des National-sozialismus an der Universität Graz', in Wolfgang Freidl and Werner Sauer (eds), *NS-Wissenschaft als Vernichtungsinstrument*, Vienna: Facultas, 2004, 61–85

Mankowski, Friedrich, *Herz, steig in den Morgen. Gedichte und Briefe eines großen Liebenden. Erläutert u herausgegeben von Irene Mertens und Georg Schaller*, Graz: Verlag Styria, 1985

Menees, T.O., J.D. Miller and L.E. Holly, 'Amniography: Preliminary report', *American Journal of Roentgenology and Radiation*, 24 (1930), pp. 363–366

Mesner, Maria, *Geburten/Kontrolle. Reproduktionspolitik im 20. Jahrhundert*, Vienna: Böhlau 2010

Müller-Hill, Benno, *Tödliche Wissenschaft*, Reinbek bei Hamburg: Rowohlt Taschenbuch Verlag, 1984

N.N., 'Ankündigung', *Physikalische Medizin und Rehabilitation*, 8.7 (1967), www.zaen.gruen.net/archiv/pdf/1967/1967-07.pdf (accessed 6 Oct 2014)

ÖCV, 'Fritz Mankowski' (2012), *www.oecv.at/Biolex/Detail/11400472* (accessed 9 Oct 2014)

ÖGA, 'Johannes Bischko Preis', *www.akupunktur.at/index.php?id=91* (accessed 7 Oct 2014)

Pauley, Bruce F., *Hahnenschwanz and Swastika. The Styrian Heimatschutz and Austrian National Socialism, 1918–1934*, PhD thesis, Rochester, NY: University of Rochester, 1966

—— *Hahnenschwanz und Hakenkreuz. Der Steirische Heimatschutz und der österreichische Nationalsozialismus 1918–1934*, Vienna: Europaverlag, 1972

Peiffer, Jürgen, 'Neuropathology in the Third Reich: Memorial to those Victims of National-Socialist Atrocities in Germany who were used by Medical Science', *Brain Pathology*, 1 (1991), pp. 125–131

Pickel, H., 'Richard Bayer (1907–1989), ein Pionier der Früherfassung des Zervixkarzinoms', *Der Gynäkologe*, 48 (2015), pp. 483–486

Pischinger, Alfred, 'Die Lage des isolelektrischen Punktes histologischer Elemente als Ursache ihrer verschiedenen Färbbarkeit', *Zeitschrift für Zellforschung und mikroskopische Anatomie*, 3 (1926), pp. 169–197

—— 'Diffusibilität und Dispersität von Farbstoffen und ihre Beziehung zur Färbung bei verschiedenen H-Ionenkonzentrationen', *Zeitschrift für Zellforschung und mikro-skopische Anatomie*, 5 (1927), pp. 347–385

—— 'Über die Anlage der vierten und fünften Schlundtasche bei der weissen Ratte', *Zeitschrift für Anatomie und Entwicklungsgeschichte*, 99 (1933), pp. 113–116

—— 'Über die Entwicklung und das Wesen des Carotislabyrinthes bei Anuren', *Zeitschrift für Anatomie und Entwicklungsgeschichte*, 103 (1934), pp. 45–52

—— 'Kiemenanlagen und ihre Schicksale bei den Amnioten. Schilddrüse und epitheliale Organe der Pharynxwand bei Tetrapoden', *Handbuch der vergleichenden Anatomie*, 3 (1937), pp. 1–70

—— 'Über das Wesen kindlicher Atembewegungen vor der Geburt', *Zentralblatt für Gynäkologie*, 65 (1941), pp. 120–124

—— 'Über die rote Pulpa der Milz, nebst Bemerkungen über das unspezifische Bindegewebe im allgemeinen', *Zeitschrift für Mikroskopisch-Anatomische Forschung*, 59 (1953), pp. 286–299

—— 'Über die Zellen des weichen Bindegewebes', *Wiener Klinische Wochenschrift*, 71.5 (1959), pp. 73–77

—— 'Krebs und Abwehreinrichungen des Organismus', *Der Krebsarzt*, 21.5 (1966), pp. 297–311

—— *Das System der Grundregulation*, Heidelberg: K.F.Haug-Verlag, 1975

—— and Hartmut Heine, *The Extracellular Matrix and Ground Regulation: Basis for a Holistic Biological Medicine*, Berkeley: North Atlantic Books, 2007

Poier, Birgit, '"Erbbiologisch unerwünscht". Die Umsetzung rassenhygienisch motivierter Gesundheits- und Sozialpolitik in der Steiermark', in Wolfgang Freidl and Werner Sauer (eds), *NS-Wissenschaft als Vernichtungsinstrument. Rassenhygiene, Zwangssterilisation, Menschenversuche und NS-Euthanasie in der Steiermark*, Vienna: Facultas, 2004, pp. 177–224

Pommerin, Rainer, *Sterilisierung der Rheinlandbastarde. Das Schicksal einer farbigen deutschen Minderheit 1918–1937*, Düsseldorf: Droste, 1979

Preuss, Johanna and Burkhard Madea, 'Gerhard Panning (1900–1944): a German forensic pathologist and his involvement in Nazi crimes during Second World War', *The American Journal of Forensic Medicine and Pathology*, 30 (2009), pp. 14–17

Prüll, Cay-Rüdiger, *Medizin am Toten oder am Lebenden. Pathologie in Berlin und in London, 1900–1945*, Basel: Schwabe & Co AG Verlag, 2003

Reifferscheid, W. and R. Schmiemann, 'Röntgenographischer Nachweis der intrauterinen Atembewegung des Fetus', *Zentralblatt für Gynäkologie*, 3 (1939), pp. 146–153

Reuter, Fritz, 'Forensische Medizin', in Josef Halban and Ludwig Seitz (eds), *Biologie und Pathologie des Weibes. Ein Handbuch der Frauenheilkunde und Geburtshilfe. VIII. Band, 3. Teil*, Berlin and Vienna: Urban und Schwarzenberg, 1929, pp. 967–1342

Scheiblechner, Petra, *". . .Politisch ist er einwandfrei. . .". Kurzbiographien der an der Medizinischen Fakultät der Universität Graz in der Zeit von 1938 bis 1945 tätigen Wissenschaftlerinnen*, Graz: Akademische Druck-u. Verlagsanstalt, 2002

Schwarzacher, Hans-Georg, 'In memoriam Prof. Dr. A. Pischinger', *Wiener Klinische Wochenschrift*, 96.2 (1984), p. 79

—— 'Nachruf auf Alfred Pischinger', *Zeitschrift für Mikroskopisch- Anatomische Forschung*, 98.6 (1984), pp. 801–804

Schwarze, Gisela, *Kinder, die nicht zählten. Ostarbeiterinnen und ihre Kinder im Zweiten Weltkrieg*, Essen: Klartext, 1997

Snyder, Franklin F. and Morris Rosenfeld, 'Intrauterine Respiratory Movements of the Human Fetus', *Journal of the American Medical Association*, 108 (1937), pp. 1946–1948

—— 'Fetal Respiration and its Relation to Abnormalities of the Newborn', *The Canadian Medical Association Journal*, 38.4 (1938), pp. 338–339

Stöhr, Philipp, *FIAT Review of German Science 1939–1945. Anatomy, Histology and Embryology*, Wiesbaden: Dieterich'sche Verlagsbuchhandlung, 1947

Taubert, H.D., 'Zwangssterilisierungen 1933 -1945: Ein Versuch der Vergangenheits-bewältigung', *Zentralblatt für Gynäkologie*, 120 (1998), pp. 21–25

Usborne, Cornelie, *The Politics of the Body in Weimar Germany: Women's Rights and Women's Duty,* London: Palgrave Macmillan, 1992

Weindling, Paul, *Victims and Survivors of Nazi Human Experiments: Science and Suffering in the Holocaust,* London: Bloomsbury, 2015

Weingartner, James J., 'Massacre at Mechterstedt: The Case of the *Marburger Studentencorps,* 1920', *The Historian,* 37.4 (1975), pp. 598–618

Wilson, Emily K., 'Ex Utero: Live Human Fetal Research and the Films of Davenport Hooker', *Bulletin of the History of Medicine,* 88 (2014), pp. 132–160

Wilson, Paul J., *The Equestrian SS: Organization, Function and Leadership,* PhD thesis, Mississippi State University, 1997

Whitehead, W.H., W.F. Windle and R.F. Becker, 'Changes in Lung Structure during Aspiration of Amniotic Fluid and during Air-Breathing at Birth', *Anatomical Record,* 83 (1942), pp. 255–265

5 August Hirt and the supply of corpses at the Anatomical Institute of the *Reichsuniversität Strassburg* (1941–44)[1]

Raphael Toledano

The crimes committed by August Hirt have been extensively studied since they were publicly exposed at the Nuremberg Medical Trial, which ran from December 1946 until Augsut 1947. Hirt's "Jewish skeleton collection" project is the emblematic case of unethical misbehaviour of a physician under National Socialism: it shows the extreme barbarities of some scientific practices under the Third Reich and it "exemplifies the horror of the Jewish condition during the Nazi period".[2] Less well known is the so-called "normal" activity of the Anatomical Institute of the *Reichsuniversität Strassburg* (RUS) directed by August Hirt between 1941 and 1944. To fulfil his duty of anatomy teacher, August Hirt had to find dead corpses for the dissection lessons. At the Nuremberg Medical Trial, his assistant testified that he "made at least 250 preservations of Russian and Polish prisoners who died under the ill treatment at [Mutzig]".[3] These bodies were used for teaching and research purposes at the Anatomical Institute of the RUS.

French Military Justice tried August Hirt in absentia during the first of the two Struthof Medical Trials (Metz, 1952 and Lyon, 1954) but the three investigating judges who were in charge of the file between 1945 and 1952 were not interested in the prisoners' bodies delivered to the Anatomical Institute. The subject was neither addressed during the investigation nor during the Metz Trial. The reason might be that August Hirt was never caught and that his individual case was hardly mentioned[4] on 18 December 1952 at the Metz trial. While the French Press believed that he hid himself in Sweden,[5] August Hirt was actually dead in 1945. After the Struthof Medical Trials, the many researchers who have been interested in August Hirt's career and crimes have focused so far on the history of the "Jewish skeleton collection"[6] and, to a lesser extent, on his mustard gas experiments. There are relatively few references to the supply of corpses in the literature, except to mention in a general way that August Hirt used to receive corpses from Mutzig[7] or that he tried to obtain dead bodies from KL Natzweiler.[8]

For several reasons, the subject of the bodies delivered to the Anatomical Institute of the RUS needs to be addressed in more detail. This topic of research is part of the study of the behaviour of the anatomists and the anatomical departments under National Socialism, which has resulted in a series of publications[9] since the 1980s. Moreover, it contributes answers to the persistent question: are there still human samples obtained under the Third Reich in the Medical Faculty of Strasbourg? A polemic erupted after the publication of a book[10] in January 2015, which quoted the testimony of Uzi Bonstein. This former anatomy instructor of Strasbourg claimed to have seen at the end of the 1970s some jars labelled *Juden* (Jews) and *Zigeuner* (Gypsies) at the Institute of Anatomy of Strasbourg.[11] The University of Strasbourg immediately issued a denial,[12] based on the recent inventory of the Anatomical Institute's museum done by 15 medical students, under the leadership of the anatomist Jean-Marie Le Minor.[13] These testimonies are old[14] and have been officially denied on numerous occasions by the Medical Faculty of Strasbourg through press releases in newspapers.[15] However, until now, no light has been shed on the body procurement during the Third Reich, on the fate of those bodies, and on what happened to the anatomical preparations made by August Hirt.

This chapter will try to answer the following questions. How did August Hirt obtain corpses during the war? How did he manage the deliveries? Where did these bodies come from? What happened to them? And, finally, is it possible to identify them? Were they the victims of National Socialism?

Until September 1939, the French anatomist André Forster headed the Anatomical Institute of Strasbourg. With the beginning of the Second World War, the Civil Hospital and the Faculty of Medicine of Strasbourg moved to Clermont-Ferrand where French professors were able to continue teaching during the war. On 19 June 1940, the Nazis entered Strasbourg (whose name was Germanised to *Strassburg* between June 1940 and November 1944) and soon decided to create a special university in the newly annexed region of Alsace (*Elsass*). This university was the third *Reichsuniversität* to be created since 1933 (the *Reichsuniversität Prag* was inaugurated in Prague/Prag on 4 November 1939, and the *Reichsuniversität Posen* was inaugurated in Poznań/Posen on 27 April 1941), with the specific task to be "the bulwark of the great warrior National Socialist German Reich against the West".[16] The *Reichsuniversität Strassburg* was inaugurated[17] on 23 November 1941. August Hirt was appointed to the new Faculty of Medicine as professor of anatomy, histology and embryology, and director[18] of the Anatomical Institute of Strasburg. He held the position until November 1944. Just before the liberation of the city, he escaped from Strassburg and served as the Dean of the Faculty of Medicine of the RUS, which was moved to Tübingen until its termination in April 1945. At Natzweiler-Struthof, about 60 kilometers from Strassburg, the Nazis had opened a concentration camp on May 1941. During the three years at the RUS, August Hirt pursued various criminal activities. He carried out experiments with mustard gas[19] on 15 prisoners of KL Natzweiler in December 1942 (three died). He tried to create a Jewish anatomical collection[20] for which 86

Jews selected in Auschwitz were gassed in the Struthof-Natzweiler gas chamber in August 1943. He was also involved in a series of gassings with phosgene[21] conducted by Otto Bickenbach at the Struthof-Natzweiler gas chamber in June and August 1944 on 16 Roma and Sinti (causing four deaths). The discovery of his crimes after the liberation of Strasbourg led to the publication of articles[22] in the newspapers in early 1945. Hirt escaped to the Black Forest and finally committed suicide[23] on 2 June 1945.

The life and career of anatomist August Hirt has been well studied since the end of the war because of the notoriety of his crimes revealed during the Nuremberg Medical Trial.[24] Born[25] in Mannheim (Germany) on 29 April 1898, August Erwin Theobald Hirt had studied[26] medicine at the University of Heidelberg, after being seriously wounded in the left jaw during the First World War. After defending his doctorate in January 1922, he began a career as an anatomist, holding various positions[27] as a professor at Heidelberg (1933), Greifswald (1936), then in Frankfurt from 1938. His biggest achievement was the development of a fluorescent microscopy method[28] for viewing living tissue. This work, conducted in collaboration with pharmacology professor Philipp Ellinger, had led to the manufacture of an intravital microscope produced from 1929 by the firm of Zeiss in Jena. With the advent of Hitler to power in 1933, laws were enacted in Germany to oust Jews from academic posts. Because of his Jewish descent, Philipp Ellinger was forced to resign his professorship at Düsseldorf. August Hirt did not support the man who had been his mentor and with whom he had published eight scientific articles between 1925 and 1931. Later, he even pretended to be the sole inventor of the microscope and claimed sole authorship.[29] A virulent anti-Semite and a fervent nationalist, August Hirt was both a member of the Nazi Party and member of the SS, which he joined[30] in April 1933. In 1941, when the new university was set up in Strassburg, he was promoted to the position of chief anatomist. On 23 November 1941, on the occasion of the inauguration of the RUS, August Hirt met Wolfram Sievers, Secretary of the *Ahnenerbe* scientific society; Sievers was active in supporting the medical experiments of August Hirt.[31]

Among the most important employees at the Strassburg Anatomical Institute were those coworkers whom Hirt brought from Frankfurt am Main: his assistants Dr Karl Wimmer and Dr Anton Kiesselbach and his chief technician Otto Bong. In June 1942 a new technical assistant was recruited at the Institute of Anatomy: Henri Henrypierre[32] (whose name was Germanised to *Heinrich Heinzpeter*). He was Alsatian, born on 23 August 1905 at Lièpvre and previously worked as a pharmaceutical employee in Paris. Categorised by the French government as a "communist person to watch", he was interned on 28 April 1942 at Camp Royallieu (*Frontstalag 122*), located at Compiegne. After two weeks of detention, he was released on condition that he would return to live in the Alsace, as he was considered by the Nazis as "German-born". After his arrival in the Alsace in June 1942, he went looking for work in the pharmacy of the civil hospital of Strasbourg. As there was no vacancy, he was sent to the Anatomical Institute, where they sought to hire an assistant. Within months,

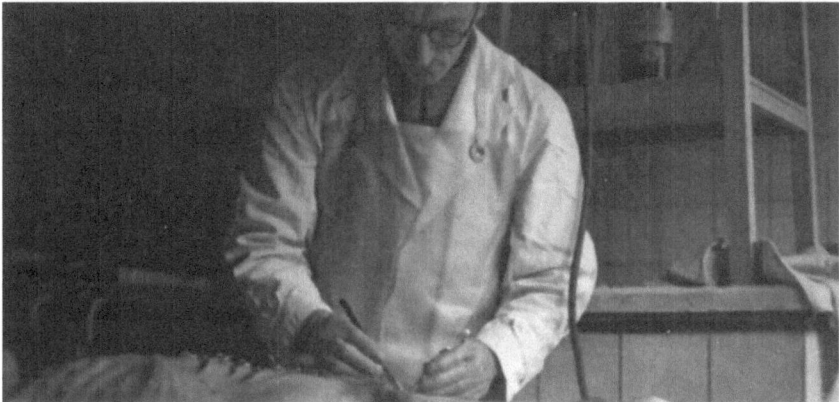

Figure 5.1 Henri Henrypierre doing the preparation of a body at the Anatomical
Institute of Strassburg

© Raphael Toledano

he was trained in the techniques of preparation and preservation of dead bodies
by Otto Bong. He remained in the anatomical department until the liberation
of Strasbourg.

As director of the Institute, August Hirt was responsible for the anatomical
education of the students at the RUS. The dissection of bodies played a central
role in his teaching during the winter semesters. When he arrived at the
Institute, Hirt encountered an inadequate body supply, due to the fact that
despite the annexation of the region of Alsace to the Reich in June 1940, the
rules in force in the *Gau* of Baden concerning deliveries of corpses to anatomical
institutes had not yet been extended to the Alsace. Thus the body storage tanks
of the Institute of Strassburg were empty in early 1942. On 21 April 1942, the
Kurator of the RUS wrote to the Civil Administrator of the Alsace in order
to have "the same rules that exist for the delivery of bodies to the Anatomical
Institute in Heidelberg and Freiburg".[33] The application was approved in the
summer of 1942 by the Ministry of Education of the Reich. However, even
before the act was made public, August Hirt confessed his impatience to the
Head of Civil Administration in the Alsace. Anton Kiesselbach met the Head
of the Civil Administration on 24 August and talked to him about the problem
of the body supply. Following this discussion, Hirt asked[34] the Head of the
Civil Administration to accelerate the process for the winter semester, which
was about to begin in late October. Teaching at the Anatomical Institute would
be in danger if it were not possible to obtain the bodies, namely: the bodies
of those who died without family and the bodies of those whose relatives did
not want to pay the funeral expenses. Hirt also insisted that a circular should
be sent to all hospitals of Alsace asking for "the bodies of those persons who
die with no relatives, or of those for which the members of the family do not
want to pay funeral expenses".[35] The note stated that the body would be used

"for teaching purposes only", that the Anatomical Institute would cover the funeral costs and that the employee who arranged for the delivery of the body would receive a remuneration of 10 Reichsmarks.

On 10 September 1942, the Head of the Civil Administration in the Alsace made public new rules for the Alsace, indicating that if a person died in public care (*Pflegling*), there was an obligation to send the body to the anatomical department.[36] This circular was complemented on 30 September 1942 by a directive reminding institutions that in case of death in "hospices and nursing homes in Alsace", with few exceptions, the welfare authority (*Fürsorgeverband*) would be in charge of determining whether the body should be sent to the anatomy rather than being buried. These new rules were also announced to the managers of psychiatric hospitals Stephansfeld and Hördt, to the care institution for the mentally retarded *Sonnenhof* (Bischweiler), to the Psychiatric Clinic of Strassburg, as well as a large number of hospitals in Alsace. Other rules were adopted, such as sending bodies of drowned[37] persons (*Wasserleichen*) to the anatomical department, although they were difficult to use from a scientific point of view. Despite all these measures, the members of the Institute of Anatomy considered, until the end of the war, the acquisition of corpses from these civil institutions insufficient to cover their needs. There is no documentation of the number of bodies sent by hospitals, clinics or nursing homes, except for a short note in a letter from Hirt indicating that between August 1942 and March 1943, he only received "eleven bodies from hospitals and hospices".[38]

Parallel to these negotiations with the civil authorities, August Hirt turned to other potential sources of corpses: the victims of National Socialism. After the start of Operation Barbarossa (Nazi Germany's invasion of the Soviet Union) on 23 June 1941, millions of soldiers and officers of the Red Army were captured by the *Wehrmacht*. These prisoners of war were sent to detention camps known as *Stalag* or *Stammlager* and *Oflag* or *Offizierslager* scattered throughout the Third Reich. Strassburg was located in the military district V where there were many Stalags: Stalag VA (Ludwigsburg), Stalag VB (Villingen), Stalag VC (Offenburg), Stalag VD (Strassburg). Two military hospitals for prisoners of war were placed in the Alsace. Prisoners of war (first Polish, then mostly Soviet, and, later, also Italian) from many prison camps were treated there. The *Reservelazarett I* was located in Strassburg[39] (in the former Hôpital Militaire Gaujot). In October 1940, the Polish prisoners were sent there for care, then, from 1941, Soviet prisoners arrived but for them, the living conditions were very difficult. After several epidemics, a second hospital for prisoners of war, the *Reservelazarett II Lazarettabteilung für Kriegsgefangene* opened, probably in 1942, in the Fort of Mutzig (renamed during the Second World War: *Feste von Witzleben*). On 29 June 1942, Hirt asked[40] the hospital of prisoners of war of Strassburg that the corpses of Soviet prisoners should be sent to him. He had to repeat his request on 5 August 1942 since he had not received any response, and then the request was granted.[41] According to our research, the first body of POW delivered to the Anatomical Institute of Strassburg was the corpse of Sergej

Kisilew. This soldier was born on 15 September 1909 in Alexejwka (USSR). He died on 11 August 1942 in the *Kgf-Laz Strassburg* (official cause of death: dysentery) and his body was sent to the "anatomy in Strassburg" on 13 August 1942. The last body transported to the Anatomical Institute we have identified was the corpse of Danijl Lugowoj. This Ukrainian soldier died in Bischheim on 24 July 1944 from a bullet trauma in the lungs. His body was sent to the Anatomical Institute on 25 July 1944. According to a laboratory assistant from the Institute of Anatomy in 1942, "each month, 30 to 60 Russian corpses [arrived] . . . all emaciated".[42] A medical student from this time remembered that there was "one corpse to dissect per six students, twice a semester".[43]

Even though prisoners of war from the *Reservelazarett* were the Anatomical Institute's main source of body procurement during the war, August Hirt also tried to obtain additional bodies in other ways. On 31 August 1942, Hirt travelled to the Natzweiler-Struthof concentration camp to discuss[44] the acquisition of bodies of prisoners who had died without family and of Soviet prisoners from the concentration camp. Following this meeting, the Secretary General of the *Ahnenerbe*, Wolfram Sievers, called the *SS-Brigadeführer* Richard Glücks, who was in charge of the economic administration of the concentration camps (*Amt D, Konzentrationslagerwesen*) in the Economic and Administrative Main Department of the SS (*SS-Wirtschafts- und Verwaltungshauptamt*, WVHA). Sievers asked for Glücks' support for Hirt's request. He told him that the Institute of Anatomy was in need of bodies and that there would be no other costs for the camp than the cost of transporting the bodies from Natzweiler. On 8 October 1942, Hirt received a list of conditions[45] issued by the WVHA.

This SS Office asked Hirt if he could comply with the following five conditions:

1 The dead had to be placed in a coffin and transferred to the cemetery of Strassburg at the expense of the Institute of Anatomy,
2 If needed, the viewing of the body must be arranged in an adequate manner with the morgue of the Institute of Pathology of the Civil Hospital and without further costs,
3 After the use of the body "for purposes of education", it must be returned to the coffin and incinerated at the crematorium of Strassburg,
4 The Anatomical Institute must inform the relevant civilian authorities of the number of the cremations, so that the burial urn could possibly be transferred to the hometown cemetery of the deceased,
5 Cremation must occur if the relatives of the dead request it within eight days after the date of dissection (which has been specified by the German administration) in the case of a German internee, or within six weeks if a foreign internee.

If the first four points were not a problem for Hirt, the last condition seemed unacceptable to Hirt who planned to use the bodies for dissection in anatomy classes throughout the winter semester. Therefore, he complained to his SS-superior, Wolfram Sievers: "A corpse that arrives during the summer semester could be incinerated at the earliest after three quarters of the year. A funeral within eight days after the viewing period would be impossible for the Institute of Anatomy".[46] Sievers shared[47] Hirt's concerns with the WVHA, but the response arrived[48] only three months later. If the WVHA was willing to amend certain requirements, it did nothing to modify the incineration time required by Hirt. Since he could not find any point of compromise, August Hirt announced to the WVHA, on 16 February 1943, that he had decided[49] to renounce the deliveries of bodies of prisoners from the KL Natzweiler. However, Sievers was not ready to accept this outcome and asked the Reich Main Security Office (*Reichssicherheitshauptamt*, RSHA) to intervene directly with the WVHA in support of Hirt. The RSHA response from 2 June 1943 apparently moved the WVHA to reconsider, as it now indicated that after "further consideration" of the issue, it finally saw "no objection" that the body of "Eastern workers who died at the concentration camp of Natzweiler, without relatives"[50] would be delivered to the Anatomical Institute of the RUS. Wolfram Sievers informed Hirt of this new decision and Hirt thanked him for his "efforts".[51] We are currently unable to find any name from an "Eastern" internee (i.e., Soviet prisoners) from the KL Natzweiler sent to the Anatomical Institute in the summer of 1943.

In March 1943, Hirt turned[52] to Professor Hans Reiter, President of the Reich Health Office (*Reichsgesundheitsamts*), complaining about the difficulties in obtaining bodies of executed people. On 15 July 1943, six French resistance fighters were shot at the shooting range of Desaix in Strassburg. Henri Henrypierre revealed in his memoirs[53] that there were not six but eight victims of this shooting. On that day, August Hirt asked Henrypierre to go with Otto Bong to the shooting range. Immediately after the execution, the first two bodies were taken by Bong and Henrypierre and transported to the Institute, where Hirt and Wimmer were waiting. The victims' bodies were dismembered and numerous tissue specimens were taken. The remains were cremated and the ashes buried on 8 November 1944. One was Joseph Bloesch who had been convicted for theft[54] in 1942. The other was a young Alsatian resistance fighter named Alfred Reiminger, member of the Fernand Schaeffer resistance group connected to "The Black Hand". A seventeen-year-old worker, he was put on trial on 16 April 1943 by the *Sondergericht* for his removing a swastika flag from a public place (the former *Place Kléber*), drawing a Cross of Lorraine in white paint on the floor, destroying the windows of several shops, stealing many bicycles, resale of food stamps, armed assault with violence and two guns found during the search. He was sentenced to death[55] by the special court of Strassburg. A new plaque was placed on his grave and inaugurated[56] on 16 June 2016 by Roland Ries, the Mayor of Strasbourg. In his memoirs, Henrypierre talks also about the execution of a Polish forced labourer, this time by hanging, which he had to attend in June 1944 in the vicinity of Metz. Again, the body was quickly taken after the death and prepared at the execution site near Metz by Dr Wimmer (injection of 60 liters of hot water in the vein).

At the beginning of the deliveries, bodies were transported by Aubry Mortuary.[57] In June, 1942 Hirt had just hired Henrypierre, who in addition to his care for the bodies now also had to learn driving. The driver's license fee was paid for by the RUS and was the answer to several of Hirt's concerns: transports by the firm Aubry were not secure and were causing additional costs. However, the Institute had at its disposal a new vehicle for the transportation of bodies: a hearse or *Leichenwagen* manufactured by Framo. Hirt wanted Henrypierre to drive it, especially for the transfer of bodies of Polish and Soviet prisoners from the Camp of Mutzig. Henri Henrypierre gave many details about the procedure used for the preparation and conservation of bodies at the Anatomical Institute. The corpse was first put on a gurney, serving as an operating table, and it was taken from the refrigerated storage room to the room where the conservation would take place. The body was washed with a large water jet and then an incision was performed from 6 to 8 cm at the groin area to access the femoral vein. In the vein, a conservation solution of 10 liters was injected. Placed about 1.50 meter above the body, this solution was infused intravenously for about 45 minutes, until the body would make the eyes close and the liquid came out from the nose and the mouth. The body was then placed in tanks containing ethyl alcohol diluted at 55 p. 100 in water and kept until its use in the class of dissection, which took place during the winter semester.

A register of deaths (or *Leichenbuch*) was held at the Institute of Anatomy of Strassburg during the Second World War. When the Allies arrived in Strassburg, Henri Henrypierre handed it to the "Military Office of General Leclerc".[58] Until now, this book was not found in the French archives. Furthermore, the municipal crematorium of Strassburg did not record the names of the incinerated corpses in its register. The bodies from the Anatomical Institute had been cremated there regularly from around 6 January 1943. But in August 1943, the Crematorium received instructions from the *Deutscher Gemeindetag* of Berlin: "I request that, in the future, you only give me a list of incinerated bodies of persons from private households. You should not consider the incinerations for the KL Natzweiler because these are specific events within the cremations. The statistics for the three months from January to March and April to June must be cleared retroactively".[59] These instructions were presumably applied also for the incineration of the bodies from the anatomical department, since they no longer appeared after March 1943. To identify the names of people whose bodies were taken to the Anatomical Institute, three other sources were used: records of Soviet prisoners of war, the unpublished manuscript of Henrypierre's memoirs and the records of the cemeteries of the city of Strasbourg.

At the Central Archive of the Russian Ministry of Defense (*Tsamo*), located in Podolsk, Russia, millions of documents are held about Soviet prisoners of war. In 2007, more than 9 million documents scanned from these records were put online and made available on the website OBD Memorial.[60] The names of hundreds of Soviet prisoners whose records indicate that they were sent to the Institute of Anatomy of Strassburg were found. In addition, we found in the Alsatian archives the files on burials of bodies from the Second World War, which held information about the burial sites of prisoners. By combining these two sources, we were able to find the names of 230 Soviet prisoners whose bodies were sent to the Anatomical Institute of Strassburg between 1942 and 1944. Their names were published in the *Annals of Anatomy*[61] in 2016. Their age at the time of death was between eighteen and 54. Sixty per cent were Russians, 27 per cent Ukrainian, 4 per cent Belarusian and the remaining were Armenian, Azerbaijani, Bashkir, Bulgarian, Chuvash, Dagestani, Georgian, Kyrgyz, Mordvin, Tatar, Udmurt and Yakut. There was also one Polish citizen. There were two main causes of death noted on the POW files: tuberculosis in 63 per cent and *Inanitio* (starvation) in 11 per cent.

The fate of the Soviet prisoners' bodies was determined by a specific note[62] from the Reich Ministry of the Interior on 27 October 1941. This decreed that the dead should be buried in the most economical way possible: no coffin but thick paper to wrap the body, mass graves in the case of simultaneous deaths, and no ceremonies or decorations on the graves. "The costs must be kept as low as possible", the note insisted. In Strassburg and Mutzig, the bodies of Soviet POWs were buried in a "wild" cemetery located in the forest. After their anatomical use, the bodies were cremated and the urns buried in a cemetery located in the Forest of Stockfeld in Neuhof. Anton Kiesselbach was in charge of organising their incineration and burial, as shown in several letters.[63] After the war, all the remains of this wild cemetery were transferred to South Cemetery of Strasbourg in a mass grave. And a plate was affixed on it with a text saying: "Here lie 208 Soviets deported by the followers of Hitler, persons who died between 1941 and 1945".

In total, the Institute of Anatomy of Strassburg has received at least 244 bodies between 1941 and 1944, among whom 232 are now clearly identified by their names. This figure is a conservative estimate, as it does not include the Polish prisoners of war from the *Reservelazarett*, internees from KL Natzweiler, other deaths from hospitals after March 1943, as well as the Soviet prisoners who have not yet been identified. This estimate of the body procurement does not include the 86 Jews killed for the project of the "Jewish skeleton collection", as these victims were not part of the "normal" body procurement.

In September 1945, Dean André Forster asked the French authorities to bury "as soon as possible" the bodies of Soviet prisoners of the Institute of Anatomy.[64] A list of 49 bodies was established. The bodies were interred[65] on 16 November 1945 in the Strasbourg South Cemetery, without any clear indication of the real identity of the persons buried. Among them was the body of a woman. A headstone was erected, but it is not accurate and, therefore, needs to be corrected. It reads: "Here lie 49 Soviet prisoners who died at the Camp of Mutzig 1941–1945". The remains of the 86 Jews transported from Auschwitz to Natzweiler were placed in 58 coffins.[66] They were buried in various cemeteries at different times. Coffins numbers 1 to 17 containing the bodies with numbers still tattooed on the arm were recognised immediately by the Jewish Community and buried in the Jewish cemetery of Cronenbourg on 28 October 1945. The coffins numbers 18 to 58 containing the remains of other bodies whose numbers had been removed, were buried in the Strasbourg North Cemetery on 23 October 1945. In 1951, the President of the Jewish Community of Strasbourg reunited[67] the bodies in a grave in the Cronenbourg Jewish Cemetery.

What happened to the anatomical specimens created by Hirt and his colleagues during this period? Hirt himself conceded in a justification letter (known as the "white paper") written in January 1945 after the publication of an article in the *Daily Mail* (London), he had worked on "some 250 new anatomical preparations"[68] during his stay in Strassburg. The current Anatomical Institute of Strasbourg indicates that there are currently no remains. As for histological preparations prepared during the Third Reich, it is likely that some slides are still present, as has been reported recently by a professor of anatomy. However, not knowing what to do with such histological slides, no audit has been undertaken so far.

During our investigation, we found a document showing that samples taken during the autopsy on the 86 gassed Jews remains were kept in the Museum of the Institute of Forensic Medicine of Strasbourg. Thus, the French forensic pathologist Camille Simonin stated in a letter written before the trial of Metz that in the Museum of the Institute of Forensic Medicine (*Institut de médecine légale*) of Strasbourg there were "two jars, one containing interesting samples of the intestine and stomach of a victim of the gas chamber and the other contains skin fragments with impressive bruises".[69] On 9 July 2015, we met Jean-Sébastien Raul, the current director of the Institute of Forensic Medicine. In the small museum of the Institute of Forensic Medicine (the so-called *Museum François Hildwein*), we found the preparations that had been described by Simonin: a jar containing five pieces of skin, immersed in Bouin solution, and two test tubes with the contents of the victim's stomach and intestine. The tattooed number of the victim was 107969. It corresponds to the name of Menachem Taffel,[70] one of Hirt's victims. In agreement with the Institute of Forensic Medicine, the Medical Faculty and the University of Strasbourg, these pieces were returned to the Jewish community and were buried[71] on 6 September 2015.

Investigations conducted in Strasbourg show that a very large number of bodies, mostly Soviet prisoners of war, were delivered to the Anatomical Institute during the Second World War. Many anatomical and histological specimens were created at that time. The body procurement at the Anatomical Institute of Strassburg was similar to many of the other German anatomical departments in the following points:[72] the anatomists lobbied with the authorities for more bodies and there was an increasing and high number of bodies of victims of the NS regime among the bodies received. The current leadership of the University of Strasbourg is aware of the need for scientific and historic research concerning this topic and has set up a scientific commission for study of medicine under National Socialism. The success of this scientific commission will depend mainly on reconstructing the activities and policies of the Nazi institutes during the war, and to guarantee the transparency of the investigations into the fate of the victim specimens left by the Nazis.

Notes

1 This chapter is based on my lecture of 5 July 2013 at the symposia "Reassessing Nazi Human Experiments and Coerced Research, 1933–1945: New Findings, Interpretations and Problems" hosted at Wadham College, Oxford and organised by Paul Weindling, Marius Turda and Volker Roelcke. A first version was published in the Annals of Anatomy on May 2016. See: Raphael Toledano, 'Anatomy in the Third Reich – The Anatomical Institute of the Reichsuniversität Strassburg and the deliveries of dead bodies', *Annals of Anatomy*, 205 (2016), pp. 128–144.

2 Jean-Claude Pressac, *The Struthof Album*, New York: The Beate Klarsfeld Foundation, 1985, p. 4.

3 Paris, Centre de recherches des Archives nationales, BB/35/215, Medical Case Transcript, Examination of Henri Henrypierre, 18 Dec 1945, p. 709.

4 Le Blanc, Dépôt central d'archives de la Justice militaire (hereafter DCAJM), TPFA Lyon, 14 May 1954, Box 202/2, Information 457, Official court records, 18 Dec 1952.

5 Jean-Toussaint Henches, 'Un acte d'accusation qui réveille l'horreur d'une tragédie', *Dernières Nouvelles d'Alsace* (17 Dec 1952), p.1; Aline Alquier, 'Les bourreaux savants du Struthof', *L'Humanité* (17 Dec 1952), p. 8.

6 Cf Paul Weindling, 'Rassenkundliche Forschung zwischen dem Getto Litzmannstadt und Auschwitz: Hans Fleischhackers Tübinger Habilitation, Juni 1943', in Jens Kolata, Richard Kühl, Henning Tümmers and Urban Wiesing (eds), *In Fleischhackers Händen. Wissenschaft, Politik und das 20. Jahrhundert. Anlässlich der Ausstellung "In Fleischhackers Händen, Tübinger Rassenforscher in Łódź 1940–1942" im Schloss Hohentübingen*, Tübingen: MUT, 2015, pp. 141–164.

7 Robert Steegmann, *Le KL-Natzweiler et ses kommandos: une nébuleuse concentrationnaire des deux côtés du Rhin*, Strasbourg: La Nuée Bleue, 2005, p. 399; Frederick H. Kasten, 'Unethical Nazi medicine in annexed Alsace-Lorraine: The strange case of Nazi anatomist, Professor Dr. August Hirt', in George O. Kent (ed.), *Historians and Archivists. Essays in Modern German History and Archival Policy*, Fairfax, VA: George Manson University Press, 1991, p. 204.

8 Edouard Conte, 'Au terme de l'horreur. La "collection de squelettes juifs" de l' "Université du Reich" de Strasbourg', in idem and Cornelia Essner (eds), *La quête de la race: Une anthropologie du nazisme*, Paris: Hachette, 1995, pp. 231–262.

9 For general overviews, see Sabine Hildebrandt, 'Anatomy in the Third Reich: an outline, part 1. National Socialist politics, anatomical institutions, and anatomists', *Clinical Anatomy*, 22 (2009), pp. 883–893; eadem, 'Anatomy in the Third Reich: an outline, part 2. Bodies for anatomy and related medical disciplines', *Clinical Anatomy*, 22 (2009), pp. 894–905; eadem, 'Anatomy in the Third Reich: an outline, part 3. The science and ethics of anatomy in National Socialist Germany and postwar consequences', *Clinical Anatomy*, 22 (2009), pp. 906–915; William E. Seidelman, 'Dissecting the history of anatomy in the Third Reich – 1989–2010: A personal account', *Annals of Anatomy*, 194 (2012), pp. 228–236; Sabine Hildebrandt, 'Anatomy in the Third Reich: Careers disrupted by National Socialist Policies', *Annals of Anatomy*, 194 (2012), pp. 251–266; Michael Viebig, '". . . the cadaver can be placed at your disposition here". – Legal, administrative basis of the transfer of cadavers in the Third Reich, its traces in archival sources', *Annals of Anatomy*, 194 (2012), pp. 267–273; Sabine Hildebrandt, 'Research on bodies of the executed in German anatomy: an accepted method that changed during

the Third Reich. Study of anatomical journals from 1924 to 1951', *Clinical Anatomy*, 26 (2013), pp. 304–326; eadem, 'Current status of identification of victims of the National Socialist regime whose bodies were used for anatomical purposes', *Clinical Anatomy*, 27 (2014), pp. 514–536; eadem, *The Anatomy of Murder: Ethical Transgressions and Anatomical Science during the Third Reich*, New York: Berghahn, 2016. **Berlin**: Brigitte Oleschinski, 'Der "Anatom der Gynäkologen". Hermann Stieve und seine Erkenntnisse über Todesangst und weiblichen Zyklus. Beiträge zur nationalsozialistischen Gesundheits- und Sozialpolitik', in H. Kahrs, A. Meyer and M.G. Esch (eds), *Modelle für ein deutsches Europa. Ökonomie und Herrschaft im Grosswirtschaftsraum*, Berlin: Rotbuch Verlag, 1992, pp. 211–218; Udo Schagen, 'Die Forschung an menschlichen Organen nach "plötzlichem Tod" und der Anatom Hermann Stieve (1886–1952)', in R. Von Bruch and R. Schaarschmidt (eds), *Die Berliner Universität in der NS-Zeit. Band 2. Fachbereiche und Fakultäten*, Stuttgart: Franz Steiner, 2005, pp. 35–54; Thorsten Noack, 'Begehrte Leichen. Der Berliner Anatom Hermann Stieve (1886–1952) und die medizinische Verwertung Hingerichteter im Natinoalsozialismus', *Medizin, Gesellschaft und Geschichte. Jahrbuch des Instituts für Geschichte der Medizin der Robert Bosch Stiftung*, 26 (2007), pp. 9–35; Sabine Hildebrandt, 'The women on Stieve's list: Victims of national socialism whose bodies were used for anatomical research', *Clinical Anatomy*, 26 (2013), pp. 3–21. **Bonn**: Ralf Forsbach, *Die Medizinische Fakultät der Universität Bonn im "Dritten Reich"*, Munich: Oldenbourg, 2006. **Danzig**: Joachim Neander, 'The Danzig Soap Case: Facts and Legends around "Professor Spanner" and the Danzig Anatomic Institute 1944–1945', *German Studies Review*, 29 (2006), pp. 63–86. **Frankfurt am Main**: Thomas Theo Brehm, Horst-Werner Korf, Udo Benzenhöfer, Christof Schomerus and Helmut Wicht, 'Notes on the history of the Dr. Senckenbergische Anatomie in Frankfurt/Main. Part I. Development of student numbers, body procurement, and gross anatomy courses from 1914 to 2013', *Annals of Anatomy*, 201 (2015), pp. 99–110; idem, 'Notes on the history of the Dr. Senckenbergische Anatomie in Frankfurt/Main. Part II. The Dr. Senckenbergische Anatomie during the Third Reich and its body supply', *Annals of Anatomy*, 201 (2015), pp. 111–119. **Freiburg im Breisgau**: Eduard Seidler, *Die Medizinische Fakültat der Albert-Ludwigs-Universität Freiburg im Breisgau*, Berlin: Springer, 1991; Sabine Hildebrandt, 'Insights into the Freiburg Anatomical Institute during National Socialism, 1933–1945', *Annals of Anatomy*, 205 (2016), pp. 90–102. **Gießen**: Sigrid Oehler-Klein, Dirk Preuss and Volker Roelcke, 'The use of executed Nazi victims in anatomy: findings from the Institute of Anatomy at Gießen University, pre- and post-1945', *Annals of Anatomy*, 194 (2012), pp. 293–297. **Göttingen**: Heinrich Becker, Hans-Joachim Dahms and Cornelia Wegeler, *Die Universität Göttingen unter dem Nationalsozialismus*, Munich: K.G. Saur, 1998; Susanne Ude-Koeller, Wilfried Knauer and Christoph Viebahn, 'Anatomical practice at Göttingen University since the Age of Enlightenment and the fate of victims from Wolfenbüttel prison under Nazi rule', *Annals of Anatomy*, 194 (2012), pp. 304–313. **Greifswald**: Dirk Alvermann, ' "Praktisch begraben" – NS-Opfer im der Greifswalder Anatomie 1935–1947', in idem (ed.), *". . . Die letzten Schranken fallen lassen"* – *Studien zur Universität Greifswald im Nationalsozialismus*, Cologne: Böhlau, 2015, pp. 311–350; idem and Jan Mittenzwei, 'The Anatomical Institute at the University of Greifswald during National Socialism: The procurement of bodies and their use for anatomical purposes', *Annals of Anatomy*, 205 (2016), pp. 103–112. **Halle**: Michael Viebig, 'Zu Problemen der Leichenversorung des Anatomischen Institutes der Universität Halle vom 19. bis Mitte des 20. Jahrhunderts', in Hermann-Josef Rupieper (ed.), *Beiträge zur Geschichte der Martin-Luther-Universität 1502–2002*, Halle: Mitteldeutscher Verlag, 2002, pp. 117–146; Rüdiger Schultka and Michael Viebig, 'The fate of the bodies of executed persons in the Anatomical Institute of Halle between 1933 and 1945', *Annals of Anatomy*, 194 (2012), pp. 274–280. **Hamburg**: Christiane Rothmaler, 'Gutachten und Dokumentation über das Anatomische Institut des Universitäts-Krankenhauses Eppendorf der Universität

Hamburg 1933–1945', 1999. *Zeitschrift für Sozialgeschichte des 20. und 21. Jahrhunderts*, 2 (1990), pp. 78–95. **Heidelberg**: Wolfgang U. Eckart, Volker Sellin and Eike Wolgast, *Die Universität Heidelberg im Nationalsozialismus*, Heidelberg: Springer, 2006. **Jena**: Christoph Redies, Michael Viebig, Susanne Zimmermann and Rosemarie Fröber, 'Origin of corpses received by the anatomical institute at the University of Jena during the Nazi regime', *The Anatomical Record Part B: The New Anatomist*, 285 (2005), pp. 6–10; idem, 'Dead bodies for the anatomical institute in the Third Reich: An investigation at the University of Jena', *Annals of Anatomy*, 194 (2012), pp. 298–303. **Innsbruck/Graz:** Herwig Czech, 'Von der Richtstätte auf den Seziertisch Zur anatomischen Verwertung von NS-Opfern in Wien, Innsbruck und Graz', *Jahrbuch des Dokumentationsarchivs des österreichischen Widerstandes*, 1 (2015), pp. 141–190. **Cologne**: Stephanie Kaiser, 'Tradition or change? Sources of body procurement for the anatomical institute of Cologne in the Third Reich', *Journal of Anatomy*, 223 (2013), pp. 410–418; eadem and Dominik Gross, 'Anatomy in Cologne – Institutional development and body supply from the Weimar Republic to the early post-war period', *Annals of Anatomy*, 200 (2015), pp. 15–23. **Marburg**: Gerhard Aumüller and Kornelia Grundmann, 'Anatomy during the third reich – The institute of anatomy at the university of Marburg, as an example', *Annals of Anatomy*, 184 (2002), pp. 295–303. **Munich**: Thorsten Noack, 'Anatomical departments in Bavaria and the corpses of executed victims of National Socialism', *Annals of Anatomy*, 194 (2012), pp. 286–292; Mathias Schütz, Jens Waschke, Georg Marckmann and Florian Steger, 'The Munich Anatomical Institute under National Socialism. First results and prospective tasks of an ongoing research project', *Annals of Anatomy*, 195 (2013), pp. 296–302. **Posen**: Götz Aly, 'Das Posener Tagebuch des Anatomen Hermann Voss', in idem, Peter Chroust and Hans-Dieter Heilmann (eds.), *Biedermann und Schreibtischtäter: Materialien zur deutschen Täter-Biographie*, Berlin: Rotbuch Verlag, 1987, pp. 15–66. **Strassburg**: Raphael Toledano, 'Anatomy in the Third Reich – The Anatomical Institute of the *Reichsuniversität Strassburg* and the deliveries of dead bodies', *Annals of Anatomy*, 205 (2016), pp. 128–144. **Tübingen**: Klaus D. Mörike, *Geschichte der Tübinger Anatomie*, Tübingen: J.C.B. Mohr (Paul Siebeck), 1988; Benigna Schönhagen, *Das Gräberfeld X. Eine Dokumentation über NS-Opfer auf dem Tübinger Stadtfriedhof*, Tübingen: Kulturamt, 1987. **Vienna**: Daniela C. Angetter, 'Anatomical science at University of Vienna 1938–45', *Lancet*, 355 (2000), pp. 1454–1457. **Würzburg**: Tim Blessing, Anna Wegener, Hermann Koepsell and Michael Stolberg, 'The Würzburg Anatomical Institute and its supply of corpses (1933–1945)', *Annals of Anatomy*, 194 (2012), pp. 281–285.

10 Michel Cymes, *Hippocrate aux enfers. Les médecins des camps de la mort*, Paris: Stock, 2015.

11 Personal file of the author, Letter from Uzi Bonstein to Raphael Toledano, 5 June 2008.

12 Strasbourg University, Le livre "Hippocrate aux enfers" met en cause notre honnêteté intellectuelle, Press release, 28 Jan 2015.

13 'Des "accusations inquiétantes et graves" dans le livre de Cymes', *Dernières Nouvelles d'Alsace* (30 Jan 2015).

14 Charles Mager, ' "Partout, autour de moi, des rafles" ', *Le Monde Diplomatique* (Aug 1993).

15 'Plus aucun reste à l'institut d'anatomie de la fac de médecine', *Dernières Nouvelles d'Alsace* (3 Feb 2005).

16 Patrick Wechsler, La Faculté de médecine de la "Reichsuniversität Strassburg" (1941–45) à l'heure nationale-socialiste, MD thesis, Strasbourg: Louis Pasteur University, 1991.

17 Tania Elias, 'La cérémonie inaugurale de la Reichsuniversität de Strasbourg (1941). L'expression du nazisme triomphant en Alsace annexée', *Revue d'Allemagne et des pays de langue allemande*, 43 (2011), pp. 341–361.

18 Universität Strassburg, *Personal- und Vorlesungs-Verzeichnis, Winter-Semester 1941/42*, Strassburg: Heitz & Co Verlag, 1941, p. 14.

19 Berlin, Bundesarchiv Berlin-Lichterfelde (hereafter BAB), NS 21/905, August Hirt, *Bericht über die mit dem übersandten L-Stoff angestellten Versuche*, 30 Nov 1942.

20 François Bayle, *Croix gammée contre caducei*, Neustadt: Imprimerie Nationale, 1950; Alexander Mitscherlich and Fred Mielke, *Medizin ohne Menschlichkeit*, Frankfurt am Main: Fischer Taschenbuch, 1960; Michael H. Kater, *Das "Ahnenerbe" der SS 1935–1945: ein Beitrag zur Kulturpolitik des Dritten Reiches*, Stuttgart: Deutsche Verlags-Anstalt, 1974; Ernest Lachman, 'Anatomist of infamy: August Hirt', *Bulletin of the history of medicine*, 51 (1977), pp. 594–602; Pressac, *The Struthof Album*; Kasten, 'Unethical Nazi medicine', pp. 173–208; Wechsler, *La Faculté de médecine*; Conte, 'Au terme de l'horreur', pp. 231–262; Jaques Heran, *Histoire de la Médecine à Strasbourg*, 2nd ed., Strasbourg: La Nuée Bleue, 1997, pp. 593–595; Ernst Klee, *La Médecine Nazie et ses Victimes*, Arles: Actes Sud, 1999, pp. 268–278; Hans-Joachim Lang, *Die Namen der Nummern. Wie es gelang, die 86 Opfer eines NS-Verbrechens zu identifizieren*, Hamburg: Hoffmann und Campe, 2004; Steegmann, *KL-Natzweiler et ses kommandos*, pp. 391–400; Heather Pringle, *Opération Ahnenerbe*, Paris: Presses de la Cité, 2007; Jean-Marie Le Minor, Franck Billmann, Henri Sick, Jean-Marie Vetter and Bertrand Ludes, *Anatomie(s) & Pathologies. Les collections morphologiques de la Faculté de Médecine de Strasbourg*, Bernardswiller: I.D. l'Edition, 2009, pp. 199–211; Paul Weindling, *Victims and Survivors of Nazi Human Experiments: Science and Suffering in the Holocaust*, London: Bloomsbury, 2014, pp. 154–157.

21 Florian Schmaltz, Kampfstoff-Forschung im Nationalsozialismus. Zur Kooperation von Kaiser-Wilhelm-Instituten, Militär und Industrie, Göttingen: Wallstein Verlag, 2005, pp. 521–562.

22 For example, see Paul Bewsher, 'SS Doctor carried out death tests on 20,000', *The Daily Mail [London]* (3 Jan 1945).

23 Personal file of the author, Letter from Erwin Wiesel to Monika Köhler, 19 Dec 1980.

24 Alexander Mitscherlich and Fred Mielke, *Das Diktat der Menschenverachtung*, Heidelberg: Verlag Lambert Schneider, 1947.

25 Mannheim, Stadtarchiv Mannheim, Familienbogen Johannes Hirt.

26 Heidelberg, Universitätsarchiv Heidelberg, PA 978, Medizinische Fakultät, Personalakten August Hirt.

27 Angelika Uhlmann, 'August Hirt und seine Mitarbeiter Kiesselbach, Wimmer und Mayer. Die Karrieren vor der Reichsuniversität Straßburg', *Revue d'Allemagne et des pays de langue allemande*, 43 (2011), pp. 333–340; eadem and Andreas Winkelmann, 'The science prior to the crime – August Hirt's career before 1941', *Annals of Anatomy*, 204 (2016), pp. 118–126.

28 Philipp Ellinger and August Hirt, 'Mikroskopische Untersuchung an lebenden Organen. I. Mitteilung. Methodik: Intravitalmikroskopie', *Zeitschrift für Anatomie und Entwicklungs-Geschichte*, 90 (1929), pp. 791–802.

29 Kasten, 'Unethical Nazi medicine', p. 180

30 BAB, NS 21/904, August Hirt, 'Lebenslauf des SS-Hauptsturmführers Prof. Dr. August Hirt', Aug 1942.

31 Ibid., BDC Ahnenerbe, DS, Sign. G0120, p. 2828, Letter from Wolfram Sievers to August Hirth (sic), 3 Jan 1942.

32 Raphael Toledano, 'Henri Henrypierre: de Lièpvre à Nuremberg, itinéraire d'un témoin des crimes du Struthof', *Société d'histoire du Val de Lièpvre*, 35 (2013), pp. 87–110.

33 Strasbourg, Archives départementales du Bas-Rhin (hereafter ADBR), 126 AL 122, Letter from the *Kurator* of the RUS to Director Sprauer of the Civil Administration, 21 Apr 1942.

34 Ibid., Letter from August Hirt to the Chief of the Civil Administration Dr Benmann, 25 Aug 1942.

35 Ibid., Annex "Entwurf" to the letter from August Hirt to the Chief of the Civil Administration, 25 Aug 1942.

36 Ibid., Letter from Civil Administration of the Alsace to the *Landkommissare*, 30 Sept 1942.

37 Ibid., Letter from Chief of the Civil Administration of the Alsace to the *Polizeipräsidenten* Strassburg, 9 Dec 1942.

38 Ibid., Letter from August Hirt to the President of the *Reichsgesundheitsamts*, 19 Mar 1943.

39 Personal file of the author, Mail from Jan Karol Szklarz to Raphael Toledano, 12 Aug 2013.

40 DCAJM, TPFA Lyon, 14 May 1954, Box 202/1, Renseignement 2, Letter from August Hirt to the *Kriegsgefangenen-Lazarett* Strassburg, 29 June 1942.

41 Ibid., Renseignement 5bis, Letter from August Hirt to the *Oberfeldarzt* Dr Schnitzler, 5 Aug 1942.

42 Ibid., Information 3, Audition of Emile Schaeffer, 26 Apr 1945.

43 Interview with Gaston Bucher, doctor and former student of August Hirt, 7 Oct 2008.

44 BAB, NS 21/904, Letter from Wolfram Sievers to Richard Glücks, 14 Sept 1942.

45 Ibid., NS 21/905, Annex to the Letter from August Hirt to Wolfram Sievers, 12 Oct 1942.

46 Ibid., Letter from August Hirt to Wolfram Sievers, 12 Oct 1942.

47 Ibid., Letter from Wolfram Sievers to the WVHA, 29 Oct 1942.

48 Ibid., NS 21/906, Letter from the *Ahnenerbe* to August Hirt, 27 Jan 1943.

49 Ibid., Letter from W. Sievers to WVHA, 16 Feb 1943.

50 Ibid., NS 21/907, Letter from the WVHA to the *Ahnenerbe*, 10 June 1943.

51 Ibid., Letter from August Hirt to Wolfram Sievers, 22 June 1943.

52 ADBR, 126 AL 122, Letter from August Hirt to the President of the *Reichsgesundheitsamts*, 19 Mar 1943.

53 Henri Henrypierre, 'Mémoire et vie d'un homme double', unpublished manuscript, 1945.

54 ADBR, 167 AL 18, So Kls 22/43, Letter from Oberstaatsanwalt Luger to the Anatomical Institute of the RUS, 12 Aug 1943.

55 Ibid., 1243 W 247, So Kls 47/43, Criminal case against Schaeffer and 12 others; 'Jugendliche Verbrecher terrorisierten die Bevölkerung', *Strassburger Neueste Nachrichten* (6 May 1943).

56 Myriam Ait-Sidhoum, 'Leurs noms retrouvés', *Dernières Nouvelles d'Alsace* (17 June 2016).

57 DCAJM, TPFA Lyon, 14 May 1954, Box 202/1, Renseignement 5bis, Letter from August Hirt to the *Oberfeldarzt* Dr Schnitzler, 5 Aug 1942.

58 Ministère de l'Information, 'Le camp de concentration de Struthof (Bas-Rhin) et l'activité de l'Institut d'Anatomie de Strasbourg pendant l'occupation allemande', *Notes Documentaires et Etudes*, 140 (8 Sept 1945), p. 5.

59 Strasbourg, Archives de la Ville et de la Communauté urbaine de Strasbourg (hereafter AVCUS), 610 MW 24, President of the *Deutscher Gemeindetag* to the Mayor of Strasbourg, Aug 1943.

60 www.obd-memorial.ru.

61 Toledano, 'Anatomy in the Third Reich', pp. 128–144.

62 ADBR, 126 AL 121, Note from the Ministry of the Interior of the Reich entitled 'Bestattung von Leichen sowjetischer Kriegsgefangener durch die Gemeinden', 27 Oct 1941.

63 For example, see DCAJM, TPFA Lyon, 14 May 1954, Box 202/1, Information 86, Letter from Fritz Beblo to the Anatomical Institute of Strasbourg, 24 Aug 1944.

64 AVCUS, 611 MW 63, Letter from Technical Adviser to the Military service corps of Strasbourg, 28 Sept 1945.

65 DCAJM, Paris, 28 May 1958, Box 575 (4/21), 1858, Forme 173, Letter from Yves Bouchard to Commandant Jadin, 15 Nov 1945.

66 AVCUS, 611 MW 64, Letter from the Mayor of Strasbourg to the President of the Jewish Community of Strasbourg, 5 Sept 1951.
67 'La réinhumation de quarante-huit corps trouvés en 1945 à l'Institut médico-légal de l'Université de Strasbourg', *Bulletin de nos Communautés, Organe du judaïsme d'Alsace et de Lorraine*, 19 (28 Sept 1951), pp. 13–14.
68 BAB, NS 19/2281, Letter from August Hirt, 25 Jan 1945.
69 DCAJM, TPFA Lyon, 14 May 1954, Box 202/1, Renseignement 88, Letter from Camille Simonin to the President of the Military Tribunal of Metz Capitaine Henriet, undated.
70 Bad Arolsed, Digital Archives of the International Tracing Service, KL Auschwitz, 1.1.2.1, 5400691, List of 89 Weil-Felix test results, 15 July 1943.
71 Anne-Camille Beckelynck, ' "Il en a fallu du temps . . ." ', *Dernières Nouvelles d'Alsace* (7 Sept 2015), p. 13.
72 Hildebrandt, *The Anatomy of Murder*.

Bibliography

Archival sources

France

Le Blanc, Dépôt central d'archives de la Justice militaire (DCAJM):
Paris, 28 May 1958, Box 575 (4/21)
TPFA Lyon, 14 May 1954, Box 202/1–2
Paris, Centre de recherches des Archives nationales, BB/35/215
Strasbourg, Archives de la Ville et de la Communauté urbaine de Strasbourg (AVCUS):
610 MW 24
611 MW 63–64
Strasbourg, Archives départementales du Bas-Rhin (ADBR):
126 AL 121–122
167 AL 18, So Kls 22/43
1243 W 247, So Kls 47/43

Germany

Bad Arolsen, Digital Archives of the International Tracing Service, KL Auschwitz, 1.1.2.1
Berlin, Bundesarchiv Berlin-Lichterfelde (BAB):
BDC Ahnenerbe, DS, Sign. G0120
NS 19/2281
NS 21/904–907
Heidelberg, Universitätsarchiv Heidelberg, PA 978, Medizinische Fakultät, Personalakten August Hirt
Mannheim, Stadtarchiv Mannheim, Familienbogen Johannes Hirt

Literature

Ait-Sidhoum, Myriam, 'Leurs noms retrouvés', *Dernières Nouvelles d'Alsace* (17 June 2016)
Alquier, Aline, 'Les bourreaux savants du Struthof', *L'Humanité* (17 Dec 1952), p. 8

Alvermann, Dirk, ' "Praktisch begraben" – NS-Opfer in der Greifswalder Anatomie 1935–1947', in Dirk Alvermann (ed.), *". . . Die letzten Schranken fallen lassen" – Studien zur Universität Greifswald im Nationalsozialismus*, Cologne: Böhlau, 2015, pp. 311–350

—— and Jan Mittenzwei, 'The Anatomical Institute at the University of Greifswald during National Socialism: The procurement of bodies and their use for anatomical purposes', *Annals of Anatomy*, 205 (2016), pp. 103–112

Aly, Götz, 'Das Posener Tagebuch des Anatomen Hermann Voss', in Götz Aly, Peter Chroust and Hans-Dieter Heilmann (eds.), *Biedermann und Schreibtischtäter: Materialien zur deutschen Täter-Biographie*, Berlin: Rotbuch Verlag, 1987, pp. 15–66

Angetter, Daniela C., 'Anatomical science at University of Vienna 1938–45', *Lancet*, 355 (2000), pp. 1454–1457

Aumüller, Gerhard and Kornelia Grundmann, 'Anatomy during the Third Reich – The institute of anatomy at the university of Marburg, as an example', *Annals of Anatomy*, 184 (2002), pp. 295–303

Bayle, François, *Croix gammée contre caducée*, Neustadt: Imprimerie Nationale, 1950

Beckelynck, Anne-Camille, ' "Il en a fallu du temps . . ." ', *Dernières Nouvelles d'Alsace* (7 Sept 2015), p. 13

Becker, Heinrich, Hans-Joachim Dahms and Cornelia Wegeler, *Die Universität Göttingen unter dem Nationalsozialismus*, Munich: K.G. Saur, 1998

Bewsher, Paul, 'SS Doctor carried out death tests on 20,000', *The Daily Mail [London]* (3 Jan 1945)

Blessing, Tim, Anna Wegener, Hermann Koepsell and Michael Stolberg, 'The Würzburg Anatomical Institute and its supply of corpses (1933–1945)', *Annals of Anatomy*, 194 (2012), pp. 281–285

Brehm, Thomas Theo, Horst-Werner Korf, Udo Benzenhöfer, Christof Schomerus and Helmut Wicht, 'Notes on the history of the Dr. Senckenbergische Anatomie in Frankfurt/Main. Part I. Development of student numbers, body procurement, and gross anatomy courses from 1914 to 2013', *Annals of Anatomy*, 201 (2015), pp. 99–110

—— 'Notes on the history of the Dr. Senckenbergische Anatomie in Frankfurt/Main. Part II. The Dr. Senckenbergische Anatomie during the Third Reich and its body supply', *Annals of Anatomy*, 201 (2015), pp. 111–119

Conte, Edouard, 'Au terme de l'horreur. La "collection de squelettes juifs" de l' "Université du Reich" de Strasbourg', in Edouard Conte and Cornelia Essner (eds), *La quête de la race: Une anthropologie du nazisme*, Paris: Hachette, 1995, pp. 231–262

Cymes, Michel, *Hippocrate aux enfers. Les médecins des camps de la mort*, Paris: Stock, 2015

Czech, Herwig, 'Von der Richtstätte auf den Seziertisch Zur anatomischen Verwertung von NS-Opfern in Wien, Innsbruck und Graz', *Jahrbuch des Dokumentationsarchivs des österreichischen Widerstandes*, 1 (2015), pp. 141–190

'Des "accusations inquiétantes et graves" dans le livre de Cymes', *Dernières Nouvelles d'Alsace* (30 Jan 2015)

Eckart, Wolfgang U., Volker Sellin and Eike Wolgast, *Die Universität Heidelberg im Nationalsozialismus*, Heidelberg: Springer, 2006

Elias, Tania, 'La cérémonie inaugurale de la Reichsuniversität de Strasbourg (1941). L'expression du nazisme triomphant en Alsace annexée', *Revue d'Allemagne et des pays de langue allemande*, 43 (2011), pp. 341–361

Ellinger, Philipp and August Hirt, 'Mikroskopische Untersuchung an lebenden Organen. I. Mitteilung. Methodik: Intravitalmikroskopie', *Zeitschrift für Anatomie und Entwicklungs-Geschichte*, 90 (1929), pp. 791–802

Forsbach, Ralf, *Die Medizinische Fakultät der Universität Bonn im "Dritten Reich"*, Munich: Oldenbourg, 2006

Henches, Jean-Toussaint, 'Un acte d'accusation qui réveille l'horreur d'une tragédie', *Dernières Nouvelles d'Alsace* (17 Dec 1952), p.1

Henrypierre, Henri, *Mémoire et vie d'un homme double*, unpublished manuscript, 1945

Heran, Jaques, *Histoire de la Médecine à Strasbourg*, 2nd ed., Strasbourg: La Nuée Bleue, 1997

Hildebrandt, Sabine, 'Anatomy in the Third Reich: an outline, part 1. National Socialist politics, anatomical institutions, and anatomists', *Clinical Anatomy*, 22 (2009), pp. 883–893

—— 'Anatomy in the Third Reich: an outline, part 2. Bodies for anatomy and related medical disciplines', *Clinical Anatomy*, 22 (2009), pp. 894–905

—— 'Anatomy in the Third Reich: an outline, part 3. The science and ethics of anatomy in National Socialist Germany and postwar consequences', *Clinical Anatomy*, 22 (2009), pp. 906–915

—— 'Anatomy in the Third Reich: Careers disrupted by National Socialist Policies', *Annals of Anatomy*, 194 (2012), pp. 251–266

—— 'The women on Stieve's list: Victims of national socialism whose bodies were used for anatomical research', *Clinical Anatomy*, 26 (2013), pp. 3–21

—— 'Research on bodies of the executed in German anatomy: an accepted method that changed during the Third Reich. Study of anatomical journals from 1924 to 1951', *Clinical Anatomy*, 26 (2013), pp. 304–326

—— 'Current status of identification of victims of the National Socialist regime whose bodies were used for anatomical purposes', *Clinical Anatomy*, 27 (2014), pp. 514–536

—— 'Insights into the Freiburg Anatomical Institute during National Socialism, 1933–1945', *Annals of Anatomy*, 205 (2016), pp. 90–102

—— *The Anatomy of Murder: Ethical Transgressions and Anatomical Science during the Third Reich*, New York: Berghahn, 2016

'Jugendliche Verbrecher terrorisierten die Bevölkerung', *Strassburger Neueste Nachrichten* (6 May 1943)

Kaiser, Stephanie, 'Tradition or change? Sources of body procurement for the anatomical institute of Cologne in the Third Reich', *Journal of Anatomy*, 223 (2013), pp. 410–418

—— and Dominik Gross, 'Anatomy in Cologne – Institutional development and body supply from the Weimar Republic to the early post-war period', *Annals of Anatomy*, 200 (2015), pp. 15–23

Kasten, Frederick H., 'Unethical Nazi medicine in annexed Alsace-Lorraine: The strange case of Nazi anatomist, Professor Dr. August Hirt', in George O. Kent (ed.), *Historians and Archivists. Essays in Modern German History and Archival Policy*, Fairfax, VA: George Manson University Press, 1991, pp. 173–208

Kater, Michael H., *Das "Ahnenerbe" der SS 1935–1945: ein Beitrag zur Kulturpolitik des Dritten Reiches*, Stuttgart: Deutsche Verlags-Anstalt, 1974

Klee, Ernst, *La Médecine Nazie et ses Victimes*, Arles: Actes Sud, 1999

Lachman, Ernest, 'Anatomist of infamy: August Hirt', *Bulletin of the History of Medicine*, 51 (1977), pp. 594–602

'La réinhumation de quarante-huit corps trouvés en 1945 à l'Institut médico-légal de l'Université de Strasbourg', *Bulletin de nos Communautés, Organe du judaïsme d'Alsace et de Lorraine*, 19 (28 Sept 1951), pp. 13–14

Lang, Hans-Joachim, *Die Namen der Nummern. Wie es gelang, die 86 Opfer eines NS-Verbrechens zu identifizieren*, Hamburg: Hoffmann und Campe, 2004

Le Minor, Jean-Marie, Franck Billmann, Henri Sick, Jean-Marie Vetter and Bertrand Ludes, *Anatomie(s) & Pathologies. Les collections morphologiques de la Faculté de Médecine de Strasbourg*, Bernardswiller: I.D. l'Edition, 2009

Mager, Charles, '"Partout, autour de moi, des rafles"', *Le Monde Diplomatique* (Aug 1993)

Ministère de l'Information, 'Le camp de concentration de Struthof (Bas-Rhin) et l'activité de l'Institut d'Anatomie de Strasbourg pendant l'occupation allemande', *Notes Documentaires et Etudes*, 140 (8 Sept 1945), p. 5

Mitscherlich, Alexander and Fred Mielke, *Das Diktat der Menschenverachtung*, Heidelberg: Verlag Lambert Schneider, 1947

—— *Medizin ohne Menschlichkeit*, Frankfurt am Main: Fischer Taschenbuch, 1960

Mörike, Klaus D., *Geschichte der Tübinger Anatomie*, Tübingen: J.C.B. Mohr (Paul Siebeck), 1988

Neander, Joachim, 'The Danzig Soap Case: Facts and Legends around "Professor Spanner" and the Danzig Anatomic Institute 1944–1945', *German Studies Review*, 29 (2006), pp. 63–86

Noack, Thorsten, 'Begehrte Leichen. Der Berliner Anatom Hermann Stieve (1886–1952) und die medizinische Verwertung Hingerichteter im Natinoalsozialismus', *Medizin, Gesellschaft und Geschichte. Jahrbuch des Instituts für Geschichte der Medizin der Robert Bosch Stiftung*, 26 (2007), pp. 9–35

—— 'Anatomical departments in Bavaria and the corpses of executed victims of National Socialism', *Annals of Anatomy*, 194 (2012), pp. 286–292

Oehler-Klein, Sigrid, Dirk Preuss and Volker Roelcke, 'The use of executed Nazi victims in anatomy: findings from the Institute of Anatomy at Gießen University, pre- and post-1945', *Annals of Anatomy*, 194 (2012), pp. 293–297

Oleschinski, Brigitte, 'Der "Anatom der Gynäkologen". Hermann Stieve und seine Erkenntnisse über Todesangst und weiblichen Zyklus. Beiträge zur nationalsozialistischen Gesundheits- und Sozialpolitik', in H. Kahrs, A. Meyer and M.G. Esch (eds), *Modelle für ein deutsches Europa. Ökonomie und Herrschaft im Grosswirtschaftsraum*, Berlin: Rotbuch Verlag, 1992, pp. 211–218

'Plus aucun reste à l'institut d'anatomie de la fac de médecine', *Dernières Nouvelles d'Alsace* (3 Feb 2005)

Pressac, Jean-Claude, *The Struthof Album*, New York: The Beate Klarsfeld Foundation, 1985

Pringle, Heather, *Opération Ahnenerbe*, Paris: Presses de la Cité, 2007

Redies, Christoph, Michael Viebig, Susanne Zimmermann and Rosemarie Fröber, 'Origin of corpses received by the anatomical institute at the University of Jena during the Nazi regime', *The Anatomical Record Part B: The New Anatomist*, 285 (2005), pp. 6–10

—— 'Dead bodies for the anatomical institute in the Third Reich: An investigation at the University of Jena', *Annals of Anatomy*, 194 (2012), pp. 298–303

Rothmaler, Christiane, 'Gutachten und Dokumentation über das Anatomische Institut des Universitäts-Krankenhauses Eppendorf der Universität Hamburg 1933–1945', *1999. Zeitschrift für Sozialgeschichte des 20. und 21. Jahrhunderts*, 2 (1990), pp. 78–95

Schagen, Udo, 'Die Forschung an menschlichen Organen nach "plötzlichem Tod" und der Anatom Hermann Stieve (1886–1952)', in R. Von Bruch and R. Schaarschmidt (eds), *Die Berliner Universität in der NS-Zeit. Band 2. Fachbereiche und Fakultäten*, Stuttgart: Franz Steiner, 2005, pp. 35–54

Schmaltz, Florian, *Kampfstoff-Forschung im Nationalsozialismus. Zur Kooperation von Kaiser-Wilhelm-Instituten, Militär und Industrie*, Göttingen: Wallstein Verlag, 2005

Schönhagen, Benigna, *Das Gräberfeld X. Eine Dokumentation über NS-Opfer auf dem Tübinger Stadtfriedhof*, Tübingen: Kulturamt, 1987

Schultka, Rüdiger and Michael Viebig, 'The fate of the bodies of executed persons in the Anatomical Institute of Halle between 1933 and 1945', *Annals of Anatomy*, 194 (2012), pp. 274–80

Schütz, Mathias, Jens Waschke, Georg Marckmann and Florian Steger, 'The Munich Anatomical Institute under National Socialism. First results and prospective tasks of an ongoing research project', *Annals of Anatomy*, 195 (2013), pp. 296–302

Seidelman, William E., 'Dissecting the history of anatomy in the Third Reich – 1989–2010: A personal account', *Annals of Anatomy*, 194 (2012), pp. 228–236

Seidler, Eduard, *Die Medizinische Fakültat der Albert-Ludwigs-Universität Freiburg im Breisgau*, Berlin: Springer, 1991

Steegmann, Robert, *Le KL-Natzweiler et ses kommandos: une nébuleuse concentrationnaire des deux côtés du Rhin*, Strasbourg: La Nuée Bleue, 2005

Strasbourg University, *Le livre "Hippocrate aux enfers" met en cause notre honnêteté intellectuelle*, Press release, 28 Jan 2015

Toledano, Raphael, 'Henri Henrypierre: de Lièpvre à Nuremberg, itinéraire d'un témoin des crimes du Struthof', *Société d'histoire du Val de Lièpvre*, 35 (2013), pp. 87–110

—— 'Anatomy in the Third Reich – The Anatomical Institute of the *Reichsuniversität Strassburg* and the deliveries of dead bodies', *Annals of Anatomy*, 205 (2016), pp. 128–144

Ude-Koeller, Susanne, Wilfried Knauer and Christoph Viebahn, 'Anatomical practice at Göttingen University since the Age of Enlightenment and the fate of victims from Wolfenbüttel prison under Nazi rule', *Annals of Anatomy*, 194 (2012), pp. 304–313

Uhlmann, Angelika, 'August Hirt und seine Mitarbeiter Kiesselbach, Wimmer und Mayer. Die Karrieren vor der Reichsuniversität Straßburg', *Revue d'Allemagne et des pays de langue allemande*, 43 (2011), pp. 333–340

—— and Andreas Winkelmann, 'The science prior to the crime – August Hirt's career before 1941', *Annals of Anatomy*, 204 (2016), pp. 118–126

Universität Strassburg, *Personal- und Vorlesungs-Verzeichnis, Winter-Semester 1941/42*, Strassburg: Heitz & Co Verlag, 1941

Viebig, Michael, 'Zu Problemen der Leichenversorung des Anatomischen Institutes der Universität Halle vom 19. bis Mitte des 20. Jahrhunderts', in Hermann-Josef Rupieper (ed.), *Beiträge zur Geschichte der Martin-Luther-Universität 1502–2002*, Halle: Mitteldeutscher Verlag, 2002, pp. 117–146

—— ' ". . . the cadaver can be placed at your disposition here". – Legal, administrative basis of the transfer of cadavers in the Third Reich, its traces in archival sources', *Annals of Anatomy*, 194 (2012), pp. 267–273

Wechsler, Patrick, *La Faculté de médecine de la "Reichsuniversität Strassburg" (1941–1945) à l'heure nationale-socialiste*, MD thesis, Strasbourg: Louis Pasteur University, 1991

Weindling, Paul, *Victims and Survivors of Nazi Human Experiments: Science and Suffering in the Holocaust,* London: Bloomsbury, 2014

—— 'Rassenkundliche Forschung zwischen dem Getto Litzmannstadt und Auschwitz: Hans Fleischhackers Tübinger Habilitation, Juni 1943', in Jens Kolata, Richard Kühl, Henning Tümmers and Urban Wiesing (eds), *In Fleischhackers Händen. Wissenschaft, Politik und das 20. Jahrhundert. Anlässlich der Ausstellung "In Fleischhackers Händen, Tübinger Rassenforscher in Łódź 1940–1942" im Schloss Hohentübingen*, Tübingen: MUT, 2015, pp. 141–164

6 Nazi anthropology and the taking of face masks

Face and death masks in the anthropological collection of the Natural History Museum, Vienna

Margit Berner

Introduction

Face and death masks have a long tradition in various historical and cultural contexts.[1] Death masks of renowned individuals can be seen on display in museums, libraries, archives and elsewhere. Many musicians, artists and politicians have been memorialised in masks. In exhibitions dedicated to the biography and life's work of a distinguished person, a mask is usually displayed as a sentimental relic, as a museological object of memorialisation.[2] In physical anthropology, casts of head and body parts have a different meaning. The tradition of taking and studying face and death masks in medical, ethnographic and physiognomic studies dates back to the eighteenth century. The process of making facial casts consists of moulding a negative and casting a positive, and requires training and learning from an instructor. Plaster casts were considered scientific objects and treated as objective and real, three-dimensional representation of specimens. Masks were seen and presented to the public as material illustrations of theoretical concepts of typology and race. In this context the identity of the studied men and women, their names and personal histories were not taken into account.

These casts are hybrid objects, not quite human remains, but still something very close, a product of physical contact with human materiality, with the physical body of the individual being represented. As a result of this contact with the face and body, these casts are imbued with a sense of intimacy. The faces held fast in the casts are not only representative of the transformation of the human into the material, but also each of these masks is witness to a human encounter between a researcher and his research object.

Plaster casts of heads and body parts can be found in most anthropological collections. However, in relation to the collections of skulls and skeletons, photographs, hair samples, measurement tables and hand, foot and finger prints, the number of such casts is comparably small. In the Natural History Museum in Vienna, all these casts were taken from the various other collections in 1990 and gathered into one collection of casts in the Department of Anthropology. This collection consists of casts of human fossils and skeletons, reconstructions and modelled busts, and casts of heads and body parts of living and in some cases of dead individuals. With few exceptions, the majority of the more than 600 casts of heads and body parts were produced during the first half of the twentieth century by "race scientists" or *Rassenforscher*. They are closely linked to the exhibition and research activities of Austrian anthropologists in the Nazi period.

The Nazi period collections

In May 1939 the Natural History Museum opened an exhibition on "The physical and spiritual appearance of the Jews" (*Das körperliche und seelische Erscheinungsbild der Juden*) conceived and realised by the then head of the Department of Anthropology Josef Wastl (1892–1968). In this display a part of the confiscated collection of the old Viennese Jewish Museum had been included.[3] Unlike the travelling exhibition "The eternal Jew" (*Der Ewige Jude*), which was organised by the Nazis in 1937 and featured virulently anti-Semitic materials, the exhibition in the Natural History Museum focused on scientific data and knowledge.[4] Anti-Semitism here was more a subtle one, deriving from tendentious and often cynical manipulation of scientific knowledge, historical events, religious tests and statistical data.[5] Based on facial photographs Jews were presented as a people of diverse racial origin, racial otherness and as racially and psychologically estranged from Germans and other Europeans. Another part of the exhibit focused on the Nuremberg Race Laws, on eugenic ideals and on the "dangers" of "miscegenation".

The anthropological projects of this period are closely linked with the name of Josef Wastl, who became a scientific associate in 1935, head in 1938 and director from 1941 onwards of the Department of Anthropology. The university assistant Robert Routil (1893–1955) who joined the museum in 1939 and was hired in 1941 was involved in all projects.

In the course of preparing the exhibition "The physical and psychological appearance of the Jews" for the department Wastl complained of a "lack of material", a circumstance that seemed to have stimulated the Museum's anthropologists' interest in racial investigations of Jews. Moreover, Wastl's preference for photography, his doctoral thesis and the Viennese anthropologists' experience with prisoners of war studies in the First World War had influenced the design and direction of the projects. Claiming collecting and research activity as war-related research, Wastl and Routil received exemption from military service at the front (*UK Stellung*).

Between 1939 and 1943 the department conducted racial investigations on Jews, prisoners of war and various Austrian populations. The collections were expanded with measurement forms, photographs, plaster masks, hair samples and hand and footprints. The department acquired skulls and death masks from concentration camp victims and undertook exhumations in a Jewish cemetery in Vienna. In addition, several hundred racial and paternity assessments were undertaken by the department for the courts or for the Reich Office of Genealogy (*Reichssippenamt*) between 1941 and 1945. A proof of paternity certificate created to serve Viennese courts in disputes on paternity in the 1920s was adopted in the Nazi period as a "genetic certificate of race and origin"; it was required of Germans of uncertain descent suspected of being "Jews" or "half-Jews" as these terms were defined in the Nuremberg Laws on Citizenship and Race. With these studies, the anthropologists contributed directly to the mass murder of the Jews. Their assessment determined the fate of the people being racially investigated.[6] In 1945, Wastl was suspended from museum service as a "minor National Socialist" and in 1948 sent into retirement. He drew up, however, like many others in his field, freelance, well-paid proofs of paternity for Austrian courts until his death in 1968. The skeletons from the Jewish cemetery were reburied in 1947, the provenance of the other collections from the Nazi period was no longer discussed, and the collection was even expanded with photographs and fingerprints from a survey in 1942 on 105 Jewish families in the Tarnow ghetto.[7]

In the course of all these activities around 350 face masks and 29 death masks were collected, the majority taken from prisoners of war. Today these collections not only bear witness to the individual interests, the careerism and entanglement in the Nazi regime of Viennese scholars, they are also a memorial to the individual victims. This article will focus on two collections of masks of the Nazi period, one collection of 29 plaster death masks of Jewish concentration camp victims and one collection of 19 face masks taken in the course of an anthropological study of Jews temporarily interned in the Vienna Stadium in 1939. These collections taken from individuals, who had not consented to these examinations, pose difficult ethical questions to the curators of the collections in terms of how to deal with and how – if at all – to exhibit them. In the case of the Stadium study, my initial historical interest quickly shifted to become a biographical study of the individuals who had been subject to racial investigation.

The Posen Collection

In 1942 the department had acquired 29 skulls and death masks of Jews and 15 skulls of Poles, concentration camp victims and Polish resistance fighters, from the Anatomical Institute of the University of Posen. The skulls and plaster masks remained in the anthropological collection until they were rediscovered in 1991. By decision of the Ministry, the skulls and death masks were handed over to the Jewish community in Vienna, which buried the skulls and passed the death masks on to Vienna's Jewish Museum.[8] The skulls of the Polish resistance fighters acquired in 1942 remained in the collection until 1999, when they were handed over to the Polish Embassy in Vienna. Two masks were later found and remained at the request of the Jewish Museum Vienna as a document of the history in the Department of Anthropology.

Already in 1987 the historian Götz Aly had published a selection of the Posen diaries of Hermann Voss, chief anatomist at the Reich University of Posen (*Reichsuniversität Posen*). This diary makes it all too clear that Posen had become a leading actor in the provision of dissected skulls and busts of executed Polish resistance fighters and Jewish concentration camp victims to institutions throughout Europe – among them the Natural History Museum in Vienna.[9] The diary and the official correspondence between Gustav von Hirschheydt, chief dissector in Posen, and Josef Wastl provides clear evidence of the racist ideology involved and the degradation of human beings to mere objects or specimens.[10] In February 1942, Wastl asked the Anatomical Institute in Posen whether they could provide several Polish skulls for the Museum. Hirschheydt offered not only "Polish skulls/males and females/for the price of 25 Reichsmarks [RM] each"; he could also provide Jewish skulls for the same price. In addition Hirschheydt wrote, "I can also provide plaster death masks of the respective individuals for a price of 15 [RM]. I can also make plaster busts of the quintessential eastern Jew for you so that you can see the form of the head and the often peculiar ears. The price would be 30–35 RM, but because of a scarcity of time and plaster I could not supply many".[11] As the budget for that fiscal year had not been exhausted, Wastl promptly ordered everything.[12] Hirschheydt sent an invoice for 15 Polish skulls, 22 Jewish skulls, 20 death masks and two busts. As fate would have it, Hirschheydt, who performed this particular work in addition to his actual duties, could not complete the order.[13] He died in June 1942 of typhus after being bitten by a louse from the body of a Jewish prisoner.[14] Voss then processed the order, adding a further seven skulls and five Jewish death masks.[15] He announced further that due to shortages of personnel, the institute would be unable to continue this business in the future.[16]

In a letter to Hirschheydt's widow, Wastl expressed his "sincere condolences" for the "loss of an important scientific worker".[17] Her late husband's plaster casts, he wrote, were "masterful". The planned museum display for the masks and skulls would be a lasting memorial to her husband's "tragic fate".[18] From the preserved documents it is not clear whether the masks were ever displayed in the museum and why, despite Wastl's order, no death masks of the murdered Poles were ever delivered. What emerges from the correspondence is that Hirschheydt was not permitted by the Gestapo and the *Sondergericht* to provide any biographical data or photographs of the executed Poles that would later allow for the identification of the individual. This fear did not hold true for the Jews, for whom, Hirschheydt could provide date and place of birth.[19] However, in the end these data were not provided, only age, sex and body measurements were documented.[20] To date the identities and biographies of all these individuals remain unknown.

The Stadium study – reconstructing biographies

Measurement sheets and photographs found during the systematic inspection of the collections in 1997 allowed for the identification of 17 uninventoried masks and two busts in the cast collection.[21] The documents and materials were from a hitherto unknown racial investigation performed by the anthropologists of the Natural History Museum. Immediately after the outbreak of the Second World War, on 10 and 11 September 1939, stateless and Polish Jews were arrested in Vienna on orders of the Chief of the Security Police, Reinhard Heydrich within the framework of a Reich-wide action. Since the prisons were already bursting at the seams, more than 1,000 men were interned temporarily in the Vienna Stadium, among them 125 residents of the Vienna Jewish Community's retirement home.[22]

In the third week of detention, on 24 September, during the Sukoth festival, an eight-member anthropological commission under the supervision of Josef Wastl started a racial investigation. They measured 440 of the imprisoned men, recorded individual data and filled out detailed survey sheets. The names of these 440 men were recorded, as were the names of their parents, their professions, places and dates of birth and the duration of their residence in Vienna. The great majority of the men were photographed; the anthropologists took over 100 hair samples and 21 of them were chosen for face masks.[23] On 30 September 1939 the prisoners in the Stadium were deported to Buchenwald concentration camp.[24] While this early wave of deportation in September 1939 was known from the literature on the history of the persecution of Austrian Jews and the Buchenwald concentration camp, the scientific instrumentalisation of the prisoners by the Viennese anthropologists and their taking of measurements had been forgotten.

In the course of an interdisciplinary research project, the historian Claudia Spring and the author tried to reconstruct the biographies of the measured men.[25] Of the 440 men who were measured, 318 died within the first few weeks of being imprisoned in Buchenwald due to malnutrition, exhaustion, severe working conditions and dysentery. Thirty men were selected in the so called 14f13 "euthanasia" programme and killed in Sonnenstein/Pirna, Bernburg/Saale and Hartheim. In spring 1940, 15 men were released and a mere 26 survived the war, either in Buchenwald or in another concentration camp.[26] The women and children imprisoned in the Vienna Stadium were deported from Vienna to various ghettos and concentration camps and were murdered there. Some children were sent away on a children's transport and survived the war abroad. With the support of the Buchenwald Memorial Foundation, the survivor's registry at the United States Holocaust Memorial Museum, the National Fund for the Victims of National Socialism and the Documentation Centre of Austrian Resistance, information was found on about 99 likely family members of the measured men.[27] More than 20 family members have been contacted with whom archival findings have been shared. Some of them had concerns and were initially hesitant, but with time they changed their minds and asked to receive the collected information as well as a photograph. Some of them refused further correspondence. For most, the information was of great interest, even if it opened or reopened many wounds. One son wrote: "I received your letter and I was shocked to hear what my father had to go through . . . I would like to hear more about the anthropological examination", and another family member: "Although your letter has reopened a very deep wound in my heart of the darkest and most painful period in my life, I appreciate the work you both do, I therefore would very much like to hear from you and discuss this matter".[28]

During the racial investigation masks of 21 men had been taken, of which 17 masks and two busts still exist in the department. Of the 17 men of whom masks were taken 11 died in Buchenwald; six in 1939 – Abraham Merker (1903–39), Jakob Biegel (1892–1939), Paul Gimpel (1890–1939), Hermann Roth (1899–1939), Ludwig Alfred Post (1896–1939) and Moses Weinstein (1892–1939); four in 1940 – Chaim Bergmann (1880–1940), Heinrich Braun (1892–1940), Israel Mayer Igelberg (1885–1940) and Otto Preminger (1923–40) and in 1941 Samuel Fried (1896–1941). Moses Max Gutmann (1892–1942) was killed in 1942 in the Bernburg "euthanasia" station. Armin Rotstein-Rosenbaum (1923–40) was released from Buchenwald in 1940; he died a few weeks after his return in the Rothschild hospital in Vienna. Gustav Pimselstein, later Gershon Evan (1923–2015) was released in 1940 and survived the war. Paul Grünberg (*1923), Heinrich Werner (1907-?) and Josef Werner (1913–?) survived Buchenwald or another concentration camp.

We are not able to answer the question "why my father would have been chosen, if only nineteen plaster masks were made?" or why particular persons were chosen for taking masks and measurements.[29] We contacted two survivors and two family members of men of whom masks are housed in the museum's collection. Gershon Evan and Paul Grünberg were both 16 years old when they were imprisoned in the Stadium. Paul Grünberg was transferred in 1942 from Buchenwald to Auschwitz and later to Monowitz. He survived the evacuation march and returned to Vienna. In 1999 he had been contacted by the Buchenwald Memorial Foundation. Although he did not remember in detail the racist investigation or the taking of the mask, he remembered being treated as an object and not as a human being.[30]

Gershon Evan, former Gustav Pimselstein was released from Buchenwald in February 1940, he returned to Vienna from where he escaped to Palestine. From 1942 to 1946 he served in the British Army and from 1948 to 1950 in the Israeli Army. In 1958 he emigrated to the United States and lived in San Francisco. In his autobiography, which was published in 2000, Evan described in detail the racial investigation and procedure of taking the mask:[31]

> Among the calipers, rulers, and unfamiliar things were a metal bowl, spatulas of different sizes, narrow flat sticks, a jar of water, and towels. A bag of plaster of Paris, its top torn open, leaned against the leg of the table. Then, as far as I was concerned, came the main feature, the highlight of my contribution to the research. . . . My head on the pillow, I stretched out on the table and closed my eyes. The man advised me to relax, while he coated my face with a greasy substance. He applied it from the top of

my forehead down to the throat and from ear to ear. The lubricant, he explained, was to prevent the hardened plaster of Paris from sticking to my skin. He instructed me to breathe naturally through my nose and not move once he started to apply the mixture. I heard scraping sounds as he stirred powder and water to the right consistency in the bowl, and then felt the creamy paste being spread over my face. From time to time he used the narrow, flat stick to keep the passage to my nostrils open. Eerie emotions and thoughts passed through my head as I waited for the plaster to harden. Perhaps I imagined it, but the soft mixture seemed to get heavier as it turned into a mask. After quite a while the man loosened the hardened cast by wiggling it from side to side. When he lifted it carefully off my face it did not hurt. The only sensation was a suction-cup effect. I would have loved to find out how I fit into their statistics. For all I know, my mask and personal details may still exist in some crates in a storage room somewhere in Germany. Before I left, he smilingly handed me a cigarette. A precious gift for a smoker, but hardly one for me. At least I made one fellow prisoner happy.[32]

The contact with Gershon Evan was of great importance, not only because of his ability to describe in detail his imprisonment in the Stadium. His memory of his feelings during the investigation is a very rare description of how these anthropological studies were perceived on the part of the research subjects.[33]

The meetings with the two survivors and sharing their memories of the racial investigation were very emotional. For family members, the contact brought new details on the fate of a close relative. Conversely, contact with survivors and family members provided details about the conditions of imprisonment in the Vienna Stadium. These details emanate from autobiographies, personal communication and documents. We had not only to inform one daughter of the existence of the mask, we also had to inform her that her father was killed in the "euthanasia" programme in Bernburg. She wrote: "The second new information to me is even more painful – that my father perished not in Buchenwald but had to go through a horrible death at Bernburg".[34] Another daughter who survived the war remembered vaguely having walked with her mother to the Stadium hoping to see her father.[35] She came to the Museum but could not abide seeing the mask. One woman whose father had been measured was very concerned about the anthropological measurements and wanted to know if they had been painful, like many of the medical experiments done in the concentration camps. This was one of the few times where the worries of family members could be calmed since the measurements were not painful, even if they were involuntary.[36] Being measured and having a mask made was not painful, although it meant discomfort and what hurt "was the vicious violence of the persecution that places life in a peril".[37] In 2003, based on an initiative by the historian David Forster, a memorial plaque was installed in the Vienna Stadium's hall of fame.[38]

Exhibition projects

Two exhibitions carried out by the Jewish Museum in Vienna initiated further exploration as well as internal and external historical investigation of the collections. In 1995 the Jewish Museum of the City of Vienna set up the exhibition "Confiscated – The Collection of the Viennese Jewish Museum after 1938" in five different locations.[39] The exhibition curated by Bernhard Purin focused on the history of the collection of the old Jewish Museum between 1938 and their restitution. The exhibition sites were identical to those where the expropriated collections of the old Jewish Museum were transferred. One of these was the Natural History Museum and focused on the exhibition "The Physical and Spiritual Appearance of the Jews" conceived and realised by Josef Wastl in 1939.[40] The 1995 exhibition confronted the institutions involved in the expropriation of the Jewish collections with a part of their own history. For the first time, the activities of the Department of Anthropology during the Nazi period were addressed.

Fifty-five years later, the Jewish Museum of the City of Vienna decided to present the death masks to the public. The 1997 exhibition curated by Felicitas Heimann-Jelinek and Hannes Sulzenbacher was entitled "Masks: Approaching the Shoah" (*Masken. Versuch über die Schoa*) was neither a historical exhibition on the Nazi policy of extermination nor a documentation of systematic and programmed mass murder. Rather, it focused on the issue of human dignity and on the relativity of ethical standards. It was an attempt to show what the Holocaust was, namely murder.[41] The exhibition presented not only the documents on the acquisition of the skulls and busts, it also presented in one room, in one long row, the 29 death masks of men, murdered in concentration camps. A part of the exhibit attempted to shift the perspective from the perpetrators to the victims. It was more than a matter of simply exhibiting the victims, but rather of exhibiting the viewer or visitor. Cameras were installed behind the masks and filmed the visitor. In the next room of the exhibition the visitors could then see themselves or others as they looked at the exhibited masks. The exhibition situation was reversed and the visitors became the objects of the exhibition. The view was focused on them and their behaviour when viewing the masks. The death masks were returned their subjectivity, the anonymous victims were returned a part of the identity and dignity that was denied them in their lives and their deaths.[42] Although their specific identities remain a mystery, the death masks became points of reference for many individual biographies.

When the author approached the Buchenwald Memorial Foundation about the fate of the Jews interned in the Vienna Stadium, they were in the process of preparing, together with the Stiftung Weimarer Klassik, a double exhibition on the occasion of Weimar being European Capital of Culture for 1999. Considering the importance of the documents and materials from the Stadium, the original plan was changed to include them. The double exhibit "From Countenance to Mask: Vienna – Weimar – Buchenwald 1939. A Sketched Place: Goethe's Views of Weimar and Thuringia" (*Vom Antlitz zur Maske. Wien –*

Weimar – Buchenwald 1939. Gezeichneter Ort. Goetheblicke auf Weimar und Thüringen) was opened in May 1999. The presentation of Goethe's sketches in Buchenwald was intended as a gesture to the victims of concentration camp, for many of whom Weimar was associated with the legacy of Goethe, Schiller and Weimar classicism. The other part of the exhibit in the Schiller Museum in Weimar narrated the fate of the 440 men from Vienna. Along the walls a frieze of the photographs and a short biography of each of the men were displayed together with their data sheet and archival documents from Buchenwald. The fact that more than two-thirds of the 440 interned men died in the first weeks of their imprisonment can be seen as one of the first mass murders of the Nazi regime on German soil.[43] The scientifically useless anthropometric images were suddenly representative of the lives that ended in Weimar. The masks were presented in the centre of the exhibition, as would have the masks of renowned persons. The goal was to find a balance between the presentation of the *corpus delicti* and a memorial context. Photographs, seven masks and one bust are now part of the newly opened historical exhibition at the Buchenwald Concentration Camp Memorial on "Ostracism and Violence 1937 to 1945".

Historical film material, together with the collections of anthropological photographs inspired another art project. In 2009 the installation entitled "Col tempo – The W. Project" formed the Hungarian contribution to the 53rd International Art Exhibition in Venice.[44] It was shown one year later in the Ernst Museum in Budapest. This installation by the media artist Peter Forgács was based predominantly on historical film and photographic material from the Nazi period, as it pertained to the Department of Anthropology. It consisted of a series of interrelated spaces arranged by dramaturgical means, so that the visitor met the same faces in various contexts. The exhibited material in "Col Tempo" was based on the motif of the human face. The installation wanted to show that human vision should reflect its own time and historicity. Depending on the context, dimension and number, the faces appeared, so András Rényi, the curator "to be live individuals, prototype idols, living dead or grotesque caricatures".[45] In one part of the installation reminiscent of a closed box or small theatre, an interview with Gershon Evan could be seen on a monitor in which he recounted his life and the process of making the mask. It was not possible to sit and one had to listen carefully if one wanted to understand anything. "By keeping viewers at an embarrassed distance, Forgács stages a form of double vision: we are unable to watch only the film, the memory alone; we are inescapably obliged to take a look at the situation of watching a film and the fragmentariness of memory. The trauma is apparent; it is not accessible".[46] In total, these different visual situations confronted the visitor with implicit practices of seeing and creating identity.

Handling today

In the last several decades, physical anthropological collections and the curating of human remains in general have become a sensitive issue.[47] Many physical anthropological collections contain human remains that were collected in the course of "racial studies" from among indigenous peoples worldwide. Requests for the return of human remains by these indigenous populations have resulted in long processes of discussion and investigation. Professional museum organisations such as, for example, the International Council of Museums (ICOM) issued ethical guidelines and collection policy suggestions for the curation, care and use of human remains in museums.[48] Most recently, the German Museum Association published suggestions, literature and recommendations for the care of human remains in museums and collections in early 2013.[49] Other sensitive collections, like photographs, casts and phonographic recordings, have been subject to less debate, their treatment and care is no less sensitive, as is the careful examination of their provenance, the history of their appropriation and the manner of their transformation into museum objects.[50]

Physical anthropological collections in Germany and Austria very often have a difficult Nazi heritage to contend with. As Robert Proctor pointed out "anthropological science flourished under the Nazis" and while certain traditions were supported and others were oppressed, the process of politicisation of scholarship was often initiated by anthropologists themselves.[51] By the end of the war, many institutions in Germany had been destroyed or closed, and large parts of their collections were lost when they were reorganised or reoriented.[52] In the case of the Vienna Museum, the physical anthropological inventory remained in the collection and remained part of the inventory after 1945, officially classified, *de facto*, as "scientific collection material", even if it was largely forgotten about – up to its rediscovery in the 1990s. Although Wastl and his co-workers began the statistical evaluation of the data collected in the Vienna Stadium, the results were never published. Only a few articles were published on the prisoner of war studies in which the provenance of the materials was concealed.[53] This was partly due to the insight that anthropological research on Jews and prisoners of war was no longer considered legitimate.[54] The anthropologists themselves considered their science to have been abused by the Nazi regime.[55] They shifted their research to archaeological skeletons.

Increasing criticism from outside and growing interest within the museum resulted in the investigation of the department's own collection. In 1991, when the collection of skulls and death masks of Jewish concentration victims and the skulls of Polish resistance fighters were rediscovered, the museum had suddenly to cope with a new situation. The lack of historical knowledge about the Nazi past of the museum or of Jewish religious and burial practice became all too obvious. In the context of research on the role of medical faculties in the Nazi era and requests from Yad Vashem and the Israeli government resulted in investigations of the anatomical, pathological and anthropological collections in Vienna by a commission from the University of Vienna.[56] At the same time, the Austrian government started a process of systematic research on the provenance of collections that had passed into the ownership of the state during or as a consequence of the National Socialist tyranny. In the course of these investigations, the Department of Anthropology undertook a systematic research of its collection.[57]

From the preserved documents and materials, the collection, research, evaluation and exhibition activities of the anthropologists employed in the museum at that time could be reconstructed. They bear witness to their individual scholarly interests, their careerism and entanglement in the Nazi regime. The anthropological data and collections are sources for the history of science as well as for the museum's purchasing and collecting policies. The context of the collections shifted from natural history to a cultural and contemporary history context. The focus shifted from the documents in the archives to other sources, material and personnel-related data in the archives of museums and academic institutions. As they relate to the discipline of physical anthropology, the findings are not only of value as a history of science, they are also witnesses of human fate, of people, who dedicated themselves voluntarily and more often were enlisted involuntarily for research purposes. The data is witness to how human beings were degraded to mere "specimens".

The reconstruction and study of the biographies of the men measured in the Vienna Stadium is an example of how it is possible to return to the victims of these studies at least a part of their human dignity. The numerous personal conversations, chronicles, letters and telephone calls that formed part of the study, but also the documents of the Vienna Stadium study itself – including a number of postcards written by internees – provided insight into the history of persecution, imprisonment and the measuring process in the Vienna Stadium. This made possible a partial reconstruction of the events, and at the same time opened the discussion on how in the future to deal with the collection. The contact with the relatives and survivors also showed that there are limits to what can be reconstructed, for example why particular persons were chosen for masks and for measurements. Moreover, it is not possible to find surviving relatives of all the measured men since many families were completely annihilated. In many cases the photographs and masks are the last witnesses of the persons' lives. For survivors and their relatives, the documents and artefacts found in the Natural History Museum are personal memories. For the museum they are a part of the institution's own history and witness of its moral obligation to tell this story. Historical research and research on the provenance of the collection, as well as the dialogue with survivors, relatives and other institutions has the potential for gaining new insights, creating new meanings and telling new histories of the museum's collections. In the last two decades, this has been done not only on the basis of the integration of individual objects into the context of the museum's exhibits but in the form of a dialogue, in the radio, on television and in the digital media. For the museum, the challenge therein has been to accept other perspectives and demands on its collections.

In the case of the Nazi period collections, exhibition projects led to increasing sensitivity and awareness on the part of the curators. Since the public, the scientific and the museum communities have became aware of the existence of these Nazi period collections, requests to loan them to other museums for their exhibits have increased.[58] Exhibitions addressing such sensitive collections can contribute to raising public awareness and stimulate debate on difficult or controversial issues. They can provide a contribution to the preservation of collective memory. Moreover, the exhibitions changed the status and meaning of the masks significantly. Once the object of racial hatred, they were transformed into witnesses of this hatred, and of the fate of the victims of the Holocaust. In the context of the Natural History Museum, the masks show that the meanings of objects are neither natural, objective or fixed – they are culturally constructed and change from one context to another.

Acknowledgement

I would like to thank Andreas Hemming for proofreading the English version of this chapter.

Notes

1 Jan Gerchow and Hans Belting (eds), *Ebenbilder, Kopien von Körpern – Modelle des Menschen*, Ostfildern-Ruit: Hatje Cantz, 2002.
2 Michael Hertl, *Totenmasken. Was vom Leben und Sterben bleibt*, Stuttgart: Thorbecke, 2002.
3 Bernhard Purin, *Beschlagnahmt. Die Sammlung des Wiener Jüdischen Museums nach 1938*, Vienna: Jüdisches Museum der Stadt Wien, 1995, pp. 11–15; Klaus Taschwer, ' "Lösung der Judenfrage". Zu einigen anthropologischen Ausstellungen im Naturhistorischen Museum Wien', in Kirstin Breitenfellner and Charlotte Kohn-Ley (eds), *Wie ein Monster entsteht. Zur Konstruktion des anderen in Rassismus und Antisemitismus*, Bodenheim: Philo, 1998, pp.161–163; Verena Pawlowsky, 'Erweiterung der Bestände. Die Anthropologische Abteilung des Naturhistorischen Museums 1938–1945', *Zeitgeschichte*, 32 (2005), pp. 72–73.
4 Taschwer, 'Lösung der Judenfrage', pp.161–163; Margit Berner, 'Judentypologisierungen in der Anthropologie am Beispiel der Bestände des Naturhistorischen Museums, Wien', *Zeitgeschichte*, 32 (2005), pp. 111–116.
5 Alan E. Steinweis, *Studying the Jew. Scholarly Antisemitism in Nazi Germany*, Cambridge, MA: Harvard University Press, 2008, p. 19.
6 Benoît Massin, 'Anthropologie und Humangenetik im Nationalsozialismus oder: Wie schreiben deutsche Wissenschaftler ihre eigene Wissenschaftsgeschichte?', in Heidrun Kaupen-Haas and Christian Saller (eds), *Wissenschaftlicher Rassismus: Analysen einer Kontinuität in den Human- und Naturwissenschaften*, Frankfurt am Main: Campus, 1999, p. 41; idem, 'The "Science of Race" ', in Dieter Kuntz (ed.), *Deadly Medicine: Creating the Master Race*, Washington, DC: United States Holocaust Memorial Museum, 2004, pp. 120–122; Hans-Peter Kröner, 'Von der Vaterschaftsbestimmung zum Rassegutachten. Der erbbiologische Ähnlichkeitsvergleich als "österreichisch-deutsches Projekt" 1926–1945', *Berichte zur Wissenschaftsgeschichte*, 22 (1999), pp. 262–263.
7 Maria Teschler-Nicola and Margit Berner, 'Die anthropologische Abteilung des Naturhistorischen Museums in der NS-Zeit. Berichte und Dokumentation von Forschungs- und Sammlungsaktivitäten 1938–1945', in Gustav Spann (ed), *Unter-suchungen zur Anatomischen Wissenschaft in Wien 1938–1945. Senatsprojekt der Universität Wien*, Vienna: Akademischer Senat der Univ. Wien, 1998, pp. 333–358.
8 Ibid., p. 334; Felicitas Heimann-Jelinek, 'Zur Geschichte einer Ausstellung. Masken. Versuch über die Schoa', in Fritz Bauer Institut (ed.), *"Beseitigung des jüdischen Einflusses . . .". Antisemitische Forschung, Eliten und Karrieren im Nationalsozialismus. Jahrbuch 1998/99*

zur Geschichte und Wirkung des Holocaust, Frankfurt am Main and New York: Campus 1999, pp.136–139.

9 Götz Aly, 'Das Posener Tagebuch des Anatomen Hermann Voss', in idem, Peter Chroust, Hans-Dieter Heilmann and Hermann Langbein (eds), *Biedermann und Schreibtischtäter. Materialien zur deutschen Täter-Biographie*, Berlin: Rotbuch, 1987, pp. 54–55.

10 Heimann-Jelinek, 'Zur Geschichte einer Ausstellung', pp. 133–137; Pawlowsky, 'Erweiterung der Bestände 2005', pp. 83–84.

11 Vienna, Natural History Museum, Department of Anthropology, Correspondence, 1941–1947, Hirschheydt to Wastl, 4 Mar 1942. The Department's correspondence includes several letters from the period February to June 1942.

12 Ibid., Wastl to Hirschheydt, 6 Mar 1942.

13 Götz Aly, 'Ein Arbeitsunfall. Rassenkunde, Nebenerwerb und Versicherungsrecht', in idem (ed), *Rasse und Klasse. Nachforschungen zum deutschen Wesen*, Frankfurt am Main: Fischer, 2003, pp. 145–154.

14 Vienna, Natural History Museum, Department of Anthropology, Correspondence, 1941–1947, Mrs. Hirschheydt to Wastl, 2 June 1942.

15 Ibid., Invoice, 19 June 1942.

16 Ibid., Voss to Wastl, 19 June 1942.

17 Ibid., Wastl to Mrs. Hirschheydt, 1 Aug 1942.

18 Ibid.

19 Ibid., Mrs. Hirschheydt to Wastl, 4 Mar 1942.

20 Ibid., List of delivered skulls and masks, 22 June 1942.

21 Teschler-Nicola and Berner, 'Die anthropologische Abteilung'.

22 Herbert Rosenkranz, *Verfolgung und Selbstbehauptung. Die Juden in Österreich 1938–1945*, Vienna and Munich: Herold, 1978, pp. 213–214; Claudia Spring, 'Staatenloses Subjekt, vermessenes Objekt: Anthropologische Untersuchungen an staatenlosen Juden', *Zeitgeschichte*, 30 (2003), p.163.

23 Vienna, Natural History Museum, Department of Anthropology, Somatologische Sammlung Inv.Nr. 2735, Tagebuch 1.

24 Harry Stein, *Juden in Buchenwald 1937–1942*, Weimar: Gedenkstätte Buchenwald, 1992, p. 85; Spring, 'Staatenloses Subjekt, vermessenes Objekt', p. 163.

25 2001–2004 FWF Project, *Anthropology in National Socialism. Projects of the Department of Anthropology of the Natural Museum in Vienna 1938–1945*.

26 Harry Stein, 'Weimar – Buchenwald', in Volkhard Knigge and Jürgen Seifert (eds), *Vom Antlitz zur Maske. Wien-Weimar-Buchenwald 1939. Gezeichneter Ort. Goetheblicke auf Weimar und Thüringen*, Weimar: Gedenkstätte Buchenwald, 1999, pp. 30–34; Claudia Spring, 'Vermessen, deklassiert und deportiert. Dokumentation zur Anthropologischen Untersuchung an 440 Juden im Wiener Stadion im September 1939 unter der Leitung von Josef Wastl vom Naturhistorischen Museum Wien', *Zeitgeschichte*, 32 (2005), pp. 99–100.

27 Ibid., pp. 99–103.

28 Claudia Spring, 'Macht und Ohnmacht vor dem musealen Bestand von einer anthropologischen Untersuchung an Juden im September 1939 in Wien: Anmerkungen und Annäherungen einer Historikerin', in Ingrid Bauer, Helga Embacher, Ernst Hanisch, Albert Lichtblau and Gerald Sprengnagel (eds), *>Kunst>Kommunikation>Macht, 6. Österreichischer Zeitgeschichtetag 2003*, Innsbruck: StudienVerlag, 2004, p. 268.

29 Email Edie R. to M. Berner and C. Spring, 27 Jan 2003.

30 Paul Grünberg and Fritz Kleinmann, 'Wien – Weimar – Buchenwald: Erinnerungen', in Knigge and Seifert, *Vom Antlitz zur Maske*, pp. 72–78. See also Margit Berner, '"Die haben uns behandelt wie Gegenstände". Anthropologische Untersuchungen an jüdischen Häftlingen im Wiener Stadion während des Nationalsozialismus', in Margit Berner, Britta Lange and Anette Hoffmann (eds), *Sensible Sammlungen. Aus dem anthropologischen Depot*, Hamburg: Philo Fine Arts, 2011, pp. 147–167.

31 Gershon Evan, *Winds of Life. The Destinies of a young Viennese Jew 1938–1958*, Riverside, CA: Ariadne, 2000, pp. 53–54.

32 Ibid.

33 Margit Berner and Claudia Spring, 'The Vienna Stadium Study', in Kuntz, *Deadly Medicine*, pp. 114–115; Spring, 'Vermessen, deklassiert und deportiert'; Berner, 'Die haben uns behandelt wie Gegenstände'.

34 Email Edie R. to M. Berner and C. Spring, 27 Jan 2003

35 Spring, 'Macht und Ohnmacht', p. 269.

36 Ibid., p. 268.

37 Paul Weindling, *Victims and Survivors of Nazi Human Experiments, Science and Suffering in the Holocaust*, London: Bloomsbury, 2015, p. 45.

38 www.davidforster.at/Initiative-Gedenktafel-im-Stadion.

39 Purin, Beschlagnahmt.

40 Ibid., pp. 11–15; Taschwer, 'Lösung der Judenfrage', pp.161–163; Pawlowsky, 'Erweiterung der Bestände', pp. 72–73.

41 Heimann-Jelinek, 'Zur Geschichte einer Ausstellung', pp. 140–142.

42 Ibid.

43 Knigge and Seifert, *Vom Antlitz zur Maske*, p. 12.

44 András Rényi (ed.), *"Col Tempo" The W. Project, Péter Forgác's Installation, 53rd International Art Exhibition in Venice*, Budapest: Műcsarnok, 2009; www.coltempo.hu/ (accessed 25 May 2016).

45 Rényi, *"Col Tempo"*, p. 12.

46 Ibid., p. 23.

47 David van Duuren, Mischa ten Kate, Micaela Pereira and Susan Legene, *Physical Anthropology Reconsidered: Human Remains at the Tropenmuseum*, Amsterdam: Koninklijk Instituut Voor de Tropen, 2007.

48 http://icom.museum/the-vision/code-of-ethics/; see also www.babao.org.uk/HumanremainsFINAL.pdf; (accessed 25 May 2016).

49 www.museumsbund.de/de/publikationen/online_publikationen/ (accessed 25 May 2016).

50 Berner, Lange and Hoffmann, *Sensible Sammlungen*; Anette Hoffmann (ed.), *What We See. Reconsidering and Anthropometrical Collection from Southern Africa: Images, Voices and Versioning*, Basel: Basler Afrika Bibliographien, 2009; Andrew Zimmerman, *Anthropology and Antihumanism in Imperial Germany*, Chicago and London: University of Chicago Press, 2001; idem, 'Adventures in the Skin Trade: German Anthropology and Colonial Corporeality', in Glenn H. Penny and Matti Bunzl (eds), *Worldly Provincialism. German Anthropology in the Age of Empire*, Ann Arbor: University of Michigan Press, 2003, pp. 156–178; Jeffrey D. Feldman, 'Contact Points: Museums and the Lost Body Problem', in Elizabeth Edwards, Chris Gosden and Ruth B. Phillips (eds), *Sensible Objects, Colonialism, Museums and Material Culture*, Oxford: Berg, 2006, pp. 245–267.

51 Robert Proctor, 'From Anthropology to Rassenkunde in the German Anthropological Tradition', in G.W. Stocking (ed.), *Bones, Bodies, Behavior. Essays on Biological Anthropology*, Madison: University of Wisconsin Press, 1988, p.140.

52 Ibid., pp. 166–174.

53 Teschler-Nicola and Berner, 'Die anthropologische Abteilung', p. 344.

54 Berner, 'Judentypologisierungen', p. 114.

55 Massin, 'Anthropologie und Humangenetik', pp. 13–14.

56 Spann, Untersuchungen.

57 Teschler-Nicola and Berner, 'Die anthropologische Abteilung'.

58 Kuntz, *Deadly Medicine*; Brigitte Kepplinger (ed.), Wert des Lebens. Gedenken, lernen – begreifen. Ausstellungskatalog Schloss Hartheim, Linz: Trauner, 2003; Felicitas Heimann-Jelinek (ed.), *Jetzt ist er bös, der Tennenbaum. Die zweite Republik und ihre Juden,*

Vienna: Jüdisches Museum der Stadt Wien, 2005; Peter Eppel (ed.), *Wo die Wuchtel fliegt. Legendäre Orte des Wiener Fußballs.* Ausstellungskatalog, Vienna: Löcker, 2008; http://gedenkstaettesteinhof.at/en/exibition/06-science-and-racism (26 May 2016).

Bibliography

Archival Sources

Austria

Vienna, Natural History Museum, Department of Anthropology: Correspondence, 1941–1947. Somatologische Sammlung, Inv.Nr. 2735

Literature

Aly, Götz, 'Das Posener Tagebuch des Anatomen Hermann Voss', in Götz Aly, Peter Chroust, Hans-Dieter Heilmann and Hermann Langbein (eds), *Biedermann und Schreibtischtäter. Materialien zur deutschen Täter-Biographie*, Berlin: Rotbuch, 1987, pp. 15–66
—— 'Ein Arbeitsunfall. Rassenkunde, Nebenerwerb und Versicherungsrecht', in Götz Aly (ed.), *Rasse und Klasse. Nachforschungen zum deutschen Wesen*, Frankfurt am Main: Fischer, 2003, pp. 145–154
Berner, Margit, 'Macht und Ohnmacht vor dem musealen Bestand: Eine anthropologische Untersuchung an Juden im September 1939 in Wien. Anmerkungen und Annäherungen einer Kuratorin', in Ingrid Bauer, Helga Embacher, Ernst Hanisch, Albert Lichtblau and Gerald Sprengnagel (eds), *>Kunst>Kommunikation>Macht, 6. Österreichischer Zeitgeschichtetag 2003*, Innsbruck: StudienVerlag, 2004, pp. 261–265
—— 'Judentypologisierungen in der Anthropologie am Beispiel der Bestände des Naturhistorischen Museums, Wien', *Zeitgeschichte*, 32 (2005), pp. 111–116
—- 'The Nazi Period Collections of Physical Anthropology in the Museum of Natural History, Vienna', in: András Rényi (ed.), *"Col Tempo" The W. Project, Péter Forgác's Installation, 53rd International Art Exhibition in Venice*, Budapest: Műcsarnok, 2009, pp. 34–48
—— ' "Die haben uns behandelt wie Gegenstände". Anthropologische Untersuchungen an jüdischen Häftlingen im Wiener Stadion während des Nationalsozialismus', in Margit Berner, Britta Lange and Anette Hoffmann (eds), *Sensible Sammlungen. Aus dem anthropologischen Depot*, Hamburg: Philo Fine Arts, 2011, pp. 147–167
—- and Claudia Spring, 'The Vienna Stadium Study', in Dieter Kuntz (ed.), *Deadly Medicine: Creating the Master Race*, Washington, DC: United States Holocaust Memorial Museum 2004, pp. 114–115
—— Britta Lange and Anette Hoffmann (eds), *Sensible Sammlungen. Aus dem anthropologischen Depot*, Hamburg: Philo Fine Arts, 2011
van Duuren, David, Mischa ten Kate, Micaela Pereira and Susan Legene, *Physical Anthropology Reconsidered: Human Remains at the Tropenmuseum*, Amsterdam: Koninklijk Instituut Voor de Tropen, 2007
Eppel, Peter (ed.), *Wo die Wuchtel fliegt. Legendäre Orte des Wiener Fußballs. Ausstellungskatalog*, Vienna: Löcker, 2008
Evan, Gershon, *Winds of Life. The Destinies of a young Viennese Jew 1938–1958*, Riverside, CA: Ariadne 2000

Feldman, Jeffrey D., 'Contact Points: Museums and the Lost Body Problem', in Elizabeth Edwards, Chris Gosden and Ruth B. Phillips (eds), *Sensible Objects, Colonialism, Museums and Material Culture*, Oxford: Berg, 2006, pp. 245–267

Gerchow, Jan, and Hans Belting (eds), *Ebenbilder, Kopien von Körpern – Modelle des Menschen*, Ostfildern-Ruit: Hatje Cantz, 2002

Grünberg, Paul, and Fritz Kleinmann, 'Wien – Weimar – Buchenwald: Erinnerungen', in Volkhard Knigge and Jürgen Seifert (eds), *Vom Antlitz zur Maske. Wien-Weimar-Buchenwald 1939. Gezeichneter Ort. Goetheblicke auf Weimar und Thüringen*, Weimar: Gedenkstätte Buchenwald, 1999, pp. 72–78

Heimann-Jelinek, Felicitas, 'Zur Geschichte einer Ausstellung. Masken. Versuch über die Schoa', in Fritz Bauer Institut (ed.), *"Beseitigung des jüdischen Einflusses . . .". Antisemitische Forschung, Eliten und Karrieren im Nationalsozialismus. Jahrbuch 1998/99 zur Geschichte und Wirkung des Holocaust*, Frankfurt am Main and New York: Campus 1999, pp. 131–146

—— (ed.), *Jetzt ist er bös, der Tennenbaum. Die zweite Republik und ihre Juden*, Vienna: Jüdisches Museum der Stadt Wien, 2005

Hertl, Michael, *Totenmasken. Was vom Leben und Sterben bleibt*, Stuttgart: Thorbecke, 2002

Hoffmann, Anette (ed.), *What We See. Reconsidering and Anthropometrical Collection from Southern Africa: Images, Voices and Versioning*, Basel: Basler Afrika Bibliographien, 2009

Kepplinger, Brigitte (ed.), *Wert des Lebens. Gedenken, lernen – begreifen. Ausstellungskatalog Schloss Hartheim*, Linz: Trauner, 2003

Knigge, Volkhard and Jürgen Seifert (eds), *Vom Antlitz zur Maske. Wien-Weimar-Buchenwald 1939. Gezeichneter Ort. Goetheblicke auf Weimar und Thüringen*, Weimar: Gedenkstätte Buchenwald, 1999

Kröner, Hans-Peter, 'Von der Vaterschaftsbestimmung zum Rassegutachten. Der erbbiologische Ähnlichkeitsvergleich als "österreichisch-deutsches Projekt" 1926–1945', *Berichte zur Wissenschaftsgeschichte*, 22 (1999), pp. 257–265

Kuntz, Dieter (ed.), *Deadly Medicine: Creating the Master Race*, Washington, DC: United States Holocaust Memorial Museum, 2004

Massin, Benoît, 'Anthropologie und Humangenetik im Nationalsozialismus oder: Wie schreiben deutsche Wissenschaftler ihre eigene Wissenschaftsgeschichte?', in Heidrun Kaupen-Haas and Christian Saller (eds), *Wissenschaftlicher Rassismus: Analysen einer Kontinuität in den Human- und Naturwissenschaften*, Frankfurt am Main: Campus, 1999, pp. 12–63

—— 'The "Science of Race"', in Dieter Kuntz (ed.), *Deadly Medicine: Creating the Master Race*, Washington, DC: United States Holocaust Memorial Museum, 2004, pp. 89–125

Pawlowsky, Verena, 'Erweiterung der Bestände. Die Anthropologische Abteilung des Naturhistorischen Museums 1938–1945', *Zeitgeschichte*, 32 (2005), pp. 69–90

Proctor, Robert, 'From Anthropology to Rassenkunde in the German Anthropological Tradition', in George W. Stocking (ed.), *Bones, Bodies, Behavior. Essays on Biological Anthropology*, Madison: University of Wisconsin Press, 1988, pp. 138–179

Purin, Bernhard, *Beschlagnahmt. Die Sammlung des Wiener Jüdischen Museums nach 1938*, Vienna: Jüdisches Museum der Stadt Wien, 1995

Rényi, András (ed) *"Col Tempo" The W. Project, Péter Forgác's Installation, 53rd International Art Exhibition in Venice*, Budapest: Műcsarnok, 2009

Rosenkranz, Herbert, *Verfolgung und Selbstbehauptung. Die Juden in Österreich 1938–1945*, Vienna and Munich: Herold, 1978

Spann, Gustav (ed.), *Untersuchungen zur Anatomischen Wissenschaft in Wien 1938–1945. Senatsprojekt der Universität Wien*, Vienna: Akademischer Senat der Univ. Wien, 1998

Spring, Claudia, 'Staatenloses Subjekt, vermessenes Objekt: Anthropologische Untersuchungen an staatenlosen Juden', *Zeitgeschichte*, 30 (2003), pp. 163–170

—— 'Macht und Ohnmacht vor dem musealen Bestand von einer anthropologischen Untersuchung an Juden im September 1939 in Wien: Anmerkungen und Annäherungen einer Historikerin', in Ingrid Bauer, Helga Embacher, Ernst Hanisch, Albert Lichtblau and Gerald Sprengnagel (eds), *>Kunst>Kommunikation>Macht, 6. Österreichischer Zeitgeschichtetag 2003*, Innsbruck: StudienVerlag, 2004, pp. 266–270

—— 'Vermessen, deklassiert und deportiert. Dokumentation zur Anthropologischen Untersuchung an 440 Juden im Wiener Stadion im September 1939 unter der Leitung von Josef Wastl vom Naturhistorischen Museum Wien', *Zeitgeschichte*, 32 (2005), pp. 91–110

Stein, Harry, *Juden in Buchenwald 1937–1942*, Weimar: Gedenkstätte Buchenwald, 1992

—— 'Weimar – Buchenwald', in Volkhard Knigge and Jürgen Seifert (eds), *Vom Antlitz zur Maske. Wien-Weimar-Buchenwald 1939. Gezeichneter Ort. Goetheblicke auf Weimar und Thüringen*, Weimar: Gedenkstätte Buchenwald, 1999, pp. 30–34

Steinweis, Alan E., *Studying the Jew. Scholarly Antisemitism in Nazi Germany*, Cambridge, MA: Harvard University Press, 2008

Taschwer, Klaus, '"Lösung der Judenfrage". Zu einigen anthropologischen Ausstellungen im Naturhistorischen Museum Wien', in Kirstin Breitenfellner and Charlotte Kohn-Ley (eds), *Wie ein Monster entsteht. Zur Konstruktion des anderen in Rassismus und Antisemitismus*, Bodenheim: Philo, 1998, pp. 153–180

Teschler-Nicola, Maria and Margit Berner, 'Die anthropologische Abteilung des Naturhistorischen Museums in der NS-Zeit. Berichte und Dokumentation von Forschungs- und Sammlungsaktivitäten 1938–1945', in Gustav Spann (ed.), *Untersuchungen zur Anatomischen Wissenschaft in Wien 1938–1945. Senatsprojekt der Universität Wien*, Vienna: Akademischer Senat der Univ. Wien, 1998, pp. 333–358

Weindling, Paul, *Victims and Survivors of Nazi Human Experiments. Science and Suffering in the Holocaust*, London: Bloomsbury, 2015

Zimmerman, Andrew, *Anthropology and Antihumanism in Imperial Germany*, Chicago and London: University of Chicago Press, 2001

—— 'Adventures in the Skin Trade: German Anthropology and Colonial Corporeality', in Glenn H. Penny and Matti Bunzl (eds.), *Worldly Provincialism. German Anthropology in the Age of Empire*, Ann Arbor: University of Michigan Press, 2003, pp. 156–178

7   Beyond Spiegelgrund and Berkatit

Human experimentation and coerced research at the Vienna School of Medicine, 1939 to 1945[1]

Herwig Czech

At the time of the *Anschluss*, Vienna University's Faculty of Medicine was the second largest medical school in the German-speaking area, and possibly worldwide. The impact of the Nazi take-over in Austria on the Faculty of Medicine was enormous, as out of 309 active and 43 retired scientists, more than half were dismissed in 1938.[2] The result was a thorough politicisation of the Faculty of Medicine, because the newly opened slots were predominantly filled with physicians connected to the NSDAP and its various organisations. However, despite the prominence of the institution, relatively little is known about the day-to-day research activities at the university during the war, including possible experimentation on humans without their consent.[3]

To date, the only concerted effort to shed light on unethical research practices at the Vienna Faculty of Medicine during National Socialism was a research project initiated by the university in 1997, after publicly voiced concerns that anatomist and former dean Eduard Pernkopf had used the body parts of Nazi victims to create his famous topographical atlas. Although the commissioned report contained detailed studies of the use of victims' body parts at various university clinics and institutes during and after the war, it was never fully published and the affair was quickly forgotten about by the public.[4] Furthermore, the mandate of the commission was limited to the question of the (mis-)use of human remains, so that the broader question of human experiments and coerced research was never properly addressed. Other instances of unethical research practices documented in the literature are the involvement of Hans Eppinger and Wilhelm Beiglböck in the seawater drinking experiments in Dachau, and the tuberculosis experiments on mentally handicapped children carried out at the Paediatric University Clinic in 1941, in collaboration with the Psychiatric-Neurological Clinic. The present chapter provides a review of the current state of our knowledge, including the results of recent research by the author into various departments of the Vienna Faculty of Medicine.

Internal medicine – the Dachau seawater drinking experiments as the tip of the iceberg?

Wilhelm Beiglböck (1905–1962), assistant at the I. Clinic of Internal Medicine under the directorship of Hans Eppinger Jr. (1879–1946), was indicted as one of 23 defendants at the Nuremberg Medical Trial for his seawater experiments on prisoners at Dachau concentration camp.[5] Eppinger himself, who had recommended his assistant for the task and personally visited Dachau on at least one occasion, initially escaped scrutiny by Allied war crimes investigators.[6] He was an internationally renowned specialist in internal medicine, who had been consulted, among others, by the Shah of Iran, and by Josef Stalin. After the war, the Austrian government went to considerable lengths to cover up his role in the Dachau experiments. In September 1946, however, Eppinger killed himself after being summoned to Nuremberg as a witness, in all likelihood out of fear of the consequences of being personally implicated.[7] With his suicide, he saved the university some embarrassment, and the latter has not proven very eager to remember this dark chapter ever since. At the same time, the research practices at Eppinger's clinic have never been properly scrutinised, although there are reasons to believe that unethical methods in the research and therapy were more widespread than hitherto acknowledged. The most striking example is the likely death of alleged serial killer Bruno Lüdke in a low-pressure chamber that had been installed on the premises of the clinic before the war in cooperation with the German Air Force. It was under the responsibility of the clinic's assistant Hermann Möschl. Apart from a single hint in a dissertation submitted at the Institute of Forensic Medicine, it is currently unknown what experiments were performed in this chamber.[8]

Publications by staff members allow insights into research practices at the clinic. In 1940, the assistant Falko Lainer published the results of human experiments he had conducted in order to study the transmission mechanism of jaundice or *icterus catarrhalis*. In one set of experiments, he performed blood transfusions from 15 patients with jaundice to healthy test subjects. In a second set, he transferred duodenum secretions from sick to healthy persons. No details are given on who the test subjects were and if they had consented to the experiments. Lainer claims that they were not harmed, since no infection was transmitted, but the fact remains that the experiments had no possible therapeutic indication and that the subjects incurred considerable risks.[9]

Another example from Eppinger's clinic concerns research on artificially induced states of shock, which was conducted in cooperation with the Psychiatric-Neurological Clinic under Otto Pötzl. In 1941, Hans Eppinger supervised a doctoral dissertation on insulin shock and salt metabolism. His interest in salt metabolism would later play a role in the seawater experiments that were carried out in Dachau. In this case, the insulin shocks were induced without any therapeutic motive. The same is true in the case of another medical dissertation written at the clinic,[10] which studied vitamin C metabolism under insulin shock. Regarding the identity of the research subjects and the question of consent, the available sources unfortunately do not provide any further information.[11] Wilhelm Beiglböck mentioned in 1942 that Pötzl and his direct superior Eppinger had instructed him "several years" before to study metabolic changes under insulin hypoglycaemia. In the course of insulin shocks, which he had induced "not for therapeutic motives", Beiglböck observed that certain patients with ailments of the digestive tract recovered after the experiments. More systematic clinical trials with insulin hypoglycaemia on more than 80 patients between 1938 and 1942 led him to recommend the treatment against ulcers.[12]

Evidence of further possible experiments at the clinic is provided by French military intelligence documents from 1946. An informant called "Alexandre" reported that Eppinger had experimented on patients with heart conditions by artificially inducing increased heart rates in order to perform certain tests. According to the source, at least two patients had died during these experiments (presumably from artificially induced heart attacks) and had been dissected afterwards. Eppinger was said to have been motivated less by his political views than by his relentless thirst for knowledge. From the document it is unclear if the informant had personally witnessed these practices, but the French rated the source's overall credibility in the medium range.[13]

On the occasion of Eppinger's suicide, the daily *Neues Österreich* reported about rumours "among Viennese physicians" alleging that he had removed tissue from the bodies of executed individuals and implanted them into patients suffering from pathological emaciation caused by malfunctioning of the pituitary glands.[14] Currently, no further details are known about these alleged experimental therapies.

"Only infants unfit to live": the Paediatric Clinic and experiments on children

With Franz Hamburger (1874–1954), the Vienna University Paediatric Clinic was directed already from 1930 by a stalwart representative of the right-wing *völkisch* camp; from 1933, he became a proponent of National Socialism and from 1934, illegally active in the NSDAP.[15] Hamburger's political stance was not without impact on the Paediatric Clinic's personnel policy and brought about its sweeping alignment with National Socialist ideology.

In the 1940 edition of their textbook of paediatrics, Franz Hamburger and Richard Priesel (Innsbruck) expressed in no uncertain terms their view on the new role doctors should assume under the Nazi regime: "At all times should you be aware of the duties of the National Socialist physician, who keeps in mind not only the individual person, but the entire *Volkskörper* [literally, people's body], in which the single person like the cell in the human organism is just a building block, just a cell of the people as a whole". In an unusually candid manner, these two authors advocated for the killing of newborn babies with malformations or mental handicaps: "For the time being, you have still the duty as a physician to preserve the child's life under any circumstances.

However, time and again, you will have to explain to the parents, at least to the less sentimental father, that it would be better for the respective child to die, that it must be sterilised to prevent hereditary-defective progeny".[16]

During the subsequent years, Hamburger's clinic routinely sent children to the Spiegelgrund, a neurological clinic and youth welfare home set up in July 1940, among other things, to serve the purposes of the "child euthanasia" programme.[17] There were further personal and institutional ties between the two establishments, for example via the Vienna Society for Curative Pedagogy, and in the person of Erwin Jekelius, the first director of the Spiegelgrund clinic, who was a former assistant of Hamburger.[18]

Another troubling aspect of the relationship between the university Paediatric Clinic and the Spiegelgrund hospital is their collaboration in vaccination experiments on children conducted by the clinic's assistant Elmar Türk (1907–2005).[19] The aim was to test the reliability of the BCG vaccine against tuberculosis. In two series of experiments in the years 1941 and 1942, Türk intentionally infected five children with virulent tuberculosis bacilli, three of them after receiving vaccinations, and two (as controls) without any protection. The results were discussed on several occasions by the Viennese paediatric community and published in two papers, in 1942 and 1944. All five were sent to the Spiegelgrund clinic after the experiments, where they died. There is evidence that some, if not all of them, were intentionally killed in order to complement the clinical observations by post-mortem examinations.[20]

The boundaries of the ethically acceptable were clearly tested and sometimes crossed in other cases of experimental research at the clinic as well, even if it is often impossible to determine with certainty if the parents had consented, and whether the children were harmed. One such example was a 1943 dissertation on the temperature regulation in children. In the most extreme of the experiments performed for the study, a six-month-old child with a mental disability was exposed to cold until his body temperature fell by several degrees Celsius. The aim of the research was to show that children, in keeping with the Nazi ideals of physical toughness, could be exposed to large temperature changes without being harmed.[21]

At least three Nazi-era publications by university lecturer Viktor Koszler, a longstanding collaborator of Franz Hamburger, must be mentioned in the context of this chapter. In 1940, Koszler published a study on "Prontosil as an influencing factor on the vaccination process".[22] It was based on a series of experiments on 20 children between the age of two months and nine years. They received a protective vaccination against smallpox and were at the same time administered high doses of Prontosil (sometimes Koszler would even try to "drown their organism" in the drug).[23] Based on his observation that Prontosil could lead to skin discoloration, Koszler wanted to find out whether Prontosil would influence skin reactions caused by the smallpox vaccination. For all the children in the experiment, this meant an unnecessary administration of drugs (since there was no therapeutic motive); moreover, Koszler established that in many cases the sulfonamide had completely cancelled out the effect of the vaccination, which therefore had to be repeated. It is unclear what therapeutic insights the experiments could have yielded since the antibacterial properties of Prontosil had to remain ineffective against viral diseases such as smallpox (*variola*). The paper provides no indication whether the parents' consent had been obtained; in any case, according to the standards of the "guidelines for new curative treatments and for the performance of scientific experiments on humans", issued in Germany in 1931, these experiments would have to be classified as inadmissible.[24]

A similar assessment applies to Koszler's experiments with Pervitin (methamphetamine), which he administered without any therapeutic motivation to examine the effect of various dosages on children of different age groups. At least some of the experimental subjects were children with mental disabilities: "Here an infant with Mongolian idiocy must be mentioned who received on three consecutive days 8, 15, resp. 18 tablets at a time; this was followed by extreme restiveness, redness of the face, occasional cyanosis, and intermittent respiration, but after many hours, the child completely regained its calm".[25]

In a 1943 paper, Koszler reported on experiments to transmit Staphylococcal scalded skin syndrome from one person to another, using the contents of the blisters characteristic for the disease; since the paper does not contain further details, it is impossible to analyse these experiments in detail. It seems clear, however, that experimental infections (even if they appear to have failed to reproduce full-fledged illness) could not possibly be justified as a therapeutic intervention in the interest of the patient.[26]

Another series of experiments by the already mentioned Elmar Türk dealt with the effect of vitamin D as a remedy and prophylaxis against rickets.[27] While the reported therapeutic attempts on 30 children seem to be unproblematic (treatment of rickets with vitamin D was already an established method), the prophylactic experiments on prematurely born infants mentioned in the same paper appear highly problematic. The reason Türk chose premature infants for his experiments was his assumption of "a practically 100 per cent susceptibility" to rickets in the absence of countermeasures.[28] For the purpose of investigating the effectiveness of the prophylactic treatment performed on 23 children, he denied 15 babies in the control group any treatment at all until 13 of them had, in fact, developed rickets that could be detected in their X-rays. To prevent parents or other physicians from distorting the research results through protective measures against rickets, he did not even shy away from deceptive manoeuvres. He misled the mothers by pretending that "further protective measures any time soon" might be "potentially hazardous" to their children; to deceive colleagues who might have been consulted, he falsified certifcates wrongly claiming that prophylactic measures had been taken. Surprisingly, Türk documented these deceptions in his publication; this clearly proves that the parents had not consented and is also indicative of the attitude toward such experiments prevailing at the hospital (and probably in the field more broadly).[29]

Another series of experiments, of an equally problematic character, concerned a total of 218 patients at the paediatric clinic. Their age ranged from infancy to seventeen years old. In this case, Türk examined skin reactions to injections either with a staphylococcal culture filtrate or with a control substance. The children, who were administered up to 15 injections in the back, derived absolutely no health benefits from these procedures.[30]

Experiments on children deemed unworthy of medical care due to their poor physical and mental condition seem to have been an acceptable practice at the Vienna Paediatric Clinic under Hamburger. Heribert Goll (1912-?), another of Hamburger's assistants, was interested in the connection between vitamin A deficiency and keratomalacia. While a general causal link between the two had already been firmly established, important questions remained unanswered. These included children's minimal vitamin A requirements or why under similar conditions of vitamin A deprivation only a small percentage of children actually developed the condition.

Goll himself described the terrible symptoms of a two and a half months old child admitted to his clinic with "typical" keratomalacia as "opacity and ulcerous decomposition of both corneas". The child responded well to treatment and recovered, but permanently lost her eyesight. In an attempt to elucidate the causation of the disease, Goll performed several series of experiments on patients at the clinic. In one instance, he kept babies on a diet as low in vitamin A as possible, inducing an artificial vitamin deficiency that lasted up to several months. The number of children subjected to this treatment is not known, but Goll's publication on this work documents that several of his experimental subjects developed xerophthalmia, the early stage of keratomalacia – a result that was neither unexpected nor original, given the existing knowledge on vitamin A deficiency at the time.[31]

In a second series of experiments, Goll wanted to find out why not all children were equally vulnerable to vitamin A deficiency. He considered the possibility that keratomalacia was caused by an infection facilitated by the vitamin deficiency, rather than by the deficiency itself. In order to test this hypothesis, he took exudate from the aforementioned girl's cornea and conjunctiva and smeared it into the eyes of four children he had chosen as human guinea pigs – three of them had been deprived of vitamin A prior to the experiment, and one child served as a control. Since this intervention failed, he repeated the experiment with *cocci* bacteria cultivated from the exudate. Fortunately for the children, the hypothesis turned out to be wrong and no transmission of the disease was possible in this way – with Goll claiming that apart from a "passing irritation of the conjunctiva" the children suffered no adverse effects. Regarding his human subjects, Goll insisted that he chose "only infants unfit to live, afflicted with meningocele and similar conditions". The fact that he openly admitted to experimenting on children with disabilities in a medical journal raises the question if such practices were generally accepted in the field, not only during the Nazi period but possibly also beyond.

A second publication by the same author, published six months later, provides further insight into his experimental studies. Again without giving exact numbers, he referred to an ongoing "larger clinical-experimental series of studies". As part of these studies, he presented the results of experiments on 20 children who had been fed a diet of fat-free milk with added carbohydrates. The children were deprived not only of vitamin A, but also of vital fats altogether. One of the children, a ten months old infant, was subjected to this regime for nearly 300 days, others for as little as five days. Goll's aim was to examine the organism's capacity to store vitamin A in the liver. In order to obtain this data, he needed autopsies of the babies' livers after their deaths. It is at this point unknown if the babies (the oldest was a little over a year old) were actively killed in order to obtain the required samples, or if they died from malnutrition or other causes.

Based on the details provided in the paper, it is possible to identify a number of Goll's research subjects. One of them was Anna Mick, who was admitted to the clinic in February 1941, aged a little over six months. Anna had been born with a hydrocephalus and suffered from severe decubitus on the back of her head, which points to a lack of adequate care. Her physical development up to this point was described as "robust", but her mental capacities were "stunted". On admission, her father gave his consent to lumbar punctures (the taking of cerebrospinal fluid from the lumbar spine), despite being warned of a possible "danger of sudden death" due to the procedure. During the 114 days she stayed at the clinic, Anna was kept on a diet of systematic malnutrition, required by Goll's experiments. Samples or probes from her eyes and from other parts of her body were sent to the Ophthalmological Clinic and other institutions for examination. It is unclear from the patient records if she was treated for her head wounds; in any case, most of the measures taken and documented were clearly motivated by diagnostic and research interests, not therapy. As for the cause of her death, the autopsy report simply states: "The child died under increasing feebleness".[32] Although Goll himself claimed in both publications that he chose infants who had no chance of survival (and who were, in his own words, "mostly idiotic"), assuming a "natural death" in this as in the other cases seems implausible at best, given the regime of systematic malnutrition to which the children had been subjected.[33]

Criminal connections: The Institute of Forensic Medicine

The Institute of Forensic Medicine's history during National Socialism is among the best documented of all the departments of the Vienna Faculty of Medicine, thanks to a book-length study dedicated to the subject.[34] The increasing importance of scientific racism in many spheres of life provided significant opportunities to open new fields of activity for the institute's members. The director Philipp Schneider (1896–1954) served as expert witness in court cases concerning the possible castration of men after sexual offences, including homosexuality, and forced sterilisations of women and men.[35] Rendering expert opinions in cases of disputed racial (mostly Jewish) origins – which could be a matter of life or death for the concerned individuals – became an important (and lucrative) part of the staff's activities. For the military, forensic doctors were engaged in identifying cases of self-harm among soldiers, which were punished with excessive harshness. The role played by the institute in critical domains of Nazi biopolitics is reflected by the fact that it was staffed with ideologically hardened Nazis, such as the director Philipp Schneider himself, an early member of the NSDAP and the SS who claimed to have participated in the Austrian Nazis' attempted putsch in July 1934.[36]

In its scientific research, the institute collaborated with the Ministry of Aviation and the Air Force. Thus, at least two doctoral dissertations were written at the suggestion of the Research Institute for Aviation Medicine of the Reich Ministry of Aviation in Berlin, headed by the physiologist Hubertus Strughold.[37] Both works dealt with the impairment of combat pilots' "high-altitude resistance" as a result of infectious diseases, particularly gonorrhoea. For the first study, 13 patients at the Air Force military hospital in Vienna had to inhale a nitrogen-oxygen mixture corresponding to an altitude of approximately 7,500 metres. Within a few minutes, they would reach the so-called "critical threshold" with increasing impairment in cognitive abilities until reaching unconsciousness.[38] While the effects of these experiments on the subjects can by no means be compared to the oftentimes deadly experiments on inmates of concentration camps, the question of consent must still be asked. The thesis fails to provide any information in this regard; as the experiments involved soldiers required to obey orders, their choices were probably limited. Since the author explicitly wished to research the effects of the respective infectious disease on high-altitude resistance (without any influence of medication administered for treatment purposes), the additional question arises whether any necessary treatment had been delayed in favour of these experiments.[39] The second dissertation investigated the effects of chemotherapeutic substances available at the time on high-altitude resistance; in this case, 14 individuals (partially identical to those in the above-mentioned experimental series) were subjected to a repeated simulation of altitude sickness up to the point of unconsciousness.[40]

In 1944, the institute was involved in a deadly human experiment taking place outside the concentration camp complex. The director (Schneider) had excellent connections with the *Reichskriminalpolizeiamt* (Reich criminal investigations department) under Arthur Nebe (1894–1945). When the latter founded a new *Kriminalmedizinisches Zentralinstitut* (Central Institute of Criminal Medicine, KMI) in 1943, it was established on the premises of the Vienna Institute of Forensic Medicine and placed under the directorship of Schneider. Due to wartime restrictions and Nebe's fall from grace in the wake of the 20 July plot against Hitler, the KMI never really took off the ground. During its short-lived existence, however, it was at the centre of one of the most bizarre – if at the time largely unreported – criminal affairs in Nazi Germany. In March 1943, the Berlin police arrested a man named Bruno Lüdke (1908–1944) under the suspicion of rape and murder. During the following interrogations, Lüdke admitted to a total of 84 murders, which corresponded to two thirds of all the unresolved murder cases in Germany at the time. This would have made him the worst serial killer in German history, but serious doubts as to the veracity of his confessions existed already at the time and have been confirmed since. The head of the German criminal police Arthur Nebe was determined, however, to close the case and charge Lüdke with the crimes. Probably in order to avoid the risk of embarrassment in a formal trial, he had Lüdke transferred to the Vienna KMI in December 1943, where the latter died in April 1944, after being subjected to a series of examinations and experiments. Forensic experts and anthropologists strived to document his bodily features as an ideal example of a "born criminal". Schneider and his assistant Ferdinand Schoen (1906–1984) forced Lüdke to drink pure alcohol in order to examine the alcohol level in the cerebrospinal fluid, which they examined via lumbar and occipital punctures. The precise circumstances of Lüdke's death on 8 April 1944 are unclear; the most likely hypothesis is that he died during an experiment in the low-pressure chamber installed at Eppinger's Clinic of Internal Medicine.[41]

Heroic measures: dangerous experiments in neurosurgery

The I. Surgical Clinic under the directorship of Leopold Schönbauer was one of the institutions designated to perform forced sterilisations (in this case on men). The interventions were carried out by Schönbauer himself or by his assistant Wolfram Sorgo (1907–1983), and later Paul Deuticke (1901–1981).[42] While forced sterilisations have been studied in some detail, so far there is no information available on possible human experiments at the surgical clinic. One hint is that Schönbauer was accused after liberation by a medical student of having transplanted tissue material from executed political prisoners to some of his patients for experimental purposes. The student gave his name and the accusations were rather specific, but so far they have not been verified on the basis of other sources.[43] There are other strong indications, however, that surgical patients at Schönbauer's clinic were subjected to rather questionable non-therapeutic experiments.

In 1942, the already mentioned assistant physician Wolfram Sorgo published a paper on his "observations on the effect of intracranial vascular ligation on the peripheral circulation". The published observations were based on five patients who had to have parts of their brains removed because of tumours (in one case, following gunshot injury). In the course of these operations, which were performed with the patients being fully conscious, Sorgo disrupted the blood flow in various cerebral vessels to study the effects on blood pressure. Hereby he was able to confirm the observation, already published by others, that ligation of the anterior cerebral artery led to unconsciousness under certain blood-pressure conditions. As was usual for medical literature at the time, there is no indication whether the patients had consented, and the further course of the surgeries is not documented. Be this as it may, tampering with cerebral circulation to the point of unconsciousness definitely constituted an additional and unnecessary risk during a procedure that was life-threatening even under the best of circumstances.[44]

Wolfram Sorgo also wrote a paper in 1940 on the diagnostic value of lumbar puncture in connection with brain tumours. He reported on 365 patients on whom he had performed this procedure, in each case shortly before brain surgery. He concluded that this method was of very limited diagnostic value while, at the same time, highly dangerous and sometimes even lethal for the patients. He therefore advised against the use of lumbar puncture in most cases.[45] In this context, the question arises whether it had, in fact, been necessary to expose such a large number of patients to danger to obtain this result, or whether it might not have been indicated to refrain much earlier on from conducting any further lumbar punctures of such limited value in connection with brain surgery.

States of shock: the Psychiatric–Neurological Clinic, experimental treatments and "euthanasia"

Considering the field's significance with regard to Nazi medical crimes, it is perhaps surprising that no comprehensive study of the Vienna Psychiatric-Neurological Clinic during the war years exists.[46] Members of the clinic contributed to the forced sterilisation programme, through active participation as expert witnesses or by expressing support in scientific papers.[47] Very little is known about the clinic's involvement in the "euthanasia" programmes or the treatment of patients in terms of therapy and clinical research.[48]

One of the clinic's key areas of research regarded states of shock induced for therapeutic purposes, using electricity, insulin or cardiazol. One such study was carried out by Walt(h)er Birkmayer, partly in cooperation with Fritz Redlich. During these experiments, patients undergoing cardiazol treatment were administered a variety of other drugs in order to identify the mechanism of the cardiazol shock. There was no identifiably therapeutic aim involved. This case is somewhat untypical in that it was not furthered by the political context of the Nazi regime, but rather the opposite. Redlich's emigration put an end to the collaboration between the two researchers, who published their results separately.[49] As in other cases of experimental research on human beings mentioned in this chapter, the boundaries of the ethically acceptable were clearly tested here, although it is impossible to determine whether patients consented and whether they were harmed.[50]

In the context of the newest and most important of the psychiatric shock treatments, electroconvulsive therapy, the clinic's assistant Wolfgang Holzer developed two types of shock devices that competed with the leading manufacturer Siemens.[51] The "T4" organisation (which was responsible for the killing of tens of thousands of mental patients in 1940 and 1941) had a strong interest in the development of electroshock treatment and provided support for its dissemination and application.[52] Holzer was in contact with the medical director of "T4", Paul Nitsche, to promote his device and his plans for a research institute in Vienna that would focus on the development of physical methods of therapy in psychiatry.[53] In a planning document submitted to "T4", he cited the window of opportunity opened by the ongoing euthanasia killings as the main motive for his project.[54]

Emil Gelny, one of the most notorious physician perpetrators in Austria, learned of Holzer's shock device during an internship at Pötzl's clinic before assuming control of Lower Austria's two psychiatric hospitals, Gugging and Mauer-Öhling, and killing hundreds of patients there. Apart from poisoning his victims, he used a modified version of Holzer's shock device for these murders. Gelny's unique contribution to the medical killing methods used in Nazi Germany was on several occasions tested before witnesses in order to demonstrate its effectiveness. On one occasion, in spring 1944, Gelny killed two female patients with this method. According to an eye witness, one of the people "experimenting" on the women with Gelny was Holzer.[55] The latter gave evidence after the war that he had been invited to Gugging on at least one other occasion by Gelny, to assist an unknown military physician in a therapeutic experiment aimed at awakening catatonic patients with infiltrations of oxygen. The procedure was tested on two female patients, according to Holzer without harmful effects (he does not mention if the treatment was successful).[56]

The institutionalisation of scientific racism at the Vienna Faculty of Medicine

One example of how "racial research" penetrated the Medical Faculty is the 1942 dissertation "Suicide with particular consideration of the Jews", supervised by Robert Stigler and submitted by Wolfgang Damus. This study aimed at explaining the differing suicide rates among Catholics, Protestants and Jews since the nineteenth century. While the author refrained from direct references to National Socialism, his explanatory attempts were nothing but a casual accumulation of classic anti-Semitic stereotypes: religious deracination of the Jews, their special exposure to the conditions in the financial sector conducive to suicide, a missing capacity for love, greater psychological instability due to the prevalence of "nervous and other diseases typical for Jews", as well as "sexual excesses" and "degeneracies". In his view, "miscegenation between Jews and non-Jews" in particular seemed to entail dangers; after all, "crossbreeds" were "often highly unstable and weak-willed", "transgressing all boundaries in the sexual, social, and other realms" and "in many cases turning individuals into psychopaths". He did not even contemplate explaining the downright explosion in the number of suicides of Jews in Vienna – from 98 cases in 1937 to 423 in 1938 – by the obvious pressures of persecution and the increasingly desperate outlook for the Jewish minority, but rather through the arguments mentioned above.[57]

As of 1 April 1939, new medical study regulations became effective; among others, mandatory courses in "Heredity and Racial Studies", "Population

Policy", "Human Heredity as the Basis for Racial Hygiene" as well as "Racial Hygiene" were introduced.[58] In this framework, the racial hygienist Lothar Löffler (1901–1983) gave a lecture in the winter semester of 1943/44 titled *Das Judentum als rassisches und soziales Problem* (Jewry as a racial and social problem).[59]

Löffler was also a central figure in attempts – observable from 1938 onward – to establish a dedicated Institute of Race Biology at the University of Vienna. Löffler's goal was to institutionalise race biology "as a science that does not serve narrow self-interests, but certain important practical and ideological tasks set by the National Socialist state". In Vienna, he saw an opportunity to realise the first institute of its kind in the German Reich. He presented his ambitious plans in a position paper of November 1938. The umbrella term "race biology" was to include not only the newly emerging fields of bio-political intervention such as "hereditary and racial hygiene", but also disciplines such as genetics, hereditary pathology and physical anthropology. The institute was intended to comprise six departments ("racial science and hereditary biology", "racial hygiene and racial policy", "psychiatric and psychological genetic research", "physical hereditary diseases", "experimental genetic research" as well as "hereditary statistics and biometry") and employ 55 people including the director.[60]

Ultimately, as a result of internal conflicts and the war, Löffler's grand plans, however, could be implemented only to a limited extent. Just a few departments had their own head and other staff by the war's end and could be described as at least partially functioning. The appointees were, besides Löffler (in Vienna from November 1942), Georg Gottschewski from Königsberg for experimental genetic research (May 1942), Horst Geyer for psychiatric, neurological and psychological genetic research (January 1943), and Hans Ritter, a pupil of Eugen Fischer in Berlin, for the Department of Anthropology (June 1943).[61] This limited realisation notwithstanding, the project of the Viennese Institute of Race Biology permits insights into how one of the leading eugenicists of the German Reich imagined the future of his discipline at the interface of academic research, training of the next generation and racial-political intervention.

Löffler was also involved in research in the context of "child euthanasia", as emerges from a report by Ernst Wentzler, one of the three "experts" responsible for selecting the victims. According to Wentzler, Löffler's research dealt with "questions of hereditary biology linked to social factors based on our card file material", which suggests an orientation toward the persecution of so-called "antisocial individuals".[62] In an application to the Reich research council in 1943, Löffler pointed out that his institute was "intimately" collaborating with the *Reichsausschuss* (the secret organisation charged with executing the "child euthanasia" programme) within the framework of "research on hereditary diseases, their genesis and spreading for the purpose [of] their control and containment".[63]

Harvesting bodies: the exploitation of Nazi victims' body parts in anatomy and histology

In November 1942, Heinrich Gross (1915–2005) presented to the Viennese Biological Society a case study on Günther Pernegger (1941–1942), who had been born with malformations and had died (allegedly from pneumonia, but in all likelihood from poison) at the Spiegelgrund "euthanasia"clinic in January 1942 at the age of 14 weeks. Gross, who was personally responsible for many of the children's deaths at Spiegelgrund, performed the post-mortem examinations at Vienna University's Anatomical Institute, jointly with the anatomist Wilhelm Wirtinger (1893–1945).[64] Gross also used this case for a publication in 1953, the first of a long list of works on specimens from nearly 800 "child euthanasia" victims.[65] Records from the Spiegelgrund and the Steinhof psychiatric hospital – where approximately 3,500 patients fell victim to what is known as "decentralised euthanasia" – indicate that altogether brain specimens from up to 114 potential euthanasia victims were delivered to the Anatomical Institute.[66]

Victims' body parts were also at the heart of the affair concerning Eduard Pernkopf's famous anatomical atlas, published in several volumes between 1937 and 1960.[67] Pernkopf (1888–1955), head of the institute from 1933, was an ardent follower of National Socialism and became dean of the Faculty of Medicine in 1938 and Rector of Vienna University in 1943. Although he was dismissed in 1945, he nevertheless was able to continue his work using the university's resources. His atlas was regarded as a masterpiece by the international medical community and used in many countries for teaching and studying anatomy. From the 1980s onwards, however, various authors voiced their suspicion that body parts from Nazi victims had been used for the atlas' drawings. Only in 1996, in the face of increasing international pressure, did the university commission an investigation into accusations about the origins of some of the source materials for the illustrations.

In 1998, the commission issued a report of more than 500 pages that unfortunately was never officially published and remains difficult to obtain.[68] Despite its limited mandate, the results of the commission were shocking enough. Nearly 4,000 unclaimed bodies had been obtained by the Anatomical Institute during the Nazi period. More disturbingly, the institute had systematically sought – and obtained – the dead bodies of people executed by the regime, all in all 1,377 individuals. This represents more than a third of the currently known deliveries of bodies of executed victims to anatomical institutes in Nazi Germany.[69] They were not only used for Pernkopf's atlas, but also for other research projects carried out during these years. Furthermore, specimens from the Nazi period were in all likelihood used in the university's teaching long after the war, and not only at the Institute of Anatomy. Among 71 institutes and clinics belonging to the Faculty of Medicine, five warranted closer scrutiny because they had problematic specimens in their collections: the Institutes of Histology and Embryology, Forensic Medicine, Neurology, History of Medicine, and the Anatomical Museum.[70] At the Institute of Histology and

Embryology, about 100 wet specimens of executed persons were found, with inscriptions that explicitly mentioned the way the involuntary donors had died: "spleen, 22-year-old executed female, February 1943" was one of many similar captions, "musculus rectus abdominis, 23-year-old executed male, May 1944" another. It seems that personnel from the institute were present at the executions and immediately afterwards removed the human tissue they wanted.[71]

One concrete result of the commission's work was the burial of all human remains from the Nazi period that remained in the university's various institutes and clinics. Unfortunately, the commission decided not to publish, the names of the victims for reasons of data protection, although they were able to obtain them. Identifying victims by their names is a precondition for individual recognition and memory.[72] While the question of human remains from the Nazi period was dealt with in a thorough fashion by the commission, there were no further attempts to dig deeper into the question of human experiments and the coerced research carried out during the war at Vienna University and its possible implications for medical ethics in post-war Austria.

"Euthanasia" crimes, brain research and the Neurological Institute

Little is known about the activities of the Vienna Neurological Institute (not to be confused with the Psychiatric-Neurological Clinic under Otto Pötzl, see above) during the war. Between 1942 and 1944, among its lecturers was Hans Bertha (1901–1964), one of the psychiatric "experts" responsible for selecting patients for the gas chambers of "action T4" and later director of the Vienna Steinhof hospital.[73] Bertha had a research interest in epileptic dementia. According to Georg Renno, one of the physicians employed at the Hartheim extermination centre (where close to 30,000 people were killed), Bertha visited the institution several times to receive specimens from "euthanasia" victims that had been preserved for him.[74]

While the fate of these body parts is unknown, in 1998 it emerged that in the 1950s, Heinrich Gross gave a considerable number of victims' tissue samples (including entire brains) to the Neurological Institute. Some of these samples were kept as part of the institute's collections until the official burial of the Spiegelgrund victims' remains in 2002.[75] These contacts resulted in publications co-authored by Gross and the institute's successive directors, Hans Hoff (1897–1969), and Franz Seitelberger (1916–2007), as well as by other researchers at the institute. Specimens were also given to the Max-Planck Institute for Brain Research, at the time in Gießen, where Julius Hallervorden was departmental head, resulting in further publications.[76]

Stories untold: grey areas and open questions

As the previous sections of this chapter illustrate, our knowledge about clinical and experimental research practices at the Vienna Faculty of Medicine (and its General Hospital) is currently limited to anecdotal evidence on a relatively small number of clinics or institutes. Relatively well-researched issues such as the scientific exploitation of the Spiegelgrund victims coexist with whole clinics and institutes about which we know next to nothing. There are several clinics not mentioned in this chapter due to limited space, but also to gaps in the scholarship. These include, but are not limited to, the II. Surgical Clinic under the direction of Wolfgang Denk (1882–1970), who was involved in testing a blood coagulant on the initiative of Sigmund Rascher at Dachau,[77] the Pharmacological Institute, which was involved in the planning of sterilisation experiments at the Roma camp Lackenbach,[78] the Institute of Pathology, where tissue samples from vaccination experiments at Mauthausen concentration camp were examined,[79] the Institute of Hygiene, where a dissertation was submitted on the health status of forced labourers,[80] and the II. Gynaecological Clinic, where forced sterilisations were performed on female patients, and pregnant forced labourers were forced into abortions or used as a teaching opportunity for students.[81]

The state of research is even more limited when it comes to Austria's two other medical faculties in Graz and Innsbruck, and if we take into account the time periods prior to 1938 and after 1945. While some of the most egregious examples of abusive research practices were clearly tied to opportunities specific to the Nazi regime (research on concentration camp inmates or victims of "euthanasia"), the possibility of unethical research outside of this time frame should not be ignored. Even if in many cases it may prove impossible to establish with certainty whether certain experiments on patients who may or may not have been informed about the risks involved and who may or may not have given their consent crossed the boundary between ethical and unethical research, a thorough investigation of these questions covering the nineteenth and twentieth centuries is long overdue.

Notes

1   The author wishes to thank Jan Tuczek for help with archival research, Colin Phillips for proofreading and Lilian Dombrowski for translating parts of this chapter. The Vienna Medical School was part of Vienna University as the Vienna Medical Faculty until it became an independent institution in 2004.

2   Michael Hubenstorf, 'Medizinische Fakultät 1938–1945', in Gernot Heiß, Siegfried Mattl, Sebastian Meissl et al. (eds), *Willfährige Wissenschaft. Die Universität Wien 1938–1945*, Vienna: Verlag für Gesellschaftskritik, 1989, p. 236; Michael Hubenstorf, ' "Der Wahrheit ins Auge sehen". Die Wiener Medizin und der Nationalsozialismus/50 Jahre danach (Teil 1)', *Wiener Arzt*, 4 (1995), p. 16.

3   On the history of the Vienna Faculty of Medicine during the Nazi period, see Hubenstorf, 'Medizinische Fakultät'; idem, 'Ende einer Tradition und Fortsetzung als Provinz. Die Medizinischen Fakultäten der Universitäten Berlin und Wien 1925–1950', in Christoph Meinel and Peter Voswinckel (eds), *Medizin, Naturwissenschaft, Technik und Nationalsozialismus. Kontinuitäten und Diskontinuitäten*, Stuttgart: 1994, pp. 33–53; further literature is quoted below.

4   Gustav Spann (ed.), *Untersuchungen zur anatomischen Wissenschaft in Wien 1938–1945. Senatsprojekt der Universität Wien*, Vienna: Akademischer Senat der Univ. Wien, 1998. See also Peter Malina, 'Eduard Pernkopf's atlas of anatomy or: The fiction of "pure

science"', *Wiener klinische Wochenschrift*, 110 (1998), pp. 193–201, and Michael Hubenstorf, 'Anatomical science in Vienna, 1938–45', *The Lancet*, 356 (2000), pp. 1385–1386. For more details on the Pernkopf affair, see below.

5 It is not necessary to go into the details of the seawater experiments here, since they are one of the best-known episodes of Nazi medical crimes – see, most recently, Paul Weindling, *Victims and Survivors of Nazi Human Experiments. Science and Suffering in the Holocaust*, London: Bloomsbury, 2015, pp. 132–135. Weindling, '"Unser eigener, österreichischer Weg": Die Meerwasser-Trinkexperimente in Dachau 1944', Herwig Czech and Weindling (eds), *DOEW Jahrbuch*, (2017), pp. 133–177.

6 Josef Tschofenig, 'Affidavit concerning the seawater experiments', 7.2.1946, NMT 01. Medical Case – USA v. Karl Brandt, *et al.*, English Transcript: p. 501 (16 Dec 1946) [http://nuremberg.law.harvard.edu, retrieved 23.5.2016]; Vienna, Documentation Centre of the Austrian Resistance (hereafter DÖW), 22848.

7 Anonymous, 'Selbstmord Professor Eppingers', *Neues Österreich* (27 Sept 1946), p. 2.

8 Ingrid Arias, *Die Wiener Gerichtsmedizin im Nationalsozialismus*, Vienna: Verlagshaus der Ärzte, 2009, pp. 110–111. Walter Stüwert, *Die Sulfonanilamidwirkungen an Gesunden und Gonorrhoekranken in Bezug auf Höhenfestigkeit*, MD thesis, Vienna: University of Vienna, 1942, p. 7. For more details on the case of Bruno Lüdke, see the section on the Institute of Forensic Medicine.

9 Falko Lainer, 'Zur Frage der Infektiosität des Ikterus', *Wiener klinische Wochenschrift*, 53 (1940), pp. 601–604.

10 Heinz Dinkloh, *Über die Salzausscheidung während der Insulinhypoglycämie*, MD thesis, Vienna: University of Vienna, 1941.

11 Helmut Haid, *Das Verhalten des Vitamin C im Insulinschock*, MD thesis, Vienna: University of Vienna, 1943. See also Thomas Dudenbostel, *Medizinische Doktorarbeiten und National-sozialismus. Ideologie und Ärzteausbildung an der Universität Wien*, Master's thesis, Bielefeld: Bielefeld University, 2013, pp. 66–67.

12 Wilhelm Beiglböck, 'Insulinschockbehandlung des Ulkus. Bemerkung zur Arbeit von Dr. med. habil. M. Gülzow', *Deutsche medizinische Wochenschrift*, 68 (1942), pp. 71–72. The mentioned cooperation on hypoglycaemia between the two clinics began in 1936, see Wilhelm Beiglböck and Karl Theo Dussik, 'Zur Physiologie des hypoglykämischen Schocks bei der Behandlung der Schizophrenie', in Anonymous (ed.), *Die Therapie der Schizophrenie. Insulinschock – Cardiazol – Dauerschlaf. Bericht über die wissenschaftlichen Verhandlungen auf der 89. Versammlung der Schweizerischen Gesellschaft für Psychiatrie in Münsingen bei Bern am 29–31 Mai 1937*, Zürich: Art. Institut Orell Füssli, 1937, p. 39. Wilhelm Beiglböck and L. M. Grisoni, 'Über das Verhalten der Lactoflavinausscheidung im Harn nach großen Insulindosen', *Wiener Archiv für innere Medizin*, 34 (1940), pp. 109–118 reports on another series of hypoglycaemia experiments, involving nine test subjects. E. Albrich and Wilhelm Beiglböck, 'Die biologische und therapeutische Wirkung des Lactoflavin', *Wiener Archiv für innere Medizin*, 34 (1940), p. 157, probably refers to the same experiments. Insulin shock therapy had been developed in Vienna by Manfred Sakel (1900–57) and was first presented to an audience of specialists in 1933: Manfred Sakel, 'Neue Behandlungsart Schizophreniker und verwirrter Erregter (O. Pötzl)', *Wiener klinische Wochenschrift*, 46 (1933), p. 1372.

13 La Courneuve, The Diplomatic Archive Center of the Ministry of Foreign and European Affairs, AUT 2590, Sécurité Militaire/Poste de Vienne, Renseignements sur Dr. Eppinger, 25 June 1946. Reliability of the information (resp. of the informant) was graded C/3, in the middle of the scale.

14 Anonymous, 'Selbstmord Professor Eppingers'.

15 Michael Hubenstorf, 'Pädiatrische Emigration und die "Hamburger-Klinik" 1930–1945', in Kurt Widhalm and Arnold Pollak (eds), *90 Jahre Universitäts-Kinderklinik am AKH in Wien. Umfassende Geschichte der Wiener Pädiatrie*, Vienna: Literas Universitätsverlag, 2005, p. 98.

16 Franz Hamburger and Richard Priesel, *Kinderheilkunde. Lehrbuch für Ärzte und Studenten*, IV, Vienna: Franz Deuticke, 1940, p. 4.

17 At least 44 of the 789 children who died at Spiegelgrund were transferred from the Paediatric University Clinic. Due to missing documentation, the real number is certainly higher, Herwig Czech, 'Der Spiegelgrund-Komplex. Kinderheilkunde, Heilpädagogik, Psychiatrie und Jugendfürsorge im Nationalsozialismus', *Österreichische Zeitschrift für Geschichtswissenschaft*, 2014, p. 203.

18 Ibid., pp. 197 and 201–203.

19 For details on Elmar Türk, see Hubenstorf, *Emigration*.

20 For more details on these experiments, see Herwig Czech, 'Abusive Medical Practices on "Euthanasia" Victims in Austria During and After World War II', in Sheldon Rubenfeld and Susan Benedict (eds), *Human Subjects Research after the Holocaust*, Cham: Springer, 2014, pp. 115–116.

21 Hariklia Dem Kawura, *Beobachtungen der Wärmeregulation der Kinder bei Abkühlung*, MD thesis, Vienna: University of Vienna, 1943.

22 Viktor Koszler, 'Die Beeinflussung des Vakzinationsprozesses durch Prontosil', *Archiv für Kinderheilkunde*, 120 (1940), pp. 113–122.

23 Prontosil, developed in 1934, was the first of the sulfonamides.

24 Anonymous, 'Rundschreiben des Reichsministers des Innern, betr. Richtlinien für neuartige Heilbehandlung und für die Vornahme wissenschaftlicher Versuche am Menschen, vom 28. Februar 1931', *Reichsgesundheitsblatt* 6 (1931), pp. 174–175. On these guidelines, see the chapter by Volker Roelcke in this volume. In the pages of the most important medical journal in Austria, the *Wiener klinische Wochenschrift*, no traces can be found of a discussion on the *Richtlinien* in Austria.

25 Viktor Koszler, 'Pervitindosierung bei Kindern', *Wiener klinische Wochenschrift*, 57 (1944), p. 398.

26 Idem, 'Zur Behandlung des Pemphigus neonatorum und der Dermatitis exfoliativa', *Münchner Medizinische Wochenschrift*, 91 (1944), pp. 74–75.

27 Elmar Türk, 'Zur oralen Stoßanwendung des Vitamin D', *Archiv für Kinderheilkunde*, 121 (1940), pp. 33–46.

28 Idem, 'Zur intramuskulären Stoßanwendung des Vitamin D', *Archiv für Kinderheilkunde*, 121 (1940), p. 51.

29 Ibid., p. 43. Türk had already started experiments with vitamin D in 1937 and until 1942, by his own account, had performed them on more than 100 children. It was the topic of his habilitation dissertation, Elmar Türk, 'Vitamin-D-Stoß-Studien', *Archiv für Kinderheilkunde*, 125 (1942), p. 1.

30 Idem, 'Untersuchungen über "Staphylotoxin"-Reaktionen bei Kindern', *Zeitschrift für Immunitätsforschung und experimentelle Therapie*, 100 (1941), pp. 209–213 and 227.

31 Heribert Goll, 'Zur Frage: Vitamin A und Keratomalazie beim Säugling', *Münchner Medizinische Wochenschrift*, 88 (1941), p. 1212.

32 Vienna, Municipal and Provincial Archives of Vienna (hereafter WStLA), 1.3.2.209.1.A46, Kinderklinik: Krankengeschichten, 255/1941, Anna Mick.

33 Heribert Goll and L. Fuchs, 'Über die Vitamin A-Reserven des Säuglings', *Münchner Medizinische Wochenschrift*, 89 (1942), pp. 397–398. A detailed study of these experiments, including the background and fate of the victims, cannot be provided here and must be deferred to a future publication.

34 Arias, *Wiener Gerichtsmedizin*.

35 Ibid., pp. 43–44; Claudia Spring, *Zwischen Krieg und Euthanasie: Zwangssterilisationen in Wien 1940–1945*, Vienna: Böhlau, 2009, pp. 84, 136, 168 and 226.

36 Ibid., pp. 14–21, 56–59 and 83–85.

37 Strughold (1898–1986) participated in a 1942 conference where results of deadly experiments in Dachau were reported, see Weindling, *Victims*, pp. 84 and 116. After the war, he was never accused of any wrongdoing and emigrated to the US in 1947, where he became the founding father of space medicine: Ernst Klee, *Das Personenlexikon*

zum Dritten Reich. Wer war was vor und nach 1945, Frankfurt am Main: Fischer Taschenbuch Verlag, 2005. On the medical dissertations submitted in Vienna during the Nazi period, see Dudenbostel, *Doktorarbeiten*.

38 Helmut Bauereiß, *Infektionskrankheiten und Höhenfestigkeit unter besonderer Berücksichtigung der Gonorrhoe*, MD thesis, Vienna: University of Vienna, 1942.

39 Bauereiß, *Infektionskrankheiten*, p. 3.

40 Stüwert, *Sulfonanilamidwirkungen*. On the dissertations by Bauereiß and Stüwert see also: Dudenbostel, *Doktorarbeiten*, pp. 65–66 and Arias, *Wiener Gerichtsmedizin*, pp. 70–75.

41 Ibid., pp. 86–114. Nebe's plan to test poisoned bullets on Lüdke was in all likelihood dropped because of Schneider's opposition, see ibid., pp. 106–107. For the low-pressure chamber, see the section on Eppinger's clinic in this chapter.

42 WStLA, 1.3.2.212.A7–7, 152.31, Abt. Erb- und Rassenpflege, "Durchführung des GzVeN", 24 July 1940; Michael Hubenstorf, 'Urologie und Nationalsozialismus in Österreich', in Matthis Krischel, Friedrich Moll, Julia Bellmann *et al.* (eds), *Urologen im Nationalsozialismus, Bd. 1: Zwischen Anpassung und Vertreibung*, Berlin: Hentrich & Hentrich, 2011, p. 161.

43 Although the Allied Denazification Bureau unanimously recommended Schönbauer's dismissal due to his former ties to the Nazi regime and his participation in forced sterilisations, see College Park, MD, National Archives and Records Administration, RG 260, 2077, Box 11, Allied Denazification Bureau to Chairman, Internal Affairs Directorate, 10 Feb 1947, he retained his positions as clinic chief and (since 1945) director of the General Hospital. He became one of the most prominent figures in Austrian medicine, see Ingrid Arias, 'Die medizinische Fakultät von 1945 bis 1955: Provinzialisierung oder Anschluss an die westliche Wissenschaft?', in Margarete Grandner, Gernot Heiß and Oliver Rathkolb (eds), *Zukunft mit Altlasten. Die Universität Wien 1945–1955*, Innsbruck: 2005, pp. 76–77.

44 Wolfram Sorgo, 'Beobachtungen über die Wirkung intrakranieller Gefäßunterbindung auf den peripheren Kreislauf', *Zeitschrift für die gesamte Neurologie und Psychiatrie*, 174 (1942), pp. 325–326. At Schönbauer's Clinic, brain surgery was performed almost exclusively under local anaesthesia, see Leopold Schönbauer, 'Zehn Jahre neurochirurgische Erfahrung', *Wiener klinische Wochenschrift*, 53 (1940), p. 834.

45 Wolfram Sorgo, 'Über den Wert und die Gefahren der Lumbalpunktion beim raumbeengenden Prozess des Schädelinnern', *Wiener klinische Wochenschrift*, 53 (1940), pp. 231–233. There is no information as to when exactly he examined these 365 cases.

46 On the post-war period, see Ingrid Arias, 'Hans Hoff (1897–1969) – Remigrant und Reformer? Neue Impulse oder Kontinuität in der Psychiatrie nach 1945?', *Virus – Beiträge zur Sozialgeschichte der Medizin*, 14 (2016), pp. 177–190; Eberhard Gabriel, 'Zum Wiederaufbau des akademischen Lehrkörpers in der Psychiatrie in Wien nach 1945', *Virus – Beiträge zur Sozialgeschichte der Medizin,* 14 (2016), pp. 35–77.

47 The clinic's head Otto Pötzl participated in a considerable proportion of all sterilisation procedures in Vienna: Spring, *Krieg*, pp. 132–133 and 200. On the (later famous) assistant Walther Birkmayer, including his scholarly support of forced sterilisation, see Herwig Czech and Lawrence A. Zeidman, 'Walther Birkmayer: The man behind L-Dopa and his ties to National Socialism', *Journal of the History of the Neurosciences*, 23 (2014), p. 169.

48 For an overview on the carrying out of the Nazi "euthanasia" programmes in Austria, see Herwig Czech, 'Nazi "Euthanasia" crimes in World War II Austria', *The Holocaust in History and Memory*, 5 (2012), pp. 51–73.

49 Fritz Redlich emigrated to the United States in 1938 where he had an impressive career as a psychiatrist. In 1967, he became dean of the Yale School of Medicine, Czech and Zeidman, *Birkmayer*, p. 170.

50 The collaboration between the Psychiatric-Neurological Clinic and Hans Eppinger's Clinic of Internal Medicine on insulin-induced comas is described above.

51 Berlin, German Federal Archives Berlin (hereafter BAB), R 96 I-12, Elektroschock-apparat "Elkra I" and "Elkra II" (Advertising brochures, ca. 1944).

52 BAB, R 96 I-12, Reichsbeauftragter Heil- und Pflegeanstalten Linden to Landes-regierungen, 24 Aug 1942.

53 BAB., R 96 I-18, Paul Nitsche to Wolfgang Holzer, 21 Sept 1944.

54 BAB, R 96 I-18, W. Holzer, 'Vorschlag zur Gründung einer Forschungsanstalt für aktive Therapie der Nerven- und Geisteskrankheiten', dated Sept 1944.

55 For a detailed account of Gelny's crimes in Gugging and Mauer-Öhling, see Herwig Czech, 'From "Action T4" to "decentralized euthanasia" in Lower Austria: The psychiatric hospitals at Gugging, Mauer-Öhling and Ybbs' (2016), [www.memorial gugging.at].

56 DÖW, 18860/82, Vernehmung Wolfgang Holzer, 23 Aug 1946.

57 Wolfgang Damus, *Der Selbstmord unter besonderer Berücksichtigung der Juden*, MD thesis, Vienna: University of Vienna, 1942, pp. 32, 54–55, 65 and 67.

58 Rektorat der Universität Wien (ed.), *Öffentliche Vorlesungen an der Universität Wien. Sommersemester 1939*, Vienna: Adolf Holzhausens Nachfolger, 1939, pp. 15–19.

59 Idem (ed.), *Personal- und Vorlesungsverzeichnis für das Wintersemester 1943/44*, Vienna: Adolf Holzhausens Nachfolger, 1943, p. 138.

60 Vienna, Austrian State Archive (ÖStA), AdR, Kurator der wissenschaftlichen Hochschulen, box 22, 'Denkschrift über die Errichtung eines Rassenbiologischen Instituts an der Universität Wien', Nov 1938. A first version exists from May 1938. On the Vienna Institute of Race Biology, see in greater detail Thomas Mayer, *Das Rassenbiologische Institut der Universität Wien 1938–1945*, PhD thesis, Vienna: University of Vienna, 2015.

61 Vienna, Vienna University Archives (hereafter AdUW), Rektoratsakten, 755 ex 1938/39.

62 Wentzler an Reichsausschuss, 17 Oct 1942, reproduced in: Götz Aly (ed.), *Aktion T4 1939–1945. Die "Euthanasie"-Zentrale in der Tiergartenstraße 4*, Berlin: Edition Hentrich, 1987, pp. 134–135.

63 AdUW, Rektoratsakten, 755 ex 1938/39, Löffler to Kriegswirtschaftsstelle im Reichsforschungsrat, 17 Feb 1943.

64 The case history was published two years later as Heinrich Gross, 'Ein Fall von Akrocephalosyndaktylie', *Wiener klinische Wochenschrift*, 57 (1944), p. 493.

65 Heinrich Gross, 'Zur Morphologie des Schädels bei der Acrocephalosyndaktylie', *Morphologisches Jahrbuch*, 92 (1953), pp. 350–372. On the post-war career of Heinrich Gross, see Czech, *Practices*, pp. 116–120.

66 WStLA, 1.3.2.209.10.B4, Wiener städtische Nervenklinik für Kinder, Totenbuch; WStLA, 1.3.2.209.2.B1001 (prov.), Otto-Wagner-Spital der Stadt Wien, Sektions-protokolle der Jahre 1940 bis 1945.

67 Eduard Pernkopf, *Topographische Anatomie des Menschen, Band 1 bis 4*, Berlin: Urban und Schwarzenberg, 1937–60.

68 Spann, *Untersuchungen*. For an overview of the findings, see William E. Seidelman and H. Israel, 'Nazi Origins of an Anatomy Text: The Pernkopf Atlas', *JAMA*, 276 (1997), p. 1633; Malina, *Pernkopf*. The Anatomical Institutes in Graz and Innsbruck evaded scrutiny at the time, although it is now clear that they also received specimens from executed prisoners, albeit on a smaller scale than in Vienna, see Herwig Czech, 'Von der Richtstätte auf den Seziertisch. Zur anatomischen Verwertung von NS-Opfern in Wien, Innsbruck und Graz', *Jahrbuch des Dokumentationsarchivs des österreichischen Widerstandes*, 1 (2015), pp. 141–190.

69 Sabine Hildebrandt, *The Anatomy of Murder. Ethical Transgressions and Anatomical Science during the Third Reich*, New York and Oxford: Berghahn, 2016, p. 189. In contrast, there were only seven voluntary body donations during the same period: Daniela Angetter, 'Untersuchungen zur Anlieferung und Bestattung der Studienleichen des

Anatomischen Instituts 1938–1946', in Spann, *Untersuchungen*, p. 69. Among the executed prisoners used for teaching and research at the Anatomical Institute, eight were Jewish: Peter Schwarz, 'NS-Justiz, Todesstrafe und Hinrichtung am Landesgericht Wien unter besonderer Berücksichtigung der zum Tode verurteilten jüdischen Opfer', in Spann, *Untersuchungen*, pp. 117–141.

70 Karl Holubar and Daniela Angetter, 'Überprüfung der medizinischen Institute und Kliniken der Universität Wien', in Spann, *Untersuchungen*, p. 264.

71 Daniela Angetter, 'Überprüfung des Histologisch-Embryologischen Instituts, Schwarzspanierstraße 17, 1090 Wien', in Spann, *Untersuchungen*, pp. 294–296.

72 By way of contrast, compare the meticulous identification of 86 individuals killed for August Hirt's "Jewish skeleton collection" at the *Reichsuniversität Straßburg*: Hans-Joachim Lang, *Die Namen der Nummern. Wie es gelang, die 86 Opfer eines NS-Verbrechens zu identifizieren*, Hamburg: Hoffmann und Campe, 2004.

73 See, for example, Rektorat der Universität Wien (ed.), *Personal- und Vorlesungsverzeichnis für das Sommersemester 1942*, Vienna: Adolf Holzhausens Nachfolger, 1942, p. 174; Peter Schwarz, 'Mord durch Hunger. "Wilde Euthanasie" und "Aktion Brandt" in Steinhof in der NS-Zeit', in Eberhard Gabriel and Wolfgang Neugebauer (eds), *Von der Zwangssterilisierung zur Ermordung. Zur Geschichte der NS-Euthanasie in Wien Teil II*, Vienna: Böhlau, 2002, pp. 113–141.

74 For more details, see Czech, *Practices*, pp. 110–111.

75 Daniela Angetter, 'Überprüfung der Sammlung des Neurologischen Instituts', in Spann, *Untersuchungen*, pp. 266–288; Herwig Czech, 'Forschen ohne Skrupel. Die wissenschaftliche Verwertung von Opfern der NS-Psychiatriemorde in Wien', in Gabriel and Neugebauer, *Von der Zwangssterilisierung zur Ermordung*, pp. 160–163.

76 Czech, *Practices*, pp. 117–118. Also see for more details on the case of Heinrich Gross and his neuropathological research on victims of "child euthanasia" in post-war Austria. Seitelberger became rector of Vienna University in the 1970s despite his Nazi past, which included membership in the SS: BAB, BDC file on Franz Seitelberger; Michael Hubenstorf, 'Tote und/oder lebendige Wissenschaft. Die intellektuellen Netzwerke der NS-Patientenmordaktion in Österreich', in Gabriel and Neugebauer, *Von der Zwangssterilisierung zur Ermordung*, p. 371.

77 Weindling, *Victims*, p. 181.

78 Hubenstorf, *Emigration*, p. 162.

79 Weindling, *Victims*, p. 107.

80 Herwig Czech, 'Zwangsarbeit, Medizin und "Rassenpolitik" in Wien. Ausländische Arbeitskräfte zwischen Ausbeutung und rassistischer Verfolgung', in Andreas Frewer and Günther Siedbürger (eds), *Medizin und Zwangsarbeit im Nationalsozialismus. Einsatz und Behandlung von "Ausländern" im Gesundheitswesen*, Frankfurt am Main and New York: Campus, 2004, p. 257.

81 WStLA, 1.3.2.212.A7–7, 152.31, 'Liste der Krankenanstalten und Ärzte, die zur Durchführung von Unfruchtbarmachungen nach dem Gesetz zur Verhütung erbkranken Nachwuchses ermächtigt sind' (as of Sept 1942).

Bibliography

Archival Sources

Austria

Vienna, Austrian State Archive (ÖStA): AdR, Kurator der wissenschaftlichen Hochschulen

Vienna, Documentation Centre of the Austrian Resistance (DÖW):
18860/82, Vernehmung Wolfgang Holzer, 23 Aug 1946
22848, documents on seawater experiments
Vienna, Municipal and Provincial Archives of Vienna (WStLA):
1.3.2.209, Vienna Anstaltenamt (hospital administration)
1.3.2.212, Vienna Main Public Health Office
1.3.2.209.1.A46, Paediatric Clinic: Medical Records, 1930–75
Vienna, Vienna University Archives (AdUW): Rektoratsakten, 755 aus 1938/39, Rassenbiologisches Institut

France

La Courneuve, The Diplomatic Archive Center of the Ministry of Foreign and European Affairs: AUT 2590, Sécurité Militaire/Poste de Vienne, Renseignements sur Dr. Eppinger, 25 June 1946

Germany

Berlin, German Federal Archives Berlin (BAB):
R 96 I, Reichsbeauftragter Heil- und Pflegeanstalten
BDC file on Franz Seitelberger

USA

Cambridge, MA, Harvard Nuremberg Trials Project: Josef Tschofenig, 'Affidavit concerning the seawater experiments', 7 Feb 1946, NMT 01. Medical Case – USA v. Karl Brandt, *et al.*, English Transcript: p. 501 (16 Dec 1946) [http://nuremberg.law.harvard.edu, retrieved 23.5.2016]
College Park, MD, National Archives and Records Administration (NARA): RG 260, 2077, Box 11, Allied Denazification Bureau to Chairman, Internal Affairs Directorate, 10 Feb 1947

Literature

Anonymous, 'Rundschreiben des Reichsministers des Innern, betr. Richtlinien für neuartige Heilbehandlung und für die Vornahme wissenschaftlicher Versuche am Menschen, vom 28. Februar 1931', *Reichsgesundheitsblatt*, 6 (1931), pp. 174–175
—— 'Selbstmord Professor Eppingers', *Neues Österreich* (27 Sept 1946), p. 2
Albrich, E., and Wilhelm Beiglböck, 'Die biologische und therapeutische Wirkung des Lactoflavin', *Wiener Archiv für innere Medizin*, 34 (1940), pp. 145–164
Aly, Götz (ed.), *Aktion T4 1939–1945. Die "Euthanasie"-Zentrale in der Tiergartenstraße 4*, Berlin: Edition Hentrich, 1987
Angetter, Daniela, 'Überprüfung der Sammlung des Neurologischen Instituts', in Gustav Spann (ed.), *Untersuchungen zur anatomischen Wissenschaft in Wien 1938–1945. Senatsprojekt der Universität Wien*, Vienna: Akademischer Senat der Univ. Wien, 1998, pp. 266–288
—— 'Überprüfung des Histologisch-Embryologischen Instituts, Schwarzspanierstraße 17, 1090 Wien', in Gustav Spann (ed.), *Untersuchungen zur anatomischen Wissenschaft*

in Wien 1938–1945. Senatsprojekt der Universität Wien, Vienna: Akademischer Senat der Univ. Wien, 1998, pp. 292–302

—— 'Untersuchungen zur Anlieferung und Bestattung der Studienleichen des Anatomischen Instituts 1938–1946', in Gustav Spann (ed.), *Untersuchungen zur anatomischen Wissenschaft in Wien 1938–1945. Senatsprojekt der Universität Wien*, Vienna: Akademischer Senat der Univ. Wien, 1998, pp. 67–80

Arias, Ingrid, 'Die medizinische Fakultät von 1945 bis 1955: Provinzialisierung oder Anschluss an die westliche Wissenschaft?', in Margarete Grandner, Gernot Heiß and Oliver Rathkolb (eds), *Zukunft mit Altlasten. Die Universität Wien 1945–1955*, Innsbruck: 2005, pp. 68–88

—— *Die Wiener Gerichtsmedizin im Nationalsozialismus*, Vienna: Verlagshaus der Ärzte, 2009

—— 'Hans Hoff (1897–1969) – Remigrant und Reformer? Neue Impulse oder Kontinuität in der Psychiatrie nach 1945?', *Virus – Beiträge zur Sozialgeschichte der Medizin*, 14 (2016), pp. 177–190

Bauereiß, Helmut, *Infektionskrankheiten und Höhenfestigkeit unter besonderer Berücksichtigung der Gonorrhoe*, MD thesis, Vienna: University of Vienna, 1942

Beiglböck, Wilhelm, 'Insulinschockbehandlung des Ulkus. Bemerkung zur Arbeit von Dr. med. habil. M. Gülzow', *Deutsche medizinische Wochenschrift*, 68 (1942), pp. 71–72

—— and Karl Theo Dussik, 'Zur Physiologie des hypoglykämischen Schocks bei der Behandlung der Schizophrenie', in Anonymous (ed.), *Die Therapie der Schizophrenie. Insulinschock – Cardiazol – Dauerschlaf. Bericht über die wissenschaftlichen Verhandlungen auf der 89. Versammlung der Schweizerischen Gesellschaft für Psychiatrie in Münsingen bei Bern am 29.-31. Mai 1937*, Zürich: Art. Institut Orell Füssli, 1937, pp. 38–44

—— and L.M. Grisoni, 'Über das Verhalten der Lactoflavinausscheidung im Harn nach großen Insulindosen', *Wiener Archiv für innere Medizin*, 34 (1940), pp. 109–118

Czech, Herwig, 'Forschen ohne Skrupel. Die wissenschaftliche Verwertung von Opfern der NS-Psychiatriemorde in Wien', in Eberhard Gabriel and Wolfgang Neugebauer (eds), *Von der Zwangssterilisierung zur Ermordung. Zur Geschichte der NS-Euthanasie in Wien Teil II*, Vienna: Böhlau, 2002, pp. 143–163

—— 'Zwangsarbeit, Medizin und "Rassenpolitik" in Wien. Ausländische Arbeitskräfte zwischen Ausbeutung und rassistischer Verfolgung', in Andreas Frewer and Günther Siedbürger (eds), *Medizin und Zwangsarbeit im Nationalsozialismus. Einsatz und Behandlung von "Ausländern" im Gesundheitswesen*, Frankfurt am Main and New York: Campus, 2004, pp. 253–280

—— 'Nazi "Euthanasia" crimes in World War II Austria', *The Holocaust in History and Memory*, 5 (2012), pp. 51–73

—— 'Abusive Medical Practices on "Euthanasia" Victims in Austria During and After World War II', in Sheldon Rubenfeld and Susan Benedict (eds), *Human Subjects Research after the Holocaust*, Cham: Springer, 2014, pp. 109–125

—— 'Der Spiegelgrund-Komplex. Kinderheilkunde, Heilpädagogik, Psychiatrie und Jugendfürsorge im Nationalsozialismus', *Österreichische Zeitschrift für Geschichtswissenschaft* (2014), pp. 189–214

—— 'Von der Richtstätte auf den Seziertisch. Zur anatomischen Verwertung von NS-Opfern in Wien, Innsbruck und Graz', *Jahrbuch des Dokumentationsarchivs des österreichischen Widerstandes*, 1 (2015), pp. 141–190

—— 'From "Action T4" to "decentralized euthanasia" in Lower Austria: The psychiatric hospitals at Gugging, Mauer-Öhling and Ybbs' (2016), [www.memorial gugging.at]

—— and Lawrence A. Zeidman, 'Walther Birkmayer: The man behind L-Dopa and his ties to National Socialism', *Journal of the History of the Neurosciences*, 23 (2014), pp. 160–191

Damus, Wolfgang, *Der Selbstmord unter besonderer Berücksichtigung der Juden*, MD thesis, Vienna: University of Vienna, 1942

Dinkloh, Heinz, *Über die Salzausscheidung während der Insulinhypoglycämie*, MD thesis, Vienna: University of Vienna, 1941

Dudenbostel, Thomas, *Medizinische Doktorarbeiten und Nationalsozialismus. Ideologie und Ärzteausbildung an der Universität Wien*, Master's thesis, Bielefeld: Bielefeld University, 2013

Gabriel, Eberhard, 'Zum Wiederaufbau des akademischen Lehrkörpers in der Psychiatrie in Wien nach 1945', *Virus – Beiträge zur Sozialgeschichte der Medizin*, 14 (2016), pp. 35–77

Goll, Heribert, 'Zur Frage: Vitamin A und Keratomalazie beim Säugling', *Münchner Medizinische Wochenschrift*, 88 (1941), pp. 1212–1214

—— and L. Fuchs, 'Über die Vitamin A-Reserven des Säuglings', *Münchner Medizinische Wochenschrift*, 89 (1942), pp. 397–400

Gross, Heinrich, 'Ein Fall von Akrocephalosyndaktylie', *Wiener klinische Wochenschrift*, 57 (1944), p. 493

—— 'Zur Morphologie des Schädels bei der Acrocephalosyndaktylie', *Morphologisches Jahrbuch*, 92 (1953), pp. 350–372

Haid, Helmut, *Das Verhalten des Vitamin C im Insulinschock*, MD thesis, Vienna: University of Vienna, 1943

Hamburger, Franz and Richard Priesel, *Kinderheilkunde. Lehrbuch für Ärzte und Studenten*, Vienna: Franz Deuticke, 1940

Hildebrandt, Sabine, *The Anatomy of Murder. Ethical Transgressions and Anatomical Science during the Third Reich*, New York and Oxford: Berghahn, 2016

Holubar, Karl and Daniela Angetter, 'Überprüfung der medizinischen Institute und Kliniken der Universität Wien', in Gustav Spann (ed.), *Untersuchungen zur anatomischen Wissenschaft in Wien 1938–1945. Senatsprojekt der Universität Wien*, Vienna: Akademischer Senat der Univ. Wien, 1998, pp. 261–265

Hubenstorf, Michael, 'Medizinische Fakultät 1938–1945', in Gernot Heiß, Siegfried Mattl, Sebastian Meissl *et al.* (eds), *Willfährige Wissenschaft. Die Universität Wien 1938–1945*, Vienna: Verlag für Gesellschaftskritik, 1989, pp. 233–282

—— 'Ende einer Tradition und Fortsetzung als Provinz. Die Medizinischen Fakultäten der Universitäten Berlin und Wien 1925–1950', in Christoph Meinel and Peter Voswinckel (eds), *Medizin, Naturwissenschaft, Technik und Nationalsozialismus. Kontinuitäten und Diskontinuitäten*, Stuttgart: 1994, pp. 33–53

—— ' "Der Wahrheit ins Auge sehen". Die Wiener Medizin und der Nationalsozialismus/50 Jahre danach (Teil 1)', *Wiener Arzt*, 4 (1995), pp. 14–27

—— 'Anatomical science in Vienna, 1938–45', *The Lancet*, 356 (2000), pp. 1385–1386

—— 'Tote und/oder lebendige Wissenschaft. Die intellektuellen Netzwerke der NS-Patientenmordaktion in Österreich', in Eberhard Gabriel and Wolfgang Neugebauer (eds.), *Von der Zwangssterilisierung zur Ermordung. Zur Geschichte der NS-Euthanasie in Wien Teil II*, Vienna: Böhlau, 2002, pp. 237–420

—— 'Pädiatrische Emigration und die "Hamburger-Klinik" 1930–1945', in Kurt Widhalm and Arnold Pollak (eds), *90 Jahre Universitäts-Kinderklinik am AKH in Wien. Umfassende Geschichte der Wiener Pädiatrie*, Vienna: Literas Universitätsverlag, 2005, pp. 69–220

—— 'Urologie und Nationalsozialismus in Österreich', in Matthis Krischel, Friedrich Moll, Julia Bellmann *et al.* (eds), *Urologen im Nationalsozialismus*, Bd. 1: Zwischen Anpassung und Vertreibung, Berlin: Hentrich & Hentrich, 2011, pp. 139–172

Dem Kawura, Hariklia, *Beobachtungen der Wärmeregulation der Kinder bei Abkühlung*, MD thesis, Vienna: University of Vienna, 1943

Klee, Ernst, *Das Personenlexikon zum Dritten Reich. Wer war was vor und nach 1945*, Frankfurt am Main: Fischer Taschenbuch Verlag, 2005

Koszler, Viktor, 'Die Beeinflussung des Vakzinationsprozesses durch Prontosil', *Archiv für Kinderheilkunde*, 120 (1940), pp. 113–122

—— 'Pervitindosierung bei Kindern', *Wiener klinische Wochenschrift*, 57 (1944), pp. 398–399

—— 'Zur Behandlung des Pemphigus neonatorum und der Dermatitis exfoliativa', *Münchner Medizinische Wochenschrift*, 91 (1944), pp. 74–75

Lang, Hans-Joachim, *Die Namen der Nummern. Wie es gelang, die 86 Opfer eines NS-Verbrechens zu identifizieren*, Hamburg: Hoffmann und Campe, 2004

Malina, Peter, 'Eduard Pernkopf's atlas of anatomy or: The fiction of "pure science"', *Wiener klinische Wochenschrift*, 110 (1998), pp. 193–201

Mayer, Thomas, *Das Rassenbiologische Institut der Universität Wien 1938–1945*, PhD thesis, Vienna: University of Vienna, 2015

Pernkopf, Eduard, *Topographische Anatomie des Menschen*, Band 1 bis 4, Berlin: Urban und Schwarzenberg, 1937–1960

Rektorat der Universität Wien (ed.), *Öffentliche Vorlesungen an der Universität Wien. Sommersemester 1939*, Vienna: Adolf Holzhausens Nachfolger, 1939

—— *Personal- und Vorlesungsverzeichnis für das Sommersemester 1942*, Vienna: Adolf Holzhausens Nachfolger, 1942

—— *Personal- und Vorlesungsverzeichnis für das Wintersemester 1943/44*, Vienna: Adolf Holzhausens Nachfolger, 1943

Sakel, Manfred, 'Neue Behandlungsart Schizophreniker und verwirrter Erregter (O. Pötzl)', *Wiener klinische Wochenschrift*, 46 (1933), p. 1372

Schönbauer, Leopold, 'Zehn Jahre neurochirurgische Erfahrung', *Wiener klinische Wochenschrift*, 53 (1940), pp. 831–835

Schwarz, Peter, 'NS-Justiz, Todesstrafe und Hinrichtung am Landesgericht Wien unter besonderer Berücksichtigung der zum Tode verurteilten jüdischen Opfer', in Gustav Spann (ed.), *Untersuchungen zur anatomischen Wissenschaft in Wien 1938–1945. Senatsprojekt der Universität Wien*, Vienna: Akademischer Senat der Univ. Wien, 1998, pp. 93–145

—— 'Mord durch Hunger. "Wilde Euthanasie" und "Aktion Brandt" in Steinhof in der NS-Zeit', in Eberhard Gabriel and Wolfgang Neugebauer (eds), *Von der Zwangssterilisierung zur Ermordung. Zur Geschichte der NS-Euthanasie in Wien Teil II*, Vienna: Böhlau, 2002, pp. 113–141

Seidelman, William E. and H. Israel, 'Nazi Origins of an Anatomy Text: The Pernkopf Atlas', *JAMA*, 276 (1997), p. 1633

Sorgo, Wolfram, 'Über den Wert und die Gefahren der Lumbalpunktion beim raumbeengenden Prozess des Schädelinnern', *Wiener klinische Wochenschrift*, 53 (1940), pp. 231–233

—— 'Beobachtungen über die Wirkung intrakranieller Gefäßunterbindung auf den peripheren Kreislauf', *Zeitschrift für die gesamte Neurologie und Psychiatrie*, 174 (1942), pp. 325–326

Spann, Gustav (ed.), *Untersuchungen zur anatomischen Wissenschaft in Wien 1938–1945. Senatsprojekt der Universität Wien*, Vienna, Akademischer Senat der Univ. Wien: 1998

Spring, Claudia, *Zwischen Krieg und Euthanasie: Zwangssterilisationen in Wien 1940–1945*, Vienna: Böhlau, 2009

Stüwert, Walter, *Die Sulfonanilamidwirkungen an Gesunden und Gonorrhoekranken in Bezug auf Höhenfestigkeit*, MD thesis, Vienna: University of Vienna, 1942

Türk, Elmar, 'Zur intramuskulären Stoßanwendung des Vitamin D', *Archiv für Kinderheilkunde*, 121 (1940), pp. 46–52

—— 'Zur oralen Stoßanwendung des Vitamin D', *Archiv für Kinderheilkunde*, 121 (1940), pp. 33–46

—— 'Untersuchungen über "Staphylotoxin"-Reaktionen bei Kindern', *Zeitschrift für Immunitätsforschung und experimentelle Therapie*, 100 (1941), pp. 198–236

—— 'Vitamin-D-Stoß-Studien', *Archiv für Kinderheilkunde*, 125 (1942), pp. 1–31

Weindling, Paul, *Victims and Survivors of Nazi Human Experiments. Science and Suffering in the Holocaust*, London: Bloomsbury, 2015

8   Murdering the sick in the name of progress?

The Heidelberg psychiatrist Carl Schneider as a brain researcher and "therapeutic idealist"[1]

Maike Rotzoll and Gerrit Hohendorf

Among the psychiatrists of the Nazi era, Carl Schneider (1891–1946), professor of psychiatry in Heidelberg in the years from 1933 to 1945, must be regarded as one of the outstanding perpetrators who committed crimes against humanity (Figure 8.1). Schneider combined political activities in psychiatry and research with his engagement for the first systematic extermination of a minority group of people under National Socialism, the murder of psychiatric patients. In the history of psychiatry, Schneider appears as an ambivalent, Janus-headed figure. For Werner Janzarik (born 1920), the professor of psychiatry in Heidelberg in the 1970s and 1980s, he was a "petit bourgeois sort of scholar, uncertain in matters of good taste, and occasionally capable of immense faux pas", full of an "uncritical sense of mission".[2] The social psychiatrist Klaus Dörner (born 1933) characterised him in 1986 as a "brilliant therapist, a modern ecological systemic theorist and a euthanasia murderer". He asked how it could be possible for "one and the same person, who was, in addition, a believing Christian, to write in 1939 this theoretically progressive, amazingly helpful and humane book, *Behandlung und Verhütung der Geisteskrankeiten* (Treatment and Prevention of Mental Illnesses),[3] and, at the same time, to be a part of the closest circle of those who planned, and organised the mass murder of psychiatric patients and profited from this?"[4]

For the American psychiatrist Robert Jay Lifton (born 1926), Schneider was a psychiatric idealist: "Despite all the conflicts that he may have experienced, he was able to combine his unusual sympathy for psychiatric patients with the National Socialist biomedical vision and its humane claim to end suffering and strengthen the race".[5] But did Carl Schneider, perceived in such contradictory ways in historical judgment, really combine such incompatible views in one person?

Leipzig, Arnsdorf, Bethel: the beginning of a psychiatric career

Schneider grew up in straitened circumstances, but he was able to attend Saxony's elite school at Grimma and complete the *Abitur* (school leaving

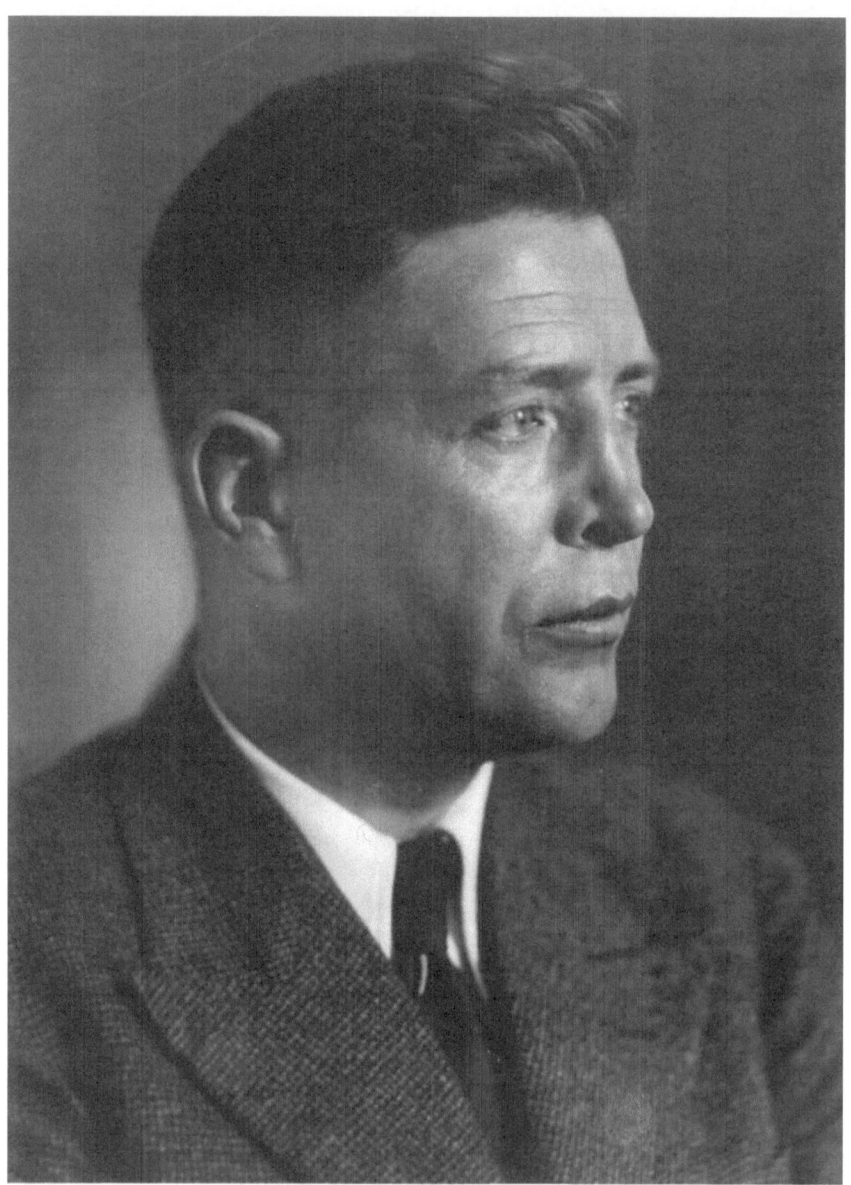

Figure 8.1 Carl Schneider

Source: Heidelberg, University Archives

certificate) there in 1911. Like many of his generation, his outlook was shaped by participation in the First World War.[6] After a period as an intern at the Neurological and Psychiatric Hospital of the University of Leipzig, under Paul Flechsig (1847–1929) and Oswald Bumke (1877–1950), Schneider went to the Saxon psychiatric asylum at Arnsdorf, where he became *Regierungsmedizinalrat* (government counsellor for medicine, a type of senior civil servant in the administration), and where he stayed until he was made Chief Physician at the Bodelschwingh Institutions at Bethel in 1930. During this period, there was an interruption in the form of a research sabbatical at the German Research Institute for Psychiatry in Munich in 1926. During the 1920s, Schneider published a number of well-received scientific works, among others on the psychology of schizophrenia.[7] In 1930, together with Paul Nitsche (1876–1948), the director of the Saxon asylum Sonnenstein, Schneider wrote the accompanying text for the psychiatric section of the hygiene exhibition in Dresden. The authors pleaded for "a comprehensively qualitative population policy that is conscious of its goals" (*eine zielbewußte und umfassende qualitative Bevölkerungspolitik*), in the sense of a "racial hygienic arrangement" of the entire economic and legal system.[8]

"A new era with new people": The national community (*Volksgemeinschaft*) and forced sterilisation

Schneider joined the NSDAP in 1932. In 1931 he was still very reserved towards the idea of sterilisation motivated by "racial hygiene", as evidenced by his position at the Symposium on Eugenics of the "Central Committee for the Internal Mission" at Treysa. However, he justified the compulsory sterilisation law passed in July 1933, "Law for the Prevention of Hereditarily Diseased Offspring", by stating that it was a "responsible attempt before God to give a new era new people".[9] Schneider saw the "moral justification" for forced sterilisation in the thinking which was founded on the Nazi concept of the "national community" (*Volksgemeinschaft*), namely that the new state could only survive in a "living community ethos of the persons belonging to the state" (*lebendig gestaltete Gesinnungsgemeinschaft der Staatsangehörigen*). The sick were not "able" enough to live in such a "community ethos". The state, in consequence, had "a right to require that only such offspring should survive, who are worthy of this living community".[10] This "communal thinking" of Schneider, which would identify all the sick, "inferior" and "abnormal", became the guideline for his psychiatric and therapeutic practice.

"Treatment and prevention": the redesign of the psychiatric clinic at Heidelberg

In November 1933, Schneider became the successor to Karl Wilmanns (1883–1945), who had been removed from office for political reasons, in the chair at Heidelberg. As far as is known, the call to the chair was not only made for reasons of party politics, but also because it corresponded to Schneider's scientific qualifications. He was not habilitated, i.e. qualified as a professor in Germany, but had proven himself to be particularly qualified in the area of schizophrenia research. In reforming the university hospital in the sense of the "new era", Schneider set three main goals. He consistently carried out the "Law for the Prevention of Hereditarily Diseased Offspring", that is to say sterilisations. In accordance with contemporary research on heredity, he carried out field research in hereditary biology in small communities in the Odenwald, a hilly region east of Heidelberg. His main area, however, was reforming the hospital in the sense of work therapy. With work therapy, Schneider wanted not only to achieve an orderly everyday course in the hospital in the sense of discipline; at the same time, he understood this as a type of therapy that intervened in, and influenced, the psychic, bodily and physiological regulatory course of the patient so as to create a "biological" therapeutic effect. Those involved, even in the most acute stages, would be torn out of their diseased forms of experience and pushed into the orderly environment of work. The background to this therapeutic and rehabilitative claim was, of course, the compulsion to adapt to a community life which Schneider saw as being essentially determined by work and productive performance.[11] Schneider's comprehensive concept of biology formed the ideological framework. "If we have read all the signs aright", began Schneider's introductory chapter of his textbook, *The Treatment and Prevention of Mental Illnesses*, "then the doctrine of mental illnesses is at a significant stage on its way to becoming a truly exact natural science".[12] He held that "a biological understanding of psychiatric facts" must be applied, which also implied the treatment of human and social relations as something biological. "Pathological art", however, did not belong among the influences "worthy of furthering" as far as Schneider was concerned. He prohibited his patients from any artistic activity. Consequently, he provided works of art from what is now known worldwide as the Prinzhorn collection, works which had been produced only a few years before, for the touring exhibition "Degenerate Art" (*Entartete Kunst*).[13]

But what happened to the patients at the Heidelberg university hospital, who proved themselves incurable as far as Schneider's therapies were concerned (from 1939 these included insulin therapy, and later electroshock therapy)? When the conclusion was reached that they could not simply be released, they were observed for a period, then transferred to asylums and nursing homes, and left to their potentially deadly fates.[14]

Curing and exterminating: two sides of a psychiatric reform programme

Carl Schneider, together with the professors Maximinian de Crinis (1889–1945) in Berlin, Werner Heyde (1902–64) in Würzburg, Berthold Kihn (1895–1964) in Jena, and prominent representatives of institutional psychiatry, in particular Paul Nitsche in Saxony, belonged from July 1939 to the inner circle of psychiatric experts for the Nazi "euthanasia" programme (Nitsche was also a member of the board of the Society of German Neurologists and Psychiatrists).[15] Already at the end of 1933, shortly after taking over the chair at Heidelberg, Schneider's close friend Nitsche had ensured that Schneider quickly gained entry to the psychiatric network around Ernst Rüdin (1874–1954), the powerful Director of the German Research Institute for Psychiatry and President of the German Professional Association of Psychiatrists.[16] Thus, Schneider became the editor of the journal of the Society of German Neurologists and Psychiatrists, the *Allgemeine Zeitschrift für Psychiatrie*, and with this, in 1935, a member of the advisory board of the Society.[17] Schneider gave up the editorship in 1937, but he remained a part of the network of the Society, which, a little later, was involved in manifold ways in the murder of the mentally ill.[18] At the invitation of the Chancellery of the Führer, leading Nazi psychiatrists came together with representatives of the Reich Ministry of the Interior at the end of July or in August 1939 to discuss the registration, selection and extermination of those considered incurably ill and economically unusable of the institutionalised patients in the German Empire.[19] In October 1939 *Aktion T4*[20] was set in motion, to which some 70,000 patients would fall victim between January 1940 and August 1941. Three psychiatric experts and a Chief Assessor, with the help of a registration form, judged patients to be "lives not worth living" (*lebensunwertes Leben*). They were murdered in one of six "killing institutions" in the German Reich with carbon monoxide gas.[21] Schneider was one of the experts who decided on the basis of the registration form on the lives of thousands of people. He was also personally involved in February 1941, when a selection committee from the department of the Chancellery of the Führer tasked with carrying out the "euthanasia" measures visited the Bodelschwingh Institutions at Bethel, which had been directed by Schneider, and selected from the patients there.[22] During the consultations for a "Law for Euthanasia for the Incurably Ill" in October 1940 (a law that was never implemented), Schneider advocated excepting from the law those incurably ill people who were in institutions and performed "socially valuable work".[23] For Schneider, actively participating in the process of the murder of ill people under National Socialism was not a necessity caused by any political circumstance or "the spirit of the time". Rather, this engagement followed his inner persuasion; in 1942, for instance, he praised the propaganda film "Existence without Life" (*Dasein ohne Leben*), which had been produced expressly to justify the "euthanasia" program, saying "I found the film in its current form particularly good, especially in view of the music. If the final words are not spoken in too elegiac a fashion, but the word 'deliverance' is spoken with the character of an uplifting duty, then the ending . . . can be left as it is".[24] If the "deliverance" of the incurably mentally ill was apparently a moral commandment for Schneider, this still did not mean that he turned aside from his therapeutic claim to do everything for the treatable patient to improve his or her condition and to enable the patient to perform socially useful work.

A report by Schneider had been planned for the minutely prepared conference of the Society of German Neurologists and Psychiatrists in October 1941, where it had been intended to treat the murder of ill people as an open secret; the conference had to be cancelled owing to the circumstances of war. The manuscript of this report, in which Schneider summarised his ideas of a modern, biologically and therapeutically orientated psychiatry, has survived:

> As it must, psychiatry is forming itself here into a decisive branch of science, decisive for all disciplines that have to do with human biology, a science of the total sum of psychophysical reactions of the human being, which has given us the means to study environmental influences in work therapy, in the other areas ways to study the internal regulatory processes of the organism. The time is no longer distant, when we will have made even the so-called incurable mental illnesses accessible to therapeutic efforts, and we can preserve the ill person from infirmity, as well as from life-long internment in an institution, so that, despite his illness ["after his sterilisation", handwritten note from Paul Nitsche at this point], he can remain an active member of the "national community" [*Volksgemeinschaft*].[25]

Prevention of mental illness by means of a consistent policy of sterilisation and the attempts at treatment of the individual patient, whose psychosis Schneider did not see as fate, but rather something that could be biologically influenced, were to come together for him to "relieve" the people, *das Volk*. Those patients would fall by the wayside, whose illness could not be treated and who could no longer seem to perform "valuable work" for the community. For them there was only medical "deliverance", which could only be justified through the claim to therapy made by psychiatry.

This connection becomes even clearer in a memorandum formulated by Schneider together with Rüdin, Nitsche, de Crinis and the director of the Brandenburg-Görden Institution, Hans Heinze (1895–1983), at the beginning of 1943 (this was based mostly on a text written by Schneider in January 1943):[26]

> But the euthanasia measures taken will find all the more general understanding and acceptance, when it is made clear that, in every case of psychic illness, every last possibility has been explored that would enable the patient to be cured or at least improve to the point where he can again be provided for economically valuable work, in his old profession or in some other form.[27]

The killing of incurable, unproductive patients is integrated as a matter of course in a comprehensive programme of psychiatric research, therapy and care. The memorandum partially anticipated demands that characterised the reform of psychiatry in the 1970s in Germany, such as setting up outpatient clinics at the mental hospitals and nursing homes, and psychiatric departments in general hospitals. However, the decisive thing was the uniform arrangement of German institutions, with a central planning office, the connection of university and institutional psychiatry, and the provision of all possible methods of diagnosis and therapy in the psychiatric asylums.[28] The requirements of research and therapy were, for Schneider, no mere matter of lip service; from 1942 he introduced advanced courses in diagnostics and therapy at the Heidelberg hospital, commissioned by "T4". He required that insulin, despite wartime rationing, should be provided for schizophrenia therapy. The close connection between healing and extermination continued to shape the period after murder by gas was interrupted in August 1941. The "T4" organisation then attempted to gain control over the killing of "unusable" patients by means of overdosing with medication in the individual mental hospitals and care homes, by delivering the anaesthetic morphine-scopalomine to the institutions. Some of this medication was probably obtained by Schneider through the offices of the clinical chemists' department at Heidelberg.[29]

Psychiatric research under National Socialism: Schneider's clinical research

In Heidelberg, Schneider was more concerned at first with managing the hospital and its new direction, which at first emphasised work therapy, and later on electric and insulin shock therapy, rather than with intensive research activity.[30] A total of 13 publications by Schneider are known from the period between 1933 and 1945, among which are two monographs.[31] Of these, the first focused entirely on psychiatric therapy and its new methods (work therapy, but also other "biological" procedures); this was what could be considered Schneider's magnum opus, the comprehensive *Behandlung und Verhütung der Geisteskrankheiten* (The Treatment and Prevention of Mental Illnesses), published in 1939. The second, *Die schizophrenen Symptomverbände* (The Collective Schizophrenic Symptoms) of 1942 reflects Schneider's strong, continual interest in schizophrenia and its clinical, psychopathological and psychological aspects.[32] Some of his shorter works are not strictly scientific, having a more propagandistic or political character, such as his contribution to the magazine *Der Wanderer* on population politics in 1933, or an essay originally intended to be a public speech for the propaganda exhibition "Degenerate Art" (*Entartete Kunst*), entitled "Degenerate Art and Mad Art" of 1940.[33] This is also the context in which a text belongs that Schneider could publish in the monthly organ of the Main Office for National Health (*Hauptamt für Volksgesundheit*) of the NSDAP in 1943, thanks to mediation by Leonardo Conti (1900–45), the Reich Health Leader (*Reichsgesundheitsführer*).[34] The other publications were mostly smaller, clinical, partly casuistic contributions, of which two published in 1934 were dedicated to the subject of epilepsy, based probably still on clinical experience at Bethel.[35] It is also known that Schneider carried out field studies on hereditary biology and epidemiology in the mid-1930s in the so-called "incest villages" in the Odenwald, supported by the "Emergency Association of German Science" (*Notgemeinschaft der Deutschen Wissenschaft*), but nothing is known of the results of these studies.[36]

The 22 doctoral theses supervised by Schneider in Heidelberg also give indications of his own scientific interests, as they may be regarded as an expression of the "normal" scientific conduct during the Nazi period.[37] Nearly a quarter of these focus on questions pertaining to schizophrenia and epilepsy.[38] Some others, too, deal with areas of interest to Schneider, for example, the "phenomena of falling asleep" and, especially, hereditary biology. Particularly worthy of note are a thesis on a "Chorea Huntingdon Clan", one on "Psychosis in the Marriages of Relatives" (referring to a village in the Palatinate, thus not directly connected to Schneider's research in the Odenwald villages), and, in particular, one on "75 cases of schizophrenia . . . carried out with regard to the Law for Prevention of Hereditarily Diseased Offspring".[39]

Nearly all of Schneider's interests were united in his research programme of 1942.[40] Within the context of the "euthanasia" programme, Schneider developed an extensive research proposal to modernise psychiatric care. He applied for 15 million Reichsmarks over 15 years with the far-ranging goal of ". . . dispel[ling] once and for all the old ideas about human beings [and] properly consider[ing] the organism as a biological unit in the development and evolution of its functions".[41] Using his biological concepts of human psychology, he intended to develop the prerequisites for therapy and for the prevention of transmission of undesirable hereditary conditions. For example, Schneider proposed four long-term studies in 1942:

1   Charting the development of 30 healthy boys and 30 healthy girls;
2   Parallel studies on children with extreme mental retardation of extrinsic and hereditary origins;
3   Examining the pathophysiological effects of shock therapy and work therapy on schizophrenics in the framework of the theory of symptom groups (*Symptomverbandslehre*);
4   Systematically examining the biology of the schizophrenic symptom group of volatile behaviours (*Sprunghaftigkeitsverband*).[42]

Concerning the fate of those he examined, he laconically wrote: "It is self-evident that histopathological and pathological-anatomical examinations not only can, but must be conducted for numerous studies, especially with regard to the [euthanasia] programme".[43] Because of the war, however, only a small part of this programme could be carried out.

Psychiatric research and "euthanasia": the Heidelberg Research Department

During the programme of murder by gassing, those within the "T4" organisation were in agreement that the opportunity provided by a mass killing action for medical, particularly psychiatric, research should not be allowed to pass by unused. However, owing to the war, only a part of the plans could ever be carried out.[44] The researcher Julius Hallervorden of the Kaiser Wilhelm

Institute for Brain Research in Berlin-Buch received brains of 1,540 persons (processed as 84,333 slides) brains mainly from "euthanasia" victims, many from the "T4" killing centres. The Institute Director Spatz had a smaller proportion of brains (still to be determined) from "euthanasia" victims.[45] Some (but not all, and in some cases the extent remains unclear) of the "special children's wards" (*Kinderfachabteilungen*) researched on children. The Spiegelgrund in Vienna is a noted example.[46] But Schneider, too, whose assistant Hans-Joachim Rauch had been trained in 1942 in histopathology at the Kaiser Wilhelm Institute for Brain Research, had brains from murdered patients sent to him from 1942, from various institutions. After the war it was possible to establish a total of 187 brains of "euthanasia" victims in the histopathological laboratory of the Heidelberg university hospital.[47] But Schneider's research interests, as he had described them in his research plan, went far beyond neuropathological questions. It was clear from the start that this research reckoned with the deaths of the patients examined. In order to carry out his research plans, Schneider was able to have recourse to a wide network of scientific contacts. Nitsche, who had been medical director of "T4" since 1941, was able to mediate for Schneider in obtaining the financial and organisational support of the "T4". The two departments of the "T4" – Schneider's department in Wiesloch and Heinze's department in the psychiatric hospital of Görden – were to remain in close contact, but the department in Wiesloch had to be closed down after only four months because of the war. From the summer of 1943, Schneider continued his researches into "problems of retardation and epilepsy" (*Probleme des Schwachsinns und der Epilepsie*) at the Heidelberg hospital.[48] In this he received support from Rüdin, the President of the Society of German Neurologists and Psychiatrists. Rüdin had called the research on mentally retarded children particularly important, in a letter written in 1942 to the *Reichsgesundheitsführer* (Reich Health Leader). The point was to develop criteria by means of which children could be recommended for "euthanasia", "both for their own sakes and for the sake of the German people", as a secure method of "countering contraselective processes in our German *Volkskörper* [literally, the collective 'body', i.e. 'race', of the people]".[49] In this light, it is understandable that Rüdin approved the employment of his assistant Julius Deussen (1906–74) at the Heidelberg research department.[50] From 1943, Deussen coordinated a wide-ranging clinical and hereditary biological programme of investigation, to which a total of 52 retarded children were subjected. The research program (Figures 8.2 and 8.3) was planned to comprise laboratory chemical examinations, radiological (encephalography) and metabolic-physiological examinations, psychological test studies to establish the intelligence age, observation in work therapy and the hereditary-biological survey of the family. In the event, innovative research methods were also applied, thus the function tests developed by Deussen, with which the children's reactions to environmental stimuli were to be systematically investigated. The goal of the research was to distinguish between exogenic and endogenic causes of "idiocy", a question that was, for Carl Schneider, "important for the war"

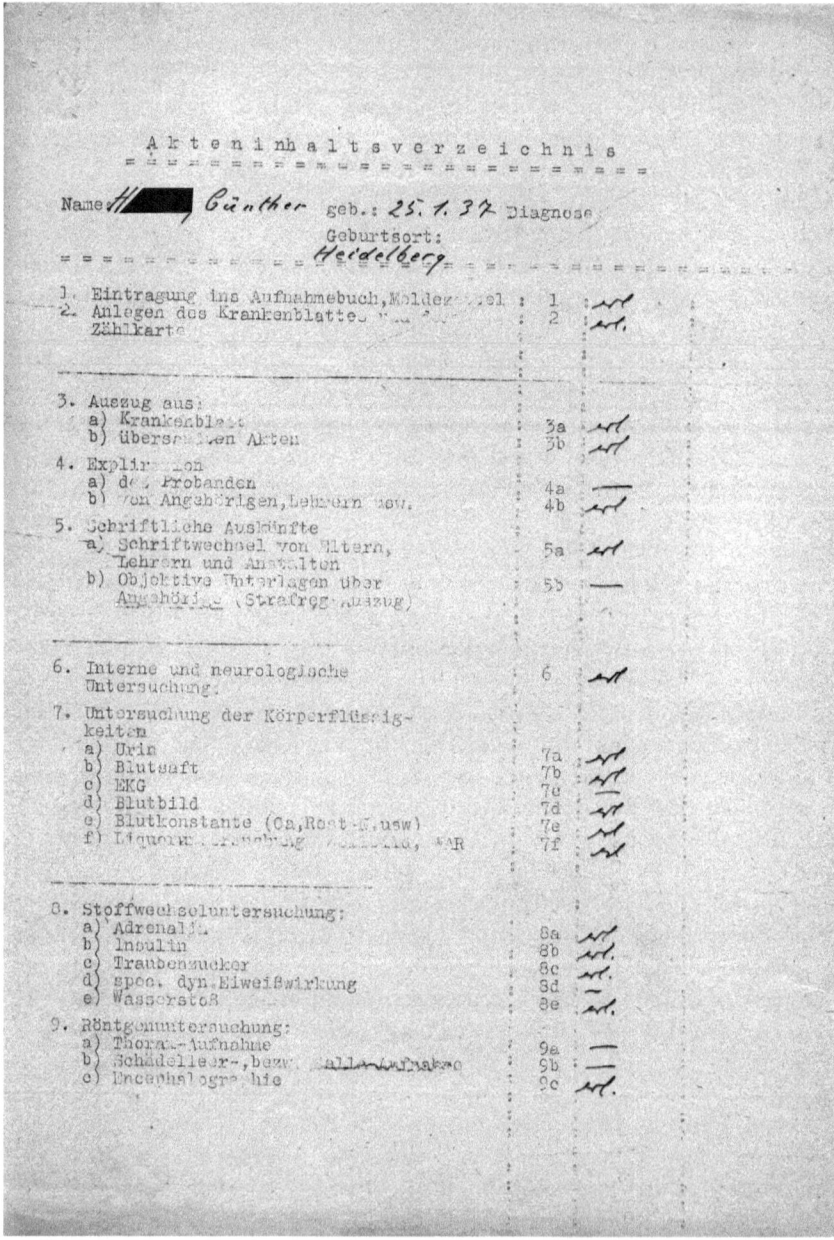

A k t e n i n h a l t s v e r z e i c h n i s
= =

Name: H█████ Günther   geb.: 25. 1. 37   Diagnose:
                        Geburtsort:
= = = = = = = = = = = = Heidelberg = = = = = = = = = = = =

1. Eintragung ins Aufnahmebuch,Meldezettel : 1
2. Anlegen des Krankenblattes, ...   : 2
   Zählkarte

3. Auszug aus:
   a) Krankenblatt   : 3a
   b) überschriebenen Akten   : 3b
4. Exploration
   a) des Probanden   : 4a
   b) von Angehörigen,Lehrern usw.   : 4b
5. Schriftliche Auskünfte
   a) Schriftwechsel von Eltern,   : 5a
      Lehrern und Anstalten
   b) Objektive Unterlagen über   : 5b
      Angehörige (Strafreg.-Auszug)

6. Interne und neurologische   : 6
   Untersuchung:

7. Untersuchung der Körperflüssig-
   keiten
   a) Urin   : 7a
   b) Blutsaft   : 7b
   c) EKG   : 7c
   d) Blutbild   : 7d
   e) Blutkonstante (Ca,Rest-N.usw)   : 7e
   f) Liquoruntersuchung /Zellzahl, WaR   : 7f

8. Stoffwechseluntersuchung:
   a) Adrenalin   : 8a
   b) Insulin   : 8b
   c) Traubenzucker   : 8c
   d) spec. dyn.Eiweißwirkung   : 8d
   e) Wasserstoß   : 8e
9. Röntgenuntersuchung:
   a) Thorax-Aufnahme   : 9a
   b) Schädelleer-,bezw. ...Aufnahme   : 9b
   c) Encephalographie   : 9c

Figures 8.2 and 8.3 Contents list/Research plan of the Heidelberg Research
        Department

Source: Heidelberg, Historical Archives of the Psychiatric University Hospital Heidelberg

10. Photographie: *Foto Akten № 1173* *Aufnahmen stehen Art noch aus*
    a) Kopf (vorn, schräg, seitlich)   : 10a
    b) Körper (stehend u. liegend)   : 10b
    c) Ohren, Hände und Fusse   : 10c
    d) Bewegungsaufnahme   : 10d :——

11. Anthropometrische Untersuchung   : *evtl.*

12. Stationsbeobachtung (Pflegebericht) 12 :——

    a) Arbeitstherapiebeobachtung   12a :——

13. Testprüfungen:
    a) Binet   : 13a :——
    b) Rorschach   : 13b
    c) Vorprüfungen   : 13c
    d) Funktionsprüfungen   : 13d
    e) Schimpansengarten   : 13e

14. Exploration durch den Arzt   14

15. Anlage der Sippentafel
    a) nach Krankenblatt und über-   : 15a :——
       sandten Akten
    b) nach Befragung des Probanden   : 15b
    c) nach Befragung der Angehöri-   : 15c
       gen usw.
    d) nach Schriftwechsel   : 15d
    e) nach eingeforderten Akten   : 15e :——

16. Sektionsbefund des Gehirns
    a) makroskopisch   : 16a
    b) histologisch   : 16b :

17. Allgemeiner Sektionsbefund   : 17

18. Kontrolle der Akten:
    a) Nach Beendigung des Klinik   : 18a
       aufenthaltes
    b) nach Eingang des Sektions-
       befundes

in view of the "struggle for existence" of the German people. Only if one were able to present clear criteria of differentiation would it be possible to prevent the parents of "feeble-minded" children from procreating, while urging other German parents to have "child rich" families.[51] The programme of investigation was concluded with the autopsy results, which required the killing of the children (in the Children's Ward for Expert Care of the state psychiatric asylum at Eichberg). Twenty-one of the "research children" were killed by medication in 1944 in Eichberg.[52] Owing to wartime transport difficulties and a lack of cooperation on the part of the Eichberg institution, "only" three brains were examined in Heidelberg.

The children and the (re)searching look

At the end of March 1944, two brothers from the Schwarzacher Hof near Mosbach were received as "research children" at the Heidelberg hospital.[53] Twelve-year-old Walter and seven-year-old Günther were regarded as "congenitally feeble-minded", and they spent about six weeks in Heidelberg (Figure 8.4).[54] They were subjected to the entire research programme, including being subjected to thorough work therapeutic observation. The older brother did better in all this. In a test involving tying bundles, he was tested both in working by hand and with a machine. "He acts quite dexterously and is industrious and enthusiastic". Günther, on the other hand, "can only barely tie the bundle by hand, with the machine he is only able to crank it". At least Günther, too, was found to be industrious and interested. Because of the involvement of her children in the research programme, the mother, too, came to the notice of the Psychiatric Hospital. In the end, it was only by good luck that she escaped forced sterilisation. Her son Walter survived the war. Günther was murdered at Eichberg on 28 December 1944, and is thus one of the last victims of the Heidelberg research project.

Conclusion

Carl Schneider was arrested by the American occupation authorities after the war and was transferred to German justice in Frankfurt on 29 November 1946. After the responsible public prosecutor had made clear to him the hopelessness of his position in the case of charges being brought against him, Carl Schneider hanged himself in his prison cell on 11 December 1946. To the last, he had believed in the correctness of his actions and had hoped that he would again have scientific and professional prospects, even after the war.[55]

If we ask, in conclusion, about the connection between the "therapeutic idealism" of Carl Schneider and his active participation in the National Socialist "euthanasia" programme, a possible answer may be found in Schneider's concept of biology. In the end, the entire world of the living human being is reduced to biology and hereditary biology. Man is understood in his interactions with the environment exclusively as a biological entity, decisive being his ability

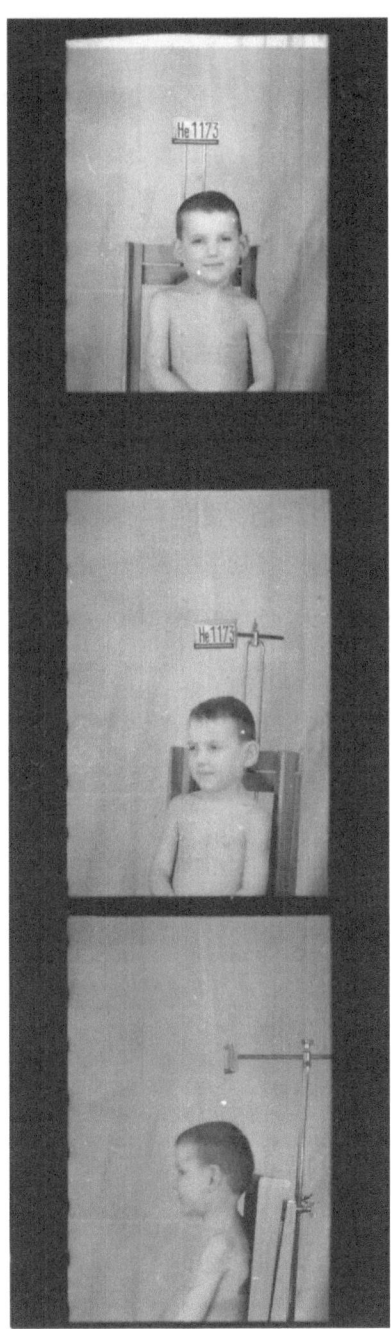

Figure 8.4 Photograph of Günther H.

Source: Heidelberg, Historical Archive of the Psychiatric University Hospital Heidelberg, "Forschungskinder", F 32

or inability to overcome the requirements of the community. If he proves unable, and cannot be integrated into the community by means of active "biological" therapy, work and shock therapy, then, in a biological sense, he has lost his right to existence.

Notes

1 This chapter is a slightly reworked version of the essay by Maike Rotzoll and Gerrit Hohendorf, 'Krankenmord im Dienst des Fortschritts? Der Heidelberger Psychiater Carl Schneider als Gehirnforscher und "therapeutischer Idealist"', *Nervenarzt*, 83 (2012), pp. 311–320.

2 Werner Janzarik, '100 Jahre Heidelberger Psychiatrie', in idem (ed.), *Psychopathologie als Grundlagenwissenschaft*, Stuttgart: Enke, 1979, p. 11.

3 Carl Schneider, *Behandlung und Verhütung der Geisteskrankheiten. Allgemeine Erfahrungen – Grundsätze – Technik – Biologie*, Berlin: Julius Springer, 1939.

4 Klaus Dörner, 'Carl Schneider: Genialer Therapeut, moderner ökologischer System-theoretiker und Euthanasiemörder. Zu Carl Schneiders "Behandlung und Verhütung der Geisteskrankheiten", Berlin: Springer 1939', *Psychiatrische Praxis*, 13 (1986), p. 114.

5 Robert J. Lifton, *Ärzte im Dritten Reich*, Stuttgart: Klett-Cotta, 1988, p. 145.

6 Christine Teller, 'Carl Schneider. Zur Biographie eines deutschen Wissenschaftlers', *Geschichte und Gesellschaft*, 16 (1990), pp. 465–467.

7 Carl Schneider, *Die Psychologie der Schizophrenen und ihre Bedeutung für die Klinik der Schizophrenie*, Leipzig: G. Thieme, 1930.

8 Paul Nitsche and Carl Schneider, *Einführung in die Abteilung seelische Hygiene der internationalen Hygieneausstellung Dresden*, Berlin and Leipzig: de Gruyter, 1930.

9 Carl Schneider, 'Die Auswirkungen der bevölkerungspolitischen und erbbiologischen Maßnahmen auf die Wandererfürsorge', *Der Wanderer*, 50 (1933), p. 234.

10 Ibid., p. 235.

11 Maike Rotzoll and Gerrit Hohendorf, 'Die Psychiatrisch-Neurologische Klinik', in Wolfgang U. Eckart, Volker Sellin and Eike Wolgast (eds), *Die Universität Heidelberg im Nationalsozialismus*, Heidelberg: Springer, 2006, pp. 914–921. For the process of coming to terms with the subject at the Heidelberg University hospital after the war, cf. Maike Rotzoll and Gerrit Hohendorf, 'Zwischen Tabu und Reformimpuls. Der Umgang mit der nationalsozialistischen Vergangenheit der Heidelberger Psychiatrischen Universitätsklinik nach 1945', in Sigrid Oehler-Klein and Volker Roelcke (eds), *Vergangenheitspolitik in der universitären Medizin nach 1945. Institutionelle und individuelle Strategien im Umgang mit dem Nationalsozialismus*, Stuttgart: Franz Steiner, 2007, pp. 307–330.

12 Schneider, *Behandlung und Verhütung*, p. 1.

13 Maike Rotzoll, Bettina Brand-Claussen and Gerrit Hohendorf, 'Carl Schneider, die Bildersammlung, die Künstler und der Mord', in Thomas Fuchs, Inge Jádi, Bettina Brand-Claussen and Christoph Mundt (eds), *Wahn Welt Bild. Die Sammlung Prinzhorn. Beiträge zur Museumseröffnung*, Berlin and Heidelberg: Springer, 2000, pp. 41–64. See Carl Schneider, 'Entartete Kunst und Irrenkunst', *Archiv für Psychiatrie*, 110 (1940), pp. 135–164.

14 Sara Bienentreu, *"Euthanasie" im Nationalsozialismus. Die Frage der Beteiligung der Universitätspsychiatrie am Beispiel der Heidelberger Klinik*, Saarbrücken: Verlag Dr. Müller, 2007.

15 Ernst Klee, *"Euthanasie" im Dritten Reich. Die "Vernichtung lebensunwerten Lebens"*, 2nd ed., Frankfurt am Main: Fischer Taschenbuch, 2010, p. 83.

16 Hans-Walter Schmuhl, *Die Gesellschaft Deutscher Neurologen und Psychiater im Nationalsozialismus*, Berlin and Heidelberg: Springer, 2016, p. 132.

17 Ibid., pp. 64–66, 110–114 and 116.

18 Ibid., pp. 192–193 and 274–275.

19 Klee, *Euthanasie*, p. 83; Schmuhl, *Die Gesellschaft*, pp. 290–291.

20 The term *Aktion T4* is first found in the prosecution files of post-war German justice. The sources from the Nazi period speak of *Aktion* or of *Geheime Reichssache* ("secret Reich matter"), using the abbreviation "T4" for the seat of the office of the Führer Chancellery at Tiergartenstrasse 4, Berlin, which was responsible for the planning and coordination of the National Socialist "euthanasia" measures. The literature on National Socialist "euthanasia" is now very extensive even for experts. To give an overview: Hans-Walter Schmuhl, ' "Euthanasie" und Krankenmord', in Robert Jütte (ed.), *Medizin und Nationalsozialismus. Bilanz und Perspektiven der Forschung*, Göttingen: Wallstein, 2011, p. 215.

21 Hans-Walter Schmuhl, *Rassenhygiene, Nationalsozialismus, Euthanasie. Von der Verhütung zur Vernichtung "lebensunwerten Lebens: 1890–1945*, Göttingen: Vandenhoeck & Ruprecht, 1992; Maike Rotzoll et al., 'Die nationalsozialistische "Euthanasie-Aktion T4". Historische Forschung, individuelle Lebensgeschichten und Erinnerungskultur', *Nervenarzt*, 81 (2010), pp. 1326–1332; Maike Rotzoll et al. (eds.), *Die nationalsozialistische "Euthanasie"-Aktion "T4" und ihre Opfer. Geschichte und ethische Konsequenzen für die Gegenwart*, Paderborn: Schöningh, 2010.

22 Hans-Walter Schmuhl, *Ärzte in der Anstalt Bethel 1870–1945*, Bielefeld: Bethel-Verlag, 1998, pp. 44–56; Klee, *"Euthanasie"*, pp. 241–244.

23 Karl Heinz Roth and Götz Aly, 'Das "Gesetz über die Sterbehilfe bei unheilbar Kranken". Protokolle der Diskussion über die Legalisierung der nationalsozialistischen Anstaltsmorde in den Jahren 1938–1941', in Karl Heinz Roth (ed.), *Erfassung zur Vernichtung. Von der Sozialhygiene zum "Gesetz über Sterbehilfe"*, Berlin: Verlagsgesellschaft Gesundheit, 1984, pp. 140–172.

24 College Park, MD, National Archives and Records Administration, US Army Europe, Record Group 549, Stack Area 290, Row 59, Comp. 17, boxes 1–5 (below cited as "Heidelberg Dokumente" = HD), p. 127 353/9, Carl Schneider (13.3.1942), Comments on the Film *Dasein ohne Leben*.

25 Carl Schneider (1941), Final comments, HD pp. 127 586–587. Schmuhl, *Die Gesellschaft*, p. 367. Schmuhl has presented this document in detail on pages 365–369 of his book; the document culminates in the idea of a "Copernican revolution" affected by the creation of a new image of the human being by psychiatry.

26 Carl Schneider, Comments on the further development of psychiatry, 28 Jan 1943, in HD, pp. 126 437–442. Schmuhl, *Die Gesellschaft*, pp. 378–379 and 385. See the chapter by Hans-Walter Schmuhl in this volume.

27 Ernst Rüdin, Maximinian de Crinis, Carl Schneider, Hans Heinze and Paul Nitsche, 1943, Reflections and propositions concerning the further development of psychiatry, in HD, p. 126 424. Cf. Schmuhl, *Die Gesellschaft*, p. 387.

28 Götz Aly, 'Der saubere und der schmutzige Fortschritt', in Götz Aly (ed.), *Reform und Gewissen. "Euthanasie" im Dienst des Fortschritts*, Berlin: Rotbuch, 1989, pp. 9–78; Hans-Walter Schmuhl, 'Reformpsychiatrie und Massenmord', in Michael Prinz and Rainer Zitelmann (eds), *Nationalsozialismus und Modernisierung*, Darmstadt: Wissenschaftliche Buchgesellschaft, 1994, pp. 239–266; Schmuhl, *Die Gesellschaft*, p. 286.

29 Letter by Carl Schneider to Nitsche, 28 Oct 1943, in HD, pp. 127 984–985.

30 Thomas Beddies, ' "Aktivere Krankenbehandlung" und "Arbeitstherapie". Anwendungsformen und Begründungszusammenhänge bei Hermann Simon und Carl Schneider', in Hans-Walter Schmuhl and Volker Roelcke (eds), *"Heroische Therapien". Die deutsche Psychiatrie im internationalen Vergleich, 1918–1945*, Göttingen: Wallstein, 2013, pp. 268–287; Maike Rotzoll, 'Rhythmus des Lebens'. Arbeit in psychiatrischen Institutionen im Nationalsozialismus zwischen Normalisierung und Selektion', in Monika Ankele and Eva Brinkschulte (eds), *Arbeitsrhythmus und Anstaltsalltag. Arbeit in der Psychiatrie vom frühen 19. Jahrhundert bis in die NS-Zeit*, Stuttgart: Steiner, 2015, pp. 193–200.

31 Bernd Laufs, *Die Psychiatrie zur Zeit des Nationalsozialismus am Beispiel der Heidelberger Universitätsklinik*, MD thesis, Homburg: Saarland University, 1989, pp. 103–104; Andreas Buck, *Psychiatrische und neurologische Dissertationen unter Carl Schneider an der Universität Heidelberg in den Jahren 1933 bis 1945. Ein Beitrag zum Wissenschaftsalltag im Nationalsozialismus*, MD thesis, Hannover: Hannover Medical School, 1993.

32 Schneider, *Behandlung und Verhütung*; idem, *Die schizophrenen Symptomverbände*, Berlin: Springer, 1942.

33 Idem, 'Die Auswirkungen'; idem, 'Entartete Kunst'.

34 Idem, 'Die moderne Behandlung der Geistesstörungen. Die Psychiatrie im Kampf um die Volksgesundheit, Gesundheitsführung', *Ziel und Weg*, 5 (1943), pp. 186–192. Schmuhl, *Die Gesellschaft*, p. 387. This essay was the consequence of a discussion with Conti on the memorandum of 1943.

35 Buck, *Psychiatrische und neurologische Dissertationen*, pp. 45–47.

36 Rotzoll and Hohendorf, 'Die Psychiatrisch-neurologische Klinik', p. 921. Schneider's research was connected to the countrywide project, supported by the Reich Ministry of the Interior, known as the "hereditary biological survey" (*erbbiologische Bestandsaufnahme*). Schneider intended to deal with the "heterozygote problem" (i.e. the problem of the non-carrier of characteristics, through whom the characteristics are, nonetheless, passed on) in his contribution on family research in the Odenwald villages. Schmuhl, *Die Gesellschaft*, pp. 241–242.

37 Volker Roelcke and Simon Duckheim, 'Medizinische Dissertationen aus der Zeit des Nationalsozialismus: Potential eines Quellenbestands und erste Ergebnisse zu "Alltag", Ethik und Mentalität der universitären medizinischen Forschung bis (und ab) 1945', *Medizinhistorisches Journal*, 49 (2014), pp. 261–262.

38 Buck, *Psychiatrische und neurologische Dissertationen*, p. 111.

39 Harald von Moers-Messmer, with regard to the "phenomena of falling asleep", the writings on hereditary biology were by Johanne Böhm, Max Vohmann and Friedrich Böttcher. Cf. Buck, *Psychiatrische und neurologische Dissertationen*, pp. 58–60; 71–78 and 86–90. The rest of the theses are distributed across the area of psychiatry and neurology, from "The Build of the Alcoholic" (*Körperbau des Alkoholikers*), through "Cellular Images in Cases of Paralysis" (*Zellbilder bei Paralyse*) to gliomas.

40 Gerrit Hohendorf and Maike Rotzoll, 'Medical Research and National Socialist Euthanasia: Carl Schneider and the Heidelberg Research children from 1942 until 1945', in Sheldon Rubenfeld and Susan Benedict (eds), *Human Subjects Research after the Holocaust,* Cham: Springer, 2014, p. 132.

41 Carl Schneider, Research proposal, 1942, in HD, pp. 127–129.

42 Schneider's concept of the psychopathology of schizophrenia is characterised by three groups of symptom called *Symptomverbände*. One of them was the *Sprunghaftigkeitsverband*; *Sprunghaftigkeit* means incoherence in thought and speech, see Schneider, *Die schizophrenen Symptomverbände*.

43 Schneider, Research proposal, 1942, in HD, pp. 127–129.

44 Schmuhl, *Die Gesellschaft*, p. 294.

45 Jürgen Peiffer, *Hirnforschung im Zwielicht: Beispiele verführbarer Wissenschaft aus der Zeit des Nationalsozialismus Julius Hallervorden – H. J. Scherer – Berthold Ostertag*, Husum: Matthiesen, 1997; Hans-Walter Schmuhl, 'Hirnforschung und Krankenmord. Das Kaiser-Wilhelm-Institut für Hirnforschung 1937–1945', *Vierteljahrshefte für Zeitgeschichte*, 50 (2002), pp. 594–605. Sascha Zoske, 'Hundert Hirnschnitte und das Rätsel der "Serie H", Heinz Wässle, ehemaliger Max-Planck-Direktor, geht der NS-Vergangenheit seines Instituts nach. Dem Rätsel um die "Serie H" ist er weiter auf der Spur', *Frankfurter Allgemeine Zeitung* (21 Apr 2015). Professor Wässle presented further impressive conclusions at the conference on brain sections at the Leopoldina, 2015, "Vom Präparat zur Person: die Wiederherstellung der Identitäten von NS-Versuchsopfern" (convenor Paul Weindling): 'SERIE H: A subjective and personal account by Heinz Wässle'. The

number of Hallervorden's brain sections accords with number buried by the Max Planck Society in 1990.

46 Paul Weindling, *Victims and Survivors of Nazi Human Experiments: Science and Suffering in the Holocaust*, London: Bloomsbury, 2014, pp. 112–117.

47 Hohendorf *et al.*, 'Innovation und Vernichtung', p. 941.

48 Schmuhl, *Die Gesellschaft*, pp. 298–303. See also Volker Roelcke, Gerrit Hohendorf and Maike Rotzoll, 'Psychiatric research and "euthanasia". The case of the psychiatric department at the University of Heidelberg, 1941–1945', *History of Psychiatry*, 5 (1994), pp. 517–532.

49 Munich, Max-Planck-Institut für Psychiatrie, Historisches Archiv, GDA 129, Letter from Rüdin to the *Reichsgesundheitsführer* Leonardo Conti, 23 Oct 1942.

50 Volker Roelcke, Gerrit Hohendorf and Maike Rotzoll, 'Erbpsychologische Forschung im Kontext der "Euthanasie": Neue Dokumente und Aspekte zu Carl Schneider, Julius Deussen und Ernst Rüdin', *Fortschritte Neurologie Psychiatrie*, 66 (1998), pp. 331–336; Volker Roelcke, 'Psychiatrische Wissenschaft im Kontext nationalsozialistischer Politik und "Euthanasie". Zur Rolle von Ernst Rüdin und der Deutschen Forschungsanstalt für Psychiatrie/Kaiser-Wilhelm-Institut', in Doris Kaufmann (ed.), *Geschichte der Kaiser-Wilhelm-Gesellschaft im Nationalsozialismus. Bestandsaufnahme und Perspektiven der Forschung*, Wallstein, Göttingen, 2000, pp. 112–150. See also Volker Roelcke, Gerrit Hohendorf, and Maike Rotzoll, 'Psychiatrische Genetik und "Erbgesundheitspolitik" im Nationalsozialismus: Zur Zusammenarbeit von Ernst Rüdin, Carl Schneider und Paul Nitsche', in Gerhardt Nissen and Frank Badura (eds), *Schriftenreihe der Deutschen Gesellschaft für Geschichte der Nervenheilkunde*, Vol. 6, Würzburg: Königshausen & Neumann, 2000, pp. 59–73.

51 Hohendorf *et al.*, 'Innovation und Vernichtung', pp. 942–943.

52 One child had already been killed at Eichberg in 1942, and was posthumously entered in the research programme. A further child was transferred to the Eichberg institution at the beginning of 1943, without being entered in the research program; but its brain was examined in Heidelberg after the murder.

53 Hans-Werner Scheuing, *". . .als Menschenleben gegen Sachwerte gewogen wurden". Die Geschichte der Erziehungs- und Pflegeanstalt für Geistesschwache Mosbach/Schwarzacher Hof und ihrer Bewohner 1933–1945*, Heidelberg: Winter, 2004, pp. 367–436.

54 Heidelberg, Historical Archive of the Psychiatric University Hospital Heidelberg, "Forschungskinder", F 32 (Günther H.) and F 33 (Walter H.). Here as well as in other publications only the first names of the children are given. This is also the case on the memorial posed in front of the Heidelberg Psychiatric Hospital in 1998. The intention of the group who initiated the memorial at that time was to put the full names. But a resolution of the hospital board made it necessary to ask all the relatives of the children who could be contacted to give their consent. It was not possible to find relatives of all the children, but unfortunately most of the persons who could be asked did not give the consent to make the full names known. Until today this makes it difficult to name the children by their full name.

55 Personal communication with a contemporary witness, Claus Schneider, in Aug 1999 in Munich.

Bibliography

Archival Sources

Germany

Heidelberg, Historical Archive of the Psychiatric University Hospital:
Contents list/Research plan of the Heidelberg Research Department

"Forschungskinder", F 32–33
Heidelberg, University Archives, photo of Carl Schneider
Munich, Max-Planck-Institut für Psychiatrie, Historisches Archiv, GDA 129

USA

College Park, MD, National Archives and Records Administration, US Army, Europe. Records of the Judge Advocate General, War Crimes Branch. Records Relating to Medical Experiments. Record Group 549 (location 290/59/17/05) ("Heidelberg Documents" = HD)

Literature

Aly, Götz, 'Der saubere und der schmutzige Fortschritt', in idem (ed.), *Reform und Gewissen. "Euthanasie" im Dienst des Fortschritts. Beiträge zur nationalsozialistischen Gesundheits- und Sozialpolitik*, Vol. 2, Berlin: Rotbuch, 1989, pp. 9–78

Beddies, Thomas, '"Aktivere Krankenbehandlung" und "Arbeitstherapie". Anwendungsformen und Begründungszusammenhänge bei Hermann Simon und Carl Schneider', in Hans-Walter Schmuhl and Volker Roelcke (eds),*"Heroische Therapien". Die deutsche Psychiatrie im internationalen Vergleich, 1918–1945,* Göttingen: Wallstein, 2013, pp. 268–287

Bienentreu, Sara, *"Euthanasie" im Nationalsozialismus. Die Frage der Beteiligung der Universitätspsychiatrie am Beispiel der Heidelberger Klinik,* Saarbrücken: Verlag Dr. Müller, 2007

Buck, Andreas, *Psychiatrische und neurologische Dissertationen unter Carl Schneider an der Universität Heidelberg in den Jahren 1933 bis 1945. Ein Beitrag zum Wissenschaftsalltag im Nationalsozialismus,* MD thesis, Hannover: Hannover Medical School, 1993

Dörner, Klaus, 'Carl Schneider: Genialer Therapeut, moderner ökologischer Systemtheoretiker und Euthanasiemörder. Zu Carl Schneiders "Behandlung und Verhütung der Geisteskrankheiten", Berlin: Springer 1939', *Psychiatrische Praxis*, 13 (1986), pp. 112–114

Hohendorf, Gerrit, Volker Roelcke and Maike Rotzoll, 'Innovation und Vernichtung – Psychiatrische Forschung und "Euthanasie" an der Heidelberger Psychiatrischen Klinik 1939–1945', *Nervenarzt*, 67 (1996), pp. 935–946

Hohendorf, Gerrit and Maike Rotzoll, 'Medical Research and National Socialist Euthanasia: Carl Schneider and the Heidelberg Research children from 1942 until 1945', in Sheldon Rubenfeld and Susan Benedict (eds), *Human Subjects Research after the Holocaust,* Cham: Springer, 2014, pp. 127–138

Janzarik, Werner, '100 Jahre Heidelberger Psychiatrie', in Werner Janzarik (ed.), *Psychopathologie als Grundlagenwissenschaft,* Stuttgart: Enke, 1979, pp. 1–18

Klee, Ernst, *"Euthanasie" im Dritten Reich. Die "Vernichtung lebensunwerten Lebens",* 2nd ed., Frankfurt am Main: Fischer Taschenbuch, 2010

Laufs, Bernd, *Psychiatrie zur Zeit des Nationalsozialismus am Beispiel der Heidelberger Universitätsklinik,* MD thesis, Homburg: Saarland University, 1989

Lifton, Robert J, *Ärzte im Dritten Reich,* Stuttgart: Klett-Cotta, 1988

Nitsche, Paul and Carl Schneider. *Einführung in die Abteilung seelische Hygiene der internationalen Hygieneausstellung Dresden,* Berlin and Leipzig: de Gruyter, 1930

Peiffer, Jürgen, *Hirnforschung im Zwielicht: Beispiele verführbarer Wissenschaft aus der Zeit des Nationalsozialismus Julius Hallervorden – H. J. Scherer – Berthold Ostertag.*

Abhandlungen zur Geschichte der Medizin und der Naturwissenschaften, Husum: Matthiesen, 1997

Roelcke, Volker, Gerrit Hohendorf and Maike Rotzoll, 'Psychiatric research and "euthanasia". The case of the psychiatric department at the University of Heidelberg, 1941–1945', *History of Psychiatry*, 5 (1994), pp. 517–532.

——— 'Erbpsychologische Forschung im Kontext der "Euthanasie": Neue Dokumente und Aspekte zu Carl Schneider, Julius Deussen und Ernst Rüdin', *Fortschritte Neurologie Psychiatrie*, 66 (1998), pp. 331–336

——— 'Psychiatrische Genetik und "Erbgesundheitspolitik" im Nationalsozialismus: Zur Zusammenarbeit von Ernst Rüdin, Carl Schneider und Paul Nitsche', in Gerhardt Nissen and Frank Badura (eds), *Schriftenreihe der Deutschen Gesellschaft für Geschichte der Nervenheilkunde*, Vol. 6, Würzburg: Königshausen & Neumann, 2000, pp. 59–73

Roelcke, Volker. 'Psychiatrische Wissenschaft im Kontext nationalsozialistischer Politik und "Euthanasie". Zur Rolle von Ernst Rüdin und der Deutschen Forschungsanstalt für Psychiatrie/Kaiser-Wilhelm-Institut', in Doris Kaufmann (ed.), *Geschichte der Kaiser-Wilhelm-Gesellschaft im Nationalsozialismus. Bestandsaufnahme und Perspektiven der Forschung*, Wallstein, Göttingen, 2000, pp. 112–150

Roelcke, Volker and Simon Duckheim, 'Medizinische Dissertationen aus der Zeit des Nationalsozialismus: Potential eines Quellenbestands und erste Ergebnisse zu "Alltag", Ethik und Mentalität der universitären medizinischen Forschung bis (und ab) 1945', *Medizinhistorisches Journal*, 49 (2014), pp. 260–271

Roth, Karl Heinz and Götz Aly. 'Das "Gesetz über die Sterbehilfe bei unheilbar Kranken". Protokolle der Diskussion über die Legalisierung der nationalsozialistischen Anstaltsmorde in den Jahren 1938–1941', in Karl Heinz Roth (ed.), *Erfassung zur Vernichtung. Von der Sozialhygiene zum "Gesetz über Sterbehilfe"*, Berlin: Verlagsgesellschaft Gesundheit, 1984, pp. 101–179

Rotzoll, Maike, Bettina Brand-Claussen and Gerrit Hohendorf, 'Carl Schneider, die Bildersammlung, die Künstler und der Mord', in Thomas Fuchs, Inge Jádi, Bettina Brand-Claussen and Christoph Mundt (eds), *Wahn Welt Bild. Die Sammlung Prinzhorn. Beiträge zur Museumseröffnung*, Berlin and Heidelberg: Springer, 2000, pp. 41–64

Rotzoll, Maike and Gerrit Hohendorf, 'Die Psychiatrisch-Neurologische Klinik', in Wolfgang U. Eckart, Volker Sellin and Eike Wolgast (eds), *Die Universität Heidelberg im Nationalsozialismus*, Heidelberg: Springer, 2006, pp. 909–939

——— 'Zwischen Tabu und Reformimpuls. Der Umgang mit der nationalsozialistischen Vergangenheit der Heidelberger Psychiatrischen Universitätsklinik nach 1945', in Sigrid Oehler-Klein and Volker Roelcke (eds), *Vergangenheitspolitik in der universitären Medizin nach 1945. Institutionelle und individuelle Strategien im Umgang mit dem Nationalsozialismus*, Stuttgart: Franz Steiner, 2007, pp. 307–330

Rotzoll, Maike, Gerrit Hohendorf, Petra Fuchs, Paul Richter, Wolfgang U. Eckart and Christoph Mundt (eds), *Die nationalsozialistische "Euthanasie"-Aktion "T4" und ihre Opfer. Geschichte und ethische Konsequenzen für die Gegenwart*, Paderborn: Schöningh, 2010

Rotzoll, Maike, Petra Fuchs, Paul Richter and Gerrit Hohendorf, 'Die nationalsozialistische "Euthanasie-Aktion T4". Historische Forschung, individuelle Lebensgeschichten und Erinnerungskultur', *Nervenarzt*, 81 (2010), pp. 1326–1332

Rotzoll, Maike and Gerrit Hohendorf, 'Krankenmord im Dienst des Fortschritts? Der Heidelberger Psychiater Carl Schneider als Gehirnforscher und "therapeutischer Idealist"', *Nervenarzt*, 83 (2012), pp. 311–320

Rotzoll, Maike, 'Rhythmus des Lebens. Arbeit in psychiatrischen Institutionen im Nationalsozialismus zwischen Normalisierung und Selektion', in Monika Ankele and Eva Brinkschulte (eds), *Arbeitsrhythmus und Anstaltsalltag. Arbeit in der Psychiatrie vom frühen 19. Jahrhundert bis in die NS-Zeit*, Stuttgart: Steiner, 2015, pp. 189–214

Scheuing, Hans-Werner, *". . .als Menschenleben gegen Sachwerte gewogen wurden". Die Geschichte der Erziehungs- und Pflegeanstalt für Geistesschwache Mosbach/Schwarzacher Hof und ihrer Bewohner 1933–1945*, Heidelberg: Winter, 2004

Schmuhl, Hans-Walter, *Rassenhygiene, Nationalsozialismus, Euthanasie. Von der Verhütung zur Vernichtung "lebensunwerten Lebens" 1890–1945*, Göttingen: Vandenhoeck & Ruprecht, 1992

—— 'Reformpsychiatrie und Massenmord', in Michael Prinz and Rainer Zitelmann (eds), *Nationalsozialismus und Modernisierung*, Darmstadt: Wissenschaftliche Buchgesellschaft, 1994, pp. 239–266

—— *Ärzte in der Anstalt Bethel 1870–1945*, Bielefeld: Bethel-Verlag, 1998

—— 'Hirnforschung und Krankenmord. Das Kaiser-Wilhelm-Institut für Hirnforschung 1937–1945', *Vierteljahrshefte für Zeitgeschichte*, 50 (2002), pp. 559–609

—— '"Euthanasie" und Krankenmord', in Robert Jütte (ed.), *Medizin und Nationalsozialismus. Bilanz und Perspektiven der Forschung*, Göttingen: Wallstein, 2011, pp. 214–255

—— *Die Gesellschaft Deutscher Neurologen und Psychiater im Nationalsozialismus*, Berlin and Heidelberg: Springer, 2016

Schneider, Carl, *Die Psychologie der Schizophrenen und ihre Bedeutung für die Klinik der Schizophrenie*, Leipzig: G. Thieme, 1930

—— 'Die Auswirkungen der bevölkerungspolitischen und erbbiologischen Maßnahmen auf die Wandererfürsorge', *Der Wanderer*, 50 (1933), p. 233–240

—— *Behandlung und Verhütung der Geisteskrankheiten. Allgemeine Erfahrungen – Grundsätze – Technik – Biologie. Monographien aus dem Gesamtgebiete der Neurologie und Psychiatrie*, Vol. 67, Berlin: Julius Springer, 1939

—— 'Entartete Kunst und Irrenkunst', *Archiv für Psychiatrie*, 110 (1940), pp. 135–164

—— *Die schizophrenen Symptomverbände*, Berlin: Springer, 1942

Teller, Christine, 'Carl Schneider. Zur Biographie eines deutschen Wissenschaftlers', *Geschichte und Gesellschaft*, 16 (1990), pp. 464–478

Weindling, Paul, *Victims and Survivors of Nazi Human Experiments: Science and Suffering in the Holocaust*, London: Bloomsbury, 2014

Zoske, Sascha, 'Hundert Hirnschnitte und das Rätsel der "Serie H", Heinz Wässle, ehemaliger Max-Planck-Direktor, geht der NS-Vergangenheit seines Instituts nach. Dem Rätsel um die "Serie H" ist er weiter auf der Spur', *Frankfurter Allgemeine Zeitung* (21 Apr 2015)

9 Der Kinderfachabteilung vorzuschlagen

The selection and elimination of children at the Youth Psychiatric Clinic Loben (1941–45)

Kamila Uzarczyk

Christa H.[1] was seven years old when in August 1944 she was admitted to the Youth Psychiatric Clinic in Loben (*Jugendpsychiatrische Klinik*) for psychological examination. Her medical history informs that she was the oldest of four children of mentally deficient parents and was both mentally and physically underdeveloped. She was able to sit, walk and run, stand and eat on her own, but she had to be assisted in all other everyday activities. She did not develop relationships with other children in the ward, was very shy with the adults, she would veil her face with her hands, grimace, suck her fingers and would not react when she was spoken to. She was a bit more trusting of the attending nurse and she followed simple orders, such as "give me your hand" or "go to the door". She could not speak or play with toys and was not interested in what the other children were doing. She was indifferent to her surroundings and revealed an extremely low intelligence level: she did not know her name, could not distinguish colours, the size or shape of various objects and showed no interest in pictures and paper figures. The X-ray picture of her brain showed no signs of organic disorders or any peculiar traits. After two weeks of observation Käthe Füssel, the physician in charge, concluded that the prognosis was unfavourable and recommended Christa's transfer to the children's care station (*Kinderpflegestation*) of the State Hospital and Nursing Home Loben (*Landes Heil- und Pflegeanstalt*).[2]

Christa is not registered on the list of 293[3] children who, in the years 1941–45, were placed in the Youth Psychiatric Clinic in Loben for psychological examination. Her medical documentation informs that at the beginning of September 1944 she was transferred to the recommended *Pflegestation*. In her medical history there are no more hints as to what happened to her, but in all likelihood she shared the fate of 297 children who were either actively killed with toxic doses of luminal or perished due to negligence.[4]

The planning

In spring 1939 a cabal of officials from Hitler's Chancellery: Viktor Brack, Hans Hefelman and Richard von Hegener worked out the procedure of the implementation of systematic killings of children with various disabilities, the programme which became known as "children's euthanasia". The planners agreed that the children would be selected on the basis of registration forms (*Meldebogen*) containing detailed medical data. These would be evaluated by a committee of experts, who would then take a decision on life and death, either by giving authorisation for so-called "treatment" (*Behandlung*) – a misleading euphemism for killing – or by ordering further observation of the educational prospects of the child.

The systematic registration process required compliance of the medical personnel that could be enforced by ministerial authority: hence Herbert Linden, in the Ministry of Interior Affairs responsible for state hospitals and nursing homes, was included in the early circle of planners. A ministerial circular, issued on 18 August 1939, obliged doctors and midwives to report children with various disabilities to the local public health officers (*Amtsärzte*). They were to pass on the documentation to Berlin to the Reich Committee for the Scientific Registration of Severe Hereditary and Congenitally Conditioned Ailments (*Reichsausschuss zur wissenschaftlichen Erfassung von erb- und anlagebedingten schweren Leiden*). Repeating the words of Henry Friedlander, "its convoluted name perfectly fitted its purported role as a scientific research institute".[5]

The registration of patients initially did not raise any suspicions. Statistical studies of the frequency of occurrence of various hereditary mental and nervous disorders were conducted during the 1930s in Silesia, Saxony, Thuringia, Bavaria and Berlin[6] and hence uninitiated physicians may have sent the formulas *bona fide*. In Berlin the trio of specialists – the psychiatrist Hans Heinze, paediatrician Ernst Wentzler and ophthalmologist Hellmuth Unger – processed the documentation and took the decision about the child's fate. It is not clear when exactly medical experts joined the inner circle of planners but, as pointed out by Udo Benzenhöfer,[7] the afflictions specified in the ministerial documents indicate a certain level of expertise in childhood diseases. Thus, physicians were undoubtedly involved in the actual decision making process from early on. Children assessed as slightly mentally deficient and educable in basic labour skills and moral habits were to be trained in special schools to perform simple, industrial jobs in the future. Children evaluated as uneducable (*Bildungsunfähig*) and socially maladjusted were to be placed in special children's units (*Kinderfachabteilung*)[8] and were subjected to "treatment" with toxic doses of barbiturates or neglected and starved to death. According to Udo Benzenhöfer, at least 30 institutions could be identified as *Kinderfachabteilungen*, and the existence of more cannot be excluded.[9] The most comprehensive list comprises 37 facilities,[10] probably including also psychiatric or paediatric wards where the children were killed although they were not included in the proceedings of the committee of experts. According to conservative estimates, 5,000 so-called *Reichausschuß children* perished. If we take into consideration unauthorised killings in various children's wards, the number of victims may be double.[11]

The first *Kinderfachabteilung* began to operate in July 1940 in Görden-Brandenburg and became a sort of a model institution and training centre for physicians who were to be heads of similar establishments. In summer 1942 Dr Ernst Buchalik (1905-?), director of the State Hospital and Nursing Home, Loben (*Landes Heil- und Pflegeanstalt Loben*), visited the facility.[12]

Scene of the killings

For many years the State Hospital and Nursing Home, Loben served mainly as a psychiatric facility for adults. In 1904 the former *Irrenanstalt* was transformed into a psychiatric hospital and over the years it gradually increased its capacity, reaching 1,500 beds in 1922. Due to territorial corrections during the eventful decades of the interwar period, the hospital was handed down from German to Polish authorities in 1922 and again to Germany in 1939. In the interwar years the Polish administration continued to use German experience in managing the hospital: the conditions for admittance, style of medical interview and formulas translated from German into Polish remained in use. In line with methods of treatment popular at the time, work therapy was the preferred therapeutic solution and the management cared enough to develop a dense network of workshops for those patients who were able to work and contribute to the hospital's economy.

It is not clear what happened to the patients after the outbreak of the war. In many other hospitals for the mentally ill in occupied Poland, the patients were killed by SS units. However, there is no known evidence that in 1939 in Loben mass killings on a large scale took place. As this part of the Polish territory was incorporated into the Third Reich, the patients may have been included in the "T-4" programme and transferred to one of the killing centres in Germany. Dietmar Schulze has proved[13] that there were transports of patients from Loben in 1941, shortly before Hitler's order of 24 August 1941 put a fake stop to the programme of the centralised killing of adults.

Schultze pointed out that, considering the capacity of the hospitals in Loben and Rybnik, registration and transports of patients began relatively late. The State Archive in Opole (Oppeln) holds a few documents that indicate that in Upper Silesia registration continued in the years 1942–43 and authorities sought to single out Polish patients. In July 1942 the president of Upper Silesia ordered registration of:

1   the mentally ill;
2   those suffering from incurable communicable diseases such as incurable tuberculosis, lues, syphilis [sic!], trachoma;
3   those afflicted with incurable diseases such as epilepsy and cancer;
4   the blind, the deaf, the handicapped unable to work of Polish origin.[14]

Remaining documentation indicates that a year after, in July 1943, the president of the Opole district (*Regierungsbezirk Oppeln*) demanded reports of registration from local health offices. Two salvaged letters from public health officials (*Amtsarzt*) from Blachownia (Blachstaedt) and Zawiercie (Warthenau) allow one to conclude that the patients – we do not know how many of them – were brought under police escort, examined again (*wieder gemustert*) and 150 persons selected, 78 and 72 respectively, were taken away (*abtransportiert*). None of these letters tell us to where. The remaining cases "of slight retardation and successfully treated schizophrenia" were released home. "There were no incidents during the whole procedure" – noted the physician from Blachstaedt – "only afterwards, did the relatives of the deported patients try to get to know about their destination and requested their release home, explaining that they should not be a burden for anyone for they would be taken care for mostly by their parents".[15] Among the deported patients there may have been relatively young individuals, including children and teenagers, although there is no hint regarding the age span.

In contrast, the killing of children continued and the years 1941–43 saw the proliferation of special youth psychiatric care units, including the one in Loben.

". . . One of the first of its kind in the Third Reich . . ."

At the beginning of December 1942 *Landes Heil- und Pflegeanstalt Loben* hosted a meeting of 35 directors of the local municipal and district Youth Offices, who met to discuss the youth care system in Upper Silesia. The location of the meeting is very telling and – as the proceedings of this gathering revealed – a particularly interesting part of the event was a visit to the Youth Psychiatric Clinic (*Jugendpsychiatrische Klinik*), Loben, directed by the specialist in child psychiatry – Dr Elisabeth Hecker (1895–1986).[16]

The facility began to operate in September 1941[17] and, as the local press proudly reported, it was one of the first of this kind in the Third Reich.[18] As the account of the meeting reveals, the clinic was to be involved in the large-scale project of the medical and psychological examination of children from various Silesian child care facilities and their further redistribution in line with Nazi eugenic policies. Participants at the meeting were unanimous that "in order to minimise bias and potential parental protests, the Youth Psychiatric Clinic should not be amalgamated with the State Hospital and Nursing Home, Loben".[19]

The report indicated how the discussants lamented the insufficient number of children's homes in the province and deplorable conditions in the existing establishments as well as the inefficient care system. They also found it intolerable that the majority of the children's homes were run by the Church and that children remained under a strong ecclesiastical influence. However, what really worried youth care officials was that in these homes all the children were raised together, regardless of their intellectual endowment and social adjustment. The situation was better only in the *NSV Jugendheimstätten*, for there eugenic selection criteria played a role in the admittance procedure. To put an end to this unacceptable situation and pick out those children promising to turn out as socially useful citizens, not only the children reported by health officials, but also the inmates from all children's homes were to be examined in the *Jugendpsychiatrische Klinik*; particularly those who suffered from nocturnal bed-wetting, more than one repeated school year, demonstrated behavioural problems such as an inclination to nibble [sic!], lie, and steal and all children with movement disorders.[20] "In this way" – noted the author of the report – "it will become clear which children are worthy of support and will be brought up in homes and families and which should be excluded from the community".[21]Cooperation between the clinic and the whole system of youth care was to ease the institutional distribution of children and provide efficient and appropriate vocational education for the inmates evaluated as "educable". Not surprisingly, the opening of the facility was considered as a "decisive step in a training of productive youth".[22]

Elisabeth Hecker cooperated closely with Dr Ernst Buchalik, director of the hospital and head of the children's care station (*Kinderpflegestation*) – known also as "Ward B" – where children were put to death. There is a bit of confusion as to when the ward began to operate.[23] It seems plausible that *Kinderpflegestation Loben* was opened in summer 1942, as suggested by the authors of earlier publications[24] and by the first recorded transfer to the unit (*Verlegung nach Kinderpflegestation*).[25] Based on the results of psychological tests and a few-weeks' observation in the Youth Psychiatric Clinic, Dr Hecker reported children to the Reich Committee and ordered their prior transfer to *Kinderpflegestation*.[26]

"Uneducable": transferred to the Children's Care Station

On average, 60 children, aged eight months to 18 years – most of them below seven – were hospitalised in the admittance station for a period of six to eight weeks.[27] During this time they were subjected to thorough medical examination and psychological observation to assess their educability and social adjustment. Based on the standard intelligence test used in various Nazi institutions for the selection of feebleminded individuals, a great majority of the patients were diagnosed with mental deficiency of various degrees, ranging from "feeblemindedness" to "idiocy".

Intelligence testing dates back to Francis Galton, who developed a series of sensory and reaction-time tasks measuring temperament rather than intelligence. His theory was based on the assumption that since people receive information via the senses, the most intelligent people must have the best developed senses. In 1905 Alfred Binet developed the first instrument to measure intelligence. Binet was influenced by the work of Hermann Ebbinghaus, who administered tests for calculation, memory for numbers and letters, and so-called cancellation tests involving the completion of the missing elements of words and letters in a sentence. Binet, however, believed that the assessment of intelligence required also the evaluation of imagination, and the ability to discuss the meaning of abstract words, construct sentences and longer stories, to express moral or aesthetic judgements. His focus was on language abilities and comprehension and tests of complex mental functions.

The tests were based on Binet-Simon and Hildegard Hetzer tests, but additionally contained questions testing the level of knowledge of the teaching curriculum in German schools. They did not contain any tasks for evaluating manual, imaginary and creative capacities in children. The criteria applied to assess children's intellectual potential were limited to the battery of linguistic exercises, which demanded good command of the German language and the ability to explain abstract ideas. For a number of children from poor family backgrounds, obtaining at least a satisfactory score was an impossible task. The children whose first or only language was Polish had obvious difficulties. Medical documentation does not contain any information regarding the nationality of the patients. Some documents, however, make remarks clearly indicating Polish origins:

> *Johann M.:*   He can name shapes and colours correctly, but in Polish . . . . He is familiar with the objects in his surrounding and knows their usage. When he cannot say something in German, he makes himself understood with drawings . . .[28]
>
> *Bruno M.:*   He understands only simple words in Polish, but responds seldom to what he is told. . . .[29]
>
> *Johanna N.:*   The girl is clean, speaks only Polish and stutters. Bad manners by the table, she is eating scruffily and with her left hand . . . .[30]
>
> *Rudolf P.:*   The boy is clean. Speech unarticulated, cannot build sentences, speaks only single words. He often talks to himself in German and Polish. . . .[31]

The Polish scholar Witold Kulesza suggested that Loben served as an annihilation centre for Polish children not fit for Germanisation.[32] However, existing documentation indicates that *Kinderfachabteilung* in Loben admitted children from the whole province and occasionally from Lower Silesia[33] and other regions of the Third Reich. Moreover, due to the eventful history of the region, distinctions between Polish and German were often blurred, with division lines sometimes going across one family. Without few doubts children from Polish families constituted a considerable contingent, though due to the lack of data regarding nationality this claim cannot be definitively established.

In the records there is one documented case of a Jewish child. The boy was admitted to the clinic from an orphanage at the age of 12. A physician from Kattowitz (Katowice), who recommended institutional care, remarked that the boy was mean (*bösartig*) and would develop into a totally asocial type. "He behaves like an ape [*affen-artig*], steals, smokes and manifests a disposition to criminality. The father is apparently Jewish",[34] added the physician. After a period of observation in the clinic, Kurt Sch. was diagnosed with an acquired mental deficiency. He could write and tell a fairy tale, count up to a thousand and calculate but, as Elisabeth Hecker remarked, he demonstrated asocial features of character linked to encephalitis. Described as impertinent, naughty, showing an inclination to threaten and with a black-hearted look, in December 1942 he was transferred to the men's ward of the hospital for further observation. After half a year he was retransferred to *Kinderpflegestation*, and died on the tenth day.[35]

The criteria of the assessment of the children's value or usefulness were not medical ones. Psychiatric discourse was based on, and at the same time strengthened, the stereotypical picture of mental disorder as a social stigma, often married to poverty. Numerous case histories show how the language of psychiatric evaluation served to stigmatise certain patterns of behaviour and formulate moral judgements, rather than to build medical diagnoses and prognoses:

> In the understanding of the Law to Prevent Hereditary Burdened Progeny [*Gesetz zur Verhütung erbkranken Nachwuchses*] the boy is feebleminded even though he demonstrates certain practical skills. Deciding [factor] in the context of further education is his constant motoric restlessness and asocial character manifested by absent-mindedness, lying, stealing, sexual excitement and general ineducability. Since these character traits are closely linked to feeblemindedness, in this case significant and fundamental progress in social adjustment is impossible. On the contrary, it can be assumed that the boy will get worse.[36]

Another example reads:

> He suffers from libidinous feeblemindedness [*triebhaften Schwachsinn*], whereupon intelligence is affected much less than character. He is sexually aggressive and often suffers severe attacks of ill humour and excitement. He is, then, unresponsive and not at all fit for the community.[37]

Remarks on cleanliness, table manners, disobedience, sexuality and educability prevail in the medical histories. Stigmatising formulations, such as "bedraggled" (*verwahrlost*), bed-wetter (*Bettnässer*) and malicious (*böswillig*) pervade the language of psychiatric judgement. As remarked by Ulrich Müller and Corina Wachsmann "the language of 'Psychiatry' was initially everyday language complemented with elements of medical terminology, whereupon socially stigmatizing associations were dragged along and integrated into psychiatric assessment".[38]

Hereditary or acquired?

Observation and psychological tests were completed by a pneumoencephalogram of the child's brain. The latter painful diagnostic method was performed in almost all the children in order to establish whether the condition was hereditary or acquired. An unclear picture[39] or unsymmetrical brain cavities[40] have been interpreted as a sign of an inflammatory process, or acquired brain disease, and not bad heredity. In the case of doubts, an examination was performed twice in a very short period of time.[41] Medical histories do not provide reports of the children's response to this highly invasive procedure. It is known, however, that two patients died as a direct consequence of this diagnostic procedure.[42]

By the year 1940 a new and less invasive diagnostic tool in neurology – electroencephalography – proved to be of help as a key diagnostic method, especially to localise organic disturbances of the brain and understand convulsive disorders. In the years 1870–1920 several researchers observed that there is electrical activity of the brain cortex and that it can be recorded with a galvanometer directly throughout the brain or even unopened skull. As early as 1875 Liverpool physician – Richard Caton (1842–1926) – reported to the British Medical Association in Edinburgh that he had used a galvanometer to record electrical impulses of the brain surface in animals. In 1924 German physician and scientist Hans Berger (1873–1941) of Jena succeeded in recording the first human electroencephalogram (EEG), but it took him five years to publish a paper, which in Germany was received with incredulity and disdain. His findings were later confirmed by the British physiologist Edgar Douglas Adrian and by 1938 the EEG was internationally recognised and widely used as a diagnostic method.

The parents, assured that the procedure was safe, had to consent in writing by signing a special formula sent from the clinic:

> Your child Walter S. is feebleminded. In order to establish whether deficiency is hereditary or acquired through some disease we have to perform a Roentgen/X-ray examination of the brain after filling [the cavities] with air. I kindly ask you to sign the attached form.[43]

The archive does not contain a copy of this document, and only few letters from family members who permitted the medical examination.[44] In one instance a parental refusal was respected;[45] however, the parents expressed their doubts extremely rarely and in such cases they were persuaded to consent for the sake of the family:

> Besides, it is not a hurtful procedure and it will only help to tell whether your daughter's disease is of a hereditary or acquired character, which is extremely important for your family. Therefore refusal would be very short-sighted.[46]
>
> As far as I understand you consider taking the Rtg/X-ray picture of the skull, previously inflated with air, as a highly invasive procedure, which, in fact, it is. Your child is to be subjected to this procedure because it helps to establish with better clarity what is the primary cause of your

child's feeblemindedness. This would serve for the benefit of the whole family if it could be determined that your child's condition is possibly the consequence of the influence of some external factors.[47]

Indeed, the results of this examination not only satisfied diagnostic curiosity but, in the context of the Nazi eugenic policies, had a practical meaning for the families. In June 1942 the father of one of the victims anxiously asked for the cause of death of his child:

> On 27 January 1942 my daughter Renata [?] was transferred from Branitz to Loben, where she died on 12 March 1943. Until now I haven't been informed about the cause of her death and I need to know it urgently. Therefore I kindly ask you to issue a medical certificate. I need to present it in the Finance Office, which, on 12 June 1942 informed me that, due to the occurrence of hereditary disease in my family, I'm not any more eligible to receive child allowance. As a father of a child-rich family I'm extremely interested in knowing the cause of death and . . . whether the conducted examinations allow for the conclusion that the illness was of a hereditary character.[48]

Roentgen/X-ray apparatus was installed in Loben not earlier than April/May 1942[49] and in this case Dr Hecker recommended a request to the local public health office for a thorough examination of the medical history of the family. In Upper Silesia the registration of hereditarily ill psychiatric patients began as early as 1934[50] and the provincial hereditary health office (*Erbgesundheitsstelle*) conducted systematic genealogical studies. Until 1941 it collected "hereditary health files" on 70 per cent of the Upper Silesian population,[51] which explains why hundreds of children could be reported and transferred to the clinic for further examination within just a few months.

Depending on the results of these coercive examinations, children were further "distributed" either to correctional institutions, the juvenile reform school in Bergstadt, recommended for *NS-Jugendheimstaetten* and family care, or transferred into the children's special unit (*Kinderfachabteilung*). According to Elisabeth Hecker's statement of 14 January 1943, the majority of children examined in the Youth Psychiatric Clinic were relocated to Bergstadt. The school was also under her supervision and through this personal union had close links to the Youth Psychiatric Clinic.[52] This model was first introduced in Brandenburg-Görden, where in early 1941 Hans Heinze organised a special school (*Lebensschule*), where children who could not follow academic instruction but, however, demonstrated sufficient practical intelligence, were to be trained in simple industrial jobs, while their susceptibility to training (*Dressurfähigkeit*) could be observed.[53]

For practical reasons, to prevent the release of the child before diagnostic procedures had been completed, the costs of hospitalisation were borne by the institution, which must have been an incentive to them to consent. Initially doctors were instructed not to use force towards those parents who opposed a child's admittance to the clinic; from September 1941,[54] in case persuasive measures failed, youth offices were entitled to initiate more radical steps, including deprivation of guardianship due to the abuse of parental rights against the child's best interests.[55]

"I would be happy if you could fix my beloved child!" (Möchte ich ja freuen wenn Sie mein liebes Kind noch mal in Ordnung bringen können)

In the majority of cases the parents did not suspect what was going to happen to their children and had no intention to oppose admittance and examination. Many of them were poorly educated and living in difficult conditions, and they were easily deceived by the promise of free treatment and the prospects for the appropriate education for their child and sometimes also by the wording of the correspondence: "Based on the decision of the Provincial Lower Silesian Authorities your little daughter [*Töchterchen*] Waltraut will be admitted to our care station. We would like to know whether we should fetch your little daughter or will you bring her yourself?"[56] – reads one of the letters from the clinic. It is not surprising that in many cases families expressed no objections and in letters full of hope inquired of their child's health, daily activities and chances to get better. "I'm kindly asking how my beloved daughter Edeltraut has been doing" – wrote her mother Anna G. in May 1942 – "Maybe you could tell me whether anything has already changed? I would be really happy if you could fix my beloved child. I'm very grateful for all the efforts that you have by now made with my beloved daughter".[57] In response, Dr Hecker reassured that the child had made certain progress and can be of help in some manual works, such as clearing the table or sweeping, and so might be useful on a farm or in gardening.[58] The girl, however, was never released from institutional care and died in Loben of flu combined with pneumonia.

Many children were transferred to the Loben facility from various institutions in Silesia, fewer from other regions of the Third Reich, and their parents often did not show any interest in their fate. In some cases, however, the transfers occasionally aroused suspicions. The father of Annelise W. from Stettin, for instance, complained that within a period of seven months she had been transferred already four times and that the "uncertain fate of his child opened hardly healed, old wounds" and affected his wife's health condition. He demanded that the transfers be stopped and in a letter to Dr Hecker of 5 May 1942 he mentioned that when the child was taken from the nursing home Bethedsa in his family town of Stettin, the minister Klütz remarked that "soon this child will be liberated from its suffering and will not exist anymore".[59]

That there were rumours circulating about Loben is suggested by documented cases, when suspicious parents took steps to take the child back home. Such instances were extremely rare but possible, and determined families could sometimes be successful in their efforts.

"I didn't know that the child would be brought here" (Ich habe nicht gewußt daß das Kind hierher gebracht würde)

Margarete B., born 1933, was admitted to the clinic for the first time on 30 November 1943 because of urine and faecal incontinence. The affliction was caused by a serious surgical intervention that the child underwent in the early weeks of its life. Due to this suffering the girl often could not attend school and was sent home because of a disgusting smell. The girl came from a poor family, living in debilitating conditions with five more children, and the mother requested immediate admittance to the institution. After a few weeks of observation in the clinic she was described as a "severe case of bed wetting . . . quiet and agreeable and gladly playing with other children. During the mock lesson, attentive but learning comes with difficulties and the girl knows surprisingly little for her age". The prognosis according to Dr Hecker was unfavourable and the child was to be transferred to the "care unit". On 26 January 1944 the child was, however, released at her parents' wishes. As Elisabeth Hecker noted, the mother took no advice and wanted only to get her daughter back, arguing that the girl would undergo another surgery. The child's condition, however, did not improve and on one occasion she was again sent home from school "because of an unbearable smell". Documentation indicates that in this case a court proceeding was initiated in order to place the girl in special care and on 2 June 1944 Margarete was again admitted to the clinic.

Loben supposedly specialised in treating bed-wetting and – as Elisabeth Hecker claimed – children who suffered for years were healed within a few days. According to Hecker, the affliction was caused by the lack of will,[60] and so she introduced simple and harsh methods of treatment, namely from 4 pm no drinks and no food.[61] Since in this case the cause of the dysfunction was muscle paralysis, this disciplining therapy was abandoned and assistant physician Dr Hildegard Stanjek remarked that "due to her condition the girl was unbearable for the surrounding" and recommended her transfer to *Kinderpflegeabteilung* as "because of her suffering she was socially unfit". Surprisingly, on 7 November 1944 Margarete was again taken home. Her mother signed a statement that she had been informed of the possible consequences and was ready to take all responsibility for her decision,[62] thus ultimately saving her life.

It is not clear whether or how much her parents knew about the programme of the killing of children. There are, however, hints indicating that their determination might have been enhanced by stories possibly circulating in the local population. As Elisabeth Hecker reported, Margarete's mother kept saying that her daughter was supposed to undergo another surgery in another hospital. When asked why she did not take her daughter there at the beginning, she answered: "I did not know the child would be brought here".[63]

In another documented case Helmut K., born 1933, was released at his mother's demand in April 1943, after around one month of observation in the

Youth Psychiatric Clinic. The boy suffered from hemiplegia and – as his school report informs – he demonstrated behavioural problems. In October 1943 his mother requested institutional care for him but indicated that she was not willing to place him in the Loben facility.[64] With four more little children at home, after a few months she surrendered and in February 1944 the boy was again admitted to the Youth Psychiatric Clinic and later, in April, transferred to the children's special unit, where he died in November that year.

In the documentation a few more cases of parents who had their child released and admitted again within a few months could be identified.[65] Apart from one, all these children were born in 1933 or 1934. It remains an open question whether – being a bit older than the others – they were more aware of what was being done to other children in the unit and more actively demanded to return home? Due to the gaps in the documentation it is also impossible to know how many families sought to get their children back. Facing difficult living conditions and often having to care for younger children and serve labour duty (*Arbeitseinsatz*), the parents, particularly single mothers, were often not able to care for those children who demanded more attention. In two cases the request for release was rejected based on the suspicion – in one case aroused by a family member[66] – that the mother sought to avoid labour duty.[67] In another unsuccessful attempt, the mother was informed that "in times of war we cannot afford it, that the child constantly destroys various objects [in his surroundings], and therefore it has to be kept in the institution".[68]

When the family insisted on a child's release, Elisabeth Hecker, who reported children to the *Reichsausschuss*, tried to prompt the experts' decision regarding the so-called treatment: "It would be advisable to issue the authorisation as soon as possible, because the mother of the child keeps saying that she will not have her child here much longer".[69] Hecker not only reported children to the *Reichsausschuss* but also ordered their transfer to the *Kinderpflegestation* beforehand, although she knew that there they would be subjected to poisonous luminal treatment.[70]

"He is on luminal"

In Loben the patients received other medicaments, such as morphine and scopolamine, only occasionally. Dr Ernst Buchalik meticulously noted the doses of luminal administered in ward B in a period from 15 August 1942 to 31 October 1944. This unique source of data, titled "Medizine-Kinder-Abteilung B", contains the names of 256 children, with a precise chronicle of the doses of the drug. Children were treated with doses of luminal ranging from 0.1 g to 0.6 g per day and some received as much as 165.9 g of luminal in the whole course of this treatment. According to the expert opinion of Polish pharmacologist Tadeusz Chruściel, the single portions were not toxic but definitely overdosed. Analysis of the data revealed that in all cases the daily dose of luminal was two- to threefold of the curative one.[71] As early as 1975 Dionizy Moska suggested that the children served as experimental subjects to test the endurance and physiological response to various quantities of luminal before they were given a lethal shot.[72] The children's responses differed, depending on their general condition. Some developed considerable resistance, like eight-year-old Margot I., who survived 14 months in the *Kinderpflegestation*.[73] The majority, however, perished within five to six months due to pulmonary diseases, heart failure and intestinal catarrh. Luminal in overdoses weakened the immune system and the children easily died of various infectious diseases. It is also well known that barbiturates in high quantities lead to dysfunctions of the cardio-vascular and respiratory system and digestive tract.

Medical documentation from the Youth Psychiatric Clinic in Loben does not contain any information on luminal treatment. In only one case, the child Withold T., did Dr Hecker provide a detailed description of luminal-induced stupefaction. On 10 August 1944 the report reads:

> The boy can speak, but speech unarticulated . . . He cannot walk, stand or sit on his own, and usually remains in bed; when trying to stand up he loses his balance (he is on luminal). He cannot eat liquid meals on his own, only a slice of bread and he eats very hastily. He shows no interest in his surroundings. Not interested in other kids, he is only looking about at what is going on around him. He moves very slowly, closes his eyes constantly and does not react when he is addressed; only when approached very energetically would he wake up and look at the person. He understands everything. When asked to show his eyes, he opens them wide. Also, he can show his mouth, ears, hands and feet, but he does not say anything, not even one word. He can correctly name some objects from his surroundings, such as a table, a ball, a pencil, a window, a lamp, a picture. He speaks with difficulties. . . . When he is given a toy he would first put it into his mouth and test whether it is something to eat and then put it aside . . . He can tell the difference between some colours, namely red, blue and white. He cannot name various shapes. Should he be asked to show three fingers, he shows his whole palm.

The relatively complete file of this child illustrates not only the results of treatment with luminal but also how important in the medical evaluation were the economic criteria and moral judgements. When he was admitted to the clinic on 21 January 1943 Dr Hecker wrote:

> In this four years old boy nocturnal bed-wetting occurs relatively often. Speech unarticulated, he can pronounce single words but cannot build a sentence. He cannot dress and undress without help. However, he can eat on his own, together with other children and he plays gladly with them. He can walk. During the mock lesson he was attentive only when individually supervised, otherwise he would play with his fingers and squirm and irritate other children . . .

A few months later, on 8 April 1943, she concluded:

> Friendly, feebleminded child, whose further development is difficult to prognose at the moment. It is, however, thinkable that thanks to his friendly openness he will develop certain manual skills in the future and will be able to earn his living. Meanwhile, due to bed-wetting, socially maladjusted [*Vorläufig steht einer sozialer Einordbarkeit Bettnässen entgegen*]

Hecker's recommendation was half a year's observation in the childcare station (*Kinderpflegestation*). After more than a year, on 19 August 1944, the diagnosis of social maladjustment was confirmed by another physician, Dr Beate Sandri, who added that most of the time the boy was sexually excited.[74] Withold T. died the next day.

It is impossible to determine how many of the inmates in *Kinderpflegestation* were actually reported to the Reich Committee before they were put on luminal. Hecker ordered the transfer of children to the care station independently of and before experts' decisions. Sources also indicate that in some reported cases the children perished before the Committee ordered the so-called "treatment".[75] It remains unclear whether they died due to negligence or were poisoned with luminal on Ernst Buchalik's decision.

"A wholly in formalin preserved brain"

Death was not the final act. Both the adult and child victims of Nazi "euthanasia" served *post mortem* as research objects. Specimens of their brains and spinal cords were sent to neurological research centres for further neuropathological examination. The goal of these studies was to confirm or repudiate the clinical diagnosis, clarify the diagnostic criteria of the hereditary or acquired character of disease – increasingly a more and more popular field of study – and to observe the various forms and courses of development of neurological disorders of interest for a given scientist. Additionally, Volker Roelcke remarks, "the studies were to provide scientific criteria for rational selection of the patients and thus scientific arguments for the euthanasia programme".[76]

The pathological tradition and the idea to prove links between the clinical form of an illness and abnormalities and lesions in the internal organs go back to the late eighteenth century and the birth of anatomical pathology. However, the launching of the "euthanasia" programme brought about new opportunities for researchers, who could not only have an unprecedented steady supply of specimens – according to Jürgen Peiffer more than 2,000 brains were examined[77] – but could also actively take part in the selection of cases, which suited their own research interests. For instance, Julius Hallervorden actively decided on occasions who was to be killed by visiting various institutions and inspecting the clinical records.[78]

Major centres of brain research were established by the "T-4" organisation in 1942 in Brandenburg-Görden, under the leadership of Hans Heinze, and in the psychiatric hospital Wiesloch, in cooperation with the University Psychiatric Clinic in Heidelberg and Carl Schneider. As Paul Weindling points out "these initiatives show that the central administration of euthanasia remained in place throughout the course of the war. . . . Both the centralized T4 organization and decentralized child killing clinics were resources for experimentation and research on the murdered children's body parts".[79] It is estimated half of these units experimented on children or sent the brains on to designated research institutes.[80] The Youth Psychiatric Clinic in Loben collaborated with the third important, but less known, centre of brain studies[81] – the Neurological Research Institute in Breslau headed by Viktor von Weizsäcker (1886–1957), formerly professor of neurology in Heidelberg.

Weizsäcker assumed his position as a director of the Institute and Chair of the Neurology Clinic in Breslau in May 1941. The Chair for Neurology had been vacant since 1939, when Otfrid Foerster (1873–1941), due to his health deterioration and under certain pressure for the fact that his wife was Jewish, resigned from the post. Weizsäcker, highly respected for his work on neuroses and work therapy,[82] seemed to have been an obvious candidate for this position, despite his disinterest in active engagement in the Nazi movement.[83] However, criticism expressed by Martin Staemmler, the Rector of the University, and war circumstances, delayed the nomination.[84]

Next to nothing is known about the circumstances of the appointment[85] of the pathologist Hans Joachim Scherer (1906–45),[86] who in the years 1942–44 examined at least 217 brains shipped from the Youth Psychiatric Clinic in Loben and possibly more.[87] He arrived in Breslau at the beginning of 1942 at Weizsäcker's invitation and ran the Neuropathological Laboratory within the Institute for Neurological Research. There are no known documents that could shed light on the background of Scherer's nomination to Breslau. In the context of the intended extensive brain studies it cannot be excluded that Scherer's reputation as a talented pathologist paved his way from Belgium back to Germany and Breslau, even though "his antifascist conviction was commonly known and therefore his situation after his comeback was difficult and threatened".[88]

It also remains unclear when exactly and who initiated cooperation between the Youth Psychiatric Clinic in Loben and the Neurological Institute in Breslau. The contact must have been established by the end of March, as indicated by the standard letter from Loben to Viktor von Weizsäcker:

> Enclosed I am sending you in accordance with your letter of 25 March 1942 fixed samples of the brain and spinal cord of (patient name follows) with the request that it be examined pathologically. I enclose a summary of the medical records.

Udo Benzenhöfer and Wilhelm Rimpau have argued that "this letter is not a proof that Weizsäcker himself knew and profited from the 'euthanasia of children'".[89] However, if we take into account that until late autumn 1944

Scherer conducted on average 60 to 80 autopsies per year,[90] the sheer quantity of specimens incoming to the Neurological Institute must have aroused suspicions as to the unprecedented mortality rate in the hospital in Loben.[91] Moreover, as suggested by Jürgen Peiffer, Scherer may have been directly instructed about "euthanasia" and planned brain research in August and September 1942, when he visited Professor Julius Hallervorden in Berlin.[92] It seems highly unlikely that the head of the institution would remain uninformed of the employees' research activities.

There are no indications that Scherer received carefully selected specimens of some very specific disorders. With few exceptions all the children were diagnosed as feebleminded, sometimes with an accompanying affliction, such as hemiplegia or epilepsy, and neuropathological examination was to clarify the hereditary or acquired character of the condition. The neuropathology of any mental deficiency was not the subject of Scherer's previous studies and it seems plausible that it was Elisabeth Hecker who requested the collaboration[93] to which Viktor von Weizsäcker "declared his willingness" (*hat sich bereit erklärt*).[94]

The scientific results of brain research of Nazi "euthanasia" victims have been questioned from the methodological point of view. Peiffer pointed out that "for all these cases the natural course of disease was interrupted by the killing of the patients. Since most of the patients were starved and their health condition seriously affected by avitaminoses, we have to consider, for example, edematous or pellagroid signs. As a result, not a single case can be compared with those findings of patients who had been examined after a 'normal course' of their illness".[95] Scherer did not publish the results of studies conducted. According to one of his contemporaries, he presented his findings in a lecture at the beginning of 1944[96] claiming that he had examined 350 brains. So far 217 victims have been identified.

Do we remember?

In 2002 a cross and a plaque in commemoration of 194 children murdered at Loben were placed at the cemetery adjacent to the hospital.[97] The text reads that it is to remember 194 victims subjected to the experiments in the clinic.[98] On 1 and 2 November each year – All Saints' and All Souls' Days – typically a few candles break up the darkness. At the same time the Internet page of the clinic states only laconically that in the years 1939–45 the hospital was under German management. And the first Youth Psychiatric Ward in Poland began to operate in Lubliniec in 1951. . .with no mention about the fate of the children.

The commemoration of "euthanasia" victims in Poland seems to be secondary as compared to events such as the annihilation of the Polish intelligentsia, the Katyń massacre or simply heroic acts and strategies of survival during the occupation. Admittedly, as pointed out by Lutz Kaelber, the very first monument dedicated to the Reich Committee children was initiated as early as 1979 in the former children's special care unit Konradstein-Kocborowo,[99] but such events do not resonate widely through the public sphere. In a history of medicine seminar, a student from Lubliniec-Loben admitted that she had never heard about "child euthanasia". With very few exceptions Polish historians and physicians have paid little attention to the medical crimes against the mentally ill and disabled, even though the first publications – mostly of a statistical character – came out relatively early (see Bibliography). Lutz Kaelber observed that "when evidence of trauma and culpability contradicts elements in a local memory culture and seems to taint the entire region or goes against the grain of the local citizenery's self-image . . . it may well be ignored, denied or repressed".[100] These processes have been at work until very recently. There is a certain inclination to present the history of medicine as a chain of heroic acts and ingenious discoveries and, in consequence, the history of the medicalised killings of the most vulnerable group of patients contradicts the popular self-image of the medical profession as being the most dignified and respectable. Suppression of the remembrance of psychiatric patients came, however, not only from within the medical profession. Quoting again Lutz Kaelber "there is evidence that families do not like to identify victims in their midst, which at least in part appears to be due to the stigma attached to psychiatric disorders and that cautions such individuals to disclose anything they believe might put a black mark on their family lines and histories". Additionally, some families may have felt guilty for not providing sufficient care to their children and did not cultivate the memory of a disabled child. In 1967 the mother of a five-year-old boy, who died in Loben, gave testimony before the Central Commission for the Investigation of Nazi Crimes against Poland. She admitted that she would not be able to find his grave. And added that her second child was healthy and developed normally.[101]

Notes

1 The names of the patients needed to be anonymised. I was instructed by the State Archive in Katowice that according to Polish regulations, introduced on 25 Feb 2016 (amendment of a law of 14 July 1983), medical data may be disclosed only 100 years after the last record. In order to obtain permission to use the documents I had to sign the statement that I would not reveal any information that may violate personal rights of the patients or be seen as such.

2 Katowice, Archiwum Państwowe w Katowicach (hereafter A.P. Katowice), Oberschlesische Provinzial-Verwaltung (hereafter O.P.V.) 118, sygn.1/34, p. 12.

3 The list contains in fact 292 names – one girl Helene F. has been listed twice under the file number 32 and 53; this is only a small proportion of the patients examined in the clinic – data are scattered in various documents and to give the overall number of children hospitalised in the clinic further research is needed.

4 Medical documentation indicates that of 292 children, who were admitted to the institution, 284 certainly died, see A.P. Katowice, Jugendpsychiatrische Klinik Loben (hereafter J.P.K. Loben) 763, sygn. 1–293, passim. Additionally K. Szwajca identified 13 more victims based on the documentation held by the hospital archive. Actually Szwajca listed 14 more children but one mistakenly: Henryk Sz. has been included in the documentation held by A.P. Katowice, J.P.K. Loben 763, sygn. 9.

5 Henry Friedlander, *The Origins of Nazi Genozide. From Euthanasia to the Final Solution*, Chapel Hill and London: The University of North Carolina Press, 1995, p. 44.

6 In Silesia psychiatrist Johanes Lange (1891–1938), director of the University Psychiatric Clinic in Bresalu, launched the study in 1936. Dorothea Boeters, *Belastungsstatistik einer schlesischen Durschnittsbevölkerung*, Breslau: 1936.

7 Udo Benzenhöfer, *Kinderfachabteilungen und NS-Kindereuthanasie*, Wetzlar: GWAB Verlag, 2000, p. 84.

8 For a detailed account of the organisation and development of special psychiatric units for children see: Sascha Topp, 'Der "Reichsausschuss zur wissenschaftlichen Erfassung erb- und anlagebedingter schwerer Leiden": Zum Organisation der der Ermordung minderjähriger Kranker im Nationalsozialismus 1939–1945', in Thomas Beddies and Kristina Hübner (eds), *Kinder in NS-Psychiatrie*, Berlin: Be.bra, 2004, pp. 17–55.

9 Benzenhöfer, *Kinderfachabteilungen*, p. 82.

10 Martin Dahl, *Endstation Spiegelgrund. Die Tötung behinderter Kinder während des Nationalsozialismus am Beispiel einer Kinderfachabteilung in Wien 1940 bis 1945*, Vienna: Erasmus, 1998, p. 29, quoted in Benzenhöfer, *Kinderfachabteilungen*, p. 59.

11 Ibid., p. 21.

12 Topp, *Der Reichsausschuss*, p. 40.

13 Schultze, 'Euthanasie Verbrechen in Oberschlesien', in Maike Rotzoll *et al.* (eds), *Die nationalsozialistische "Euthanasie" – Aktion "T4" und ihre Opfer. Geschichte und ethische Konsequenzen für die Gegenwart*, Paderborn: Ferdinand Schöningh, 2010, p. 183.

14 Opole, Archiwum Państwowe w Opolu, Rejencja Opolska I, sygn. 13 701, p. 34.

15 Ibid., pp. 41–43.

16 On Hecker's biography see: Wilfried Huck, 'Wunden der Erinnerung. Eine künstlerischeAnnäherung an das Phänomenon Kindereuthansie am Beispiel vom Elisabeth Hecker, erste Direktorin der Westphälischen Klinik für Jugendpszchiatrie, Gütersloh ab 1965 Hamm', *Mitteilungen des Landesjugendamtes*, 146 (2001), pp. 67–77; Matthias Dahl, 'Dr Elisabeth Hecker (1895–1986): Verdienste als Kinder- und Psychiaterin einerseits – Beteiligungan der Ausmerzung Behinderter andererseits', *Kinderpsychologie und Kinderpsychiatrie*, 52 (2003), pp. 98–108.

17 On 3 Dec 1942 Elisabeth Hecker reported that the "clinic's capacity of 60 beds allowed one to examine 400 children within fourteen months" which may suggest that the facility had operated since late Sept 1941, see A.P. Katowice, O.P.V. 118, sygn. 5266, p. 98. K. Szwajca dates the opening to 25 Sept 1941, when the first transport of children from Lower Silesia arrived in Loben, se K. Szwajca, 'Eksterminacja dzieci w Szpitalu Psychiatrycznym w Lublińcu w latach 1942–1945', *Szkice Lublinieckie*, 5 (2000), p. 25; the first so-called *Reichsausschuss* child was admitted in December 1941, see Udo Benzenhoeffer, *Der Arztphilosoph Viktor von Weizsäcker*, Göttingen: Vandenhoeck-Ruprecht, 2007, p. 154.

18 A.P. Katowice, O.P.V. 118, sygn. 5266, pp. 67–82; one document held in the Archive in Katowice suggests that there were plans to open one more *Jugendpsychiatrische Klinik* in Kęty (Liebenswerde) – in Nov 1944 Dr Hecker requested the nomination of Dr Paula Werth as head (*Oberarztin*) in Kęty. It is not clear whether another killing station was also planned, see A.P. Katowice, O.P.V. 118, sygn. 656, p. 8.

19 Ibid., sygn. 5266, p.101.

20 Ibid., sygn. 5767, p. 1.

21 Ibid., sygn. 5266, p. 100/101.

22 Ibid., p. 26.

23 The authors of the first publications suggested Nov 1941 – the first recorded death, see Kazimiera Marxen and Hipolit Latyński, 'Dane ze sposobów leczenia dzieci upośledzonych umysłowo, na oddziale B przy Klinice Dziecięcej w Zakładzie Psychiatrycznym w Lublińcu, które to leczenie można traktować jako eutanazję', *Rocznik Psychiatryczny*, 1 (1949), p. 63. E. Hecker dated the opening to 1941/1942, see Huck, 'Wunden der Erinnerung', p. 71.

24 Paweł Lisiewicz, ' "Casus Buchalik" jako zagadnienie unicestwiania dzieci w zakładzie psychiatrycznym na terenie Lublińca', in Andrzej Szefer (ed.), *Śląsk i Zagłębie Dąbrowskie w walce z okupantem hitlerowskim 1939–1945: Materiały z sesji naukowej zorganizowanej w 30 rocznicę najazdu hitlerowskiego na Polskę*, Katowice: Śląski Instytut Naukowy, 1969, p. 187; Dionizy Moska, 'Eksterminacja w zakładzie "Loben" ', *Przegląd Lekarski*, 1 (1975), p. 112.

25 The first record in medical documentation regarding transfer to *Kinderpflegestation* ("verlegt nach Kinderpflegestation") can be dated to July 1942, see A.P. Katowice, J.P.K. Loben 763, sygn. 38; it should also be noted that Aug 1942 saw a dramatic increase in the mortality rate – 23 children died compared to 6–7 deaths per month from Jan to July. Later the mortality rate was on average 9–11 deaths per month, see A.P. Katowice, J.P.K. Loben 763, passim.

26 A similar situation was in Vienna, see Martin Dahl, *Endstation Spiegelgrund*, quoted in Herwig Czech, 'Nazi Euthanasia Crimes in Second-World War Austria', *The Holocaust in History and Memory*, 5 (2012), p. 59.

27 A.P. Katowice, O.P.V. 118, sygn. 5266, p. 98.

28 Ibid., J.P.K. Loben 763, sygn. 231.

29 Ibid., sygn. 225.

30 Ibid., sygn. 123.

31 Ibid., sygn.131.

32 W. Kulesza, ' "Euthanasie" – Morde an polnischen Psychiatriepatient/innen während des zweiten Weltkriegs', in Rotzoll *et al.*, *Die nationalsozialistische "Euthanasie"*, p. 177.

33 "The child Emma S. has been brought here on the order of the Reich Committee, despite that she is from Lower Silesia, and whose admittance to our special care unit we tried to avoid until now", see A.P. Katowice, J.P.K. Loben 763, sygn. 167, p. 6.

34 This information is underlined in the document, see ibid., sygn. 35, p. 23.

35 Ibid., pp. 22–27.

36 Ibid., sygn. 41, p. 12.

37 Ibid., sygn. 31, p. 10

38 Ulrich Müller and Corina Wachsman, 'Krankenakten als Lebensgeschichten', in Rotzoll *et al.*, *Die nationalsozialistische "Euthanasie"*, p. 193.

39 A.P. Katowice, J.P.K. Loben 763, sygn. 63, p.4.

40 Ibid., sygn. 24, p.15

41 Ibid., sygn. 162, p.6

42 Ibid., sygn. 171 and 226

43 Ibid., sygn. 121, p.18

44 Ibid., sygn. 205; and Berlin, Bundesarchiv Berlin (hereafter BAB), R 96 I/Anhang, Bd. 1, Akte 95.

45 At the end of Aug 1942 the mother of Hans Sch. investigated the cause of his death, suspecting some kind of invasive operation. In response she was informed that no surgical treatment was performed on her child and that the Roentgen/X-ray picture could not be taken because she did not consent, see A.P. Katowice, J.P.K. Loben 763, sygn. 254.

46 Ibid., sygn. 218, p. 20.

47 A month later the mother received the results of the examination, see ibid., sygn. 24, pp. 15 and 22.

48 Ibid., sygn. 277, p. 9.

49 Ibid., sygn. 203, p. 24; sygn. 277, p. 9.

50 Kamila Uzarczyk, *Podstawy ideologiczne higieny ras i ich realizacja na Śląsku w latach 1924–44*, Toruń: Marszałek, 2002, pp. 144–151.

51 'Auf den Spuren des Sippenforschers', *Schlesische Tageszeitung* (16 Apr 1941) in Wrocław, Archiwum Państwowe we Wrocławiu, Zbiór Wycinków Prasowych, sygn. 283, p. 3, quoted in Uzarczyk, *Podstawy higieny ras*, p. 147. See also eadem, 'Rassenpolitik und "Erbgesundheit" ', in Axel C. Hüntelmann, Johannes Vossen and Herwig Czech (eds),

Gesundheit und Staat. Studien zur Geschichte der Gesundheitsämter in Deutschland,
1870–1950, Husum: Matthiesen Verlag, 2006, pp. 228–231.

52 A.P. Katowice, O.P.V. 118, sygn. 5767, p.7.

53 Hans-Walther Schmuhl, 'Hirnforschung und Krankenmord. Kaiser-Wilhelm- Institut
für Hirnforschung 1937–1945', *Vorabdrucke aus dem Forschungsprogramm Geschichte des
KWG im NS, Ergebnisse 1,* Berlin: 2000, p. 44.

54 Idem, 'Die Patientenmorde', in Angelika Ebbinghaus and Klaus Dörner (eds), *Vernichten
und Heilen. Der Nürnberg Ärzteprozeß und seine Folgen,* Berlin: AtV, 2000, p. 302.

55 A.P. Katowice, O.P.V. 118, sygn. 5266, p. 62.

56 Ibid., sygn. 169, p. 55.

57 Ibid., sygn. 174, p. 23.

58 Ibid., p. 22.

59 Ibid., sygn. 205, p. 15.

60 Ibid., sygn. 5266, p. 98.

61 Ibid., sygn. 5763, p. 105.

62 Ibid., J.P.K. Loben 763, sygn. 265, passim.

63 Ibid., p. 12.

64 Ibid., sygn. 185, p. 53

65 Ibid., sygn. 44, 79, 225, 227

66 Ibid., sygn. 15, p.4

67 Ibid., sygn. 10, p. 5.

68 Ibid., sygn. 104, p. 9.

69 Matthias Dahl, 'Dr Elisabeth Hecker', p. 105.

70 Ibid., p. 102.

71 Paweł Lisiewicz, 'Zbrodnie na dzieciach i młodzieży popełnione w szpitalu
psychiatrycznym w Lublińcu', in Czesław Pilichowski (ed.), *Zbrodnie i sprawcy.
Ludobójstwo hitlerowskie przed sądem ludzkości i historii,* Warsaw: PWN, 1980, p. 591.

72 Moska, 'Eksterminacja', p. 114.

73 A.P. Katowice, J.P.K. Loben 763, sygn. 147.

74 BAB, R 96 I/Anhang, Bd. 1, nr 94.

75 For example: A.P. Katowice, J.P.K. Loben 763, sygn. 8, 9, 100 and 120.

76 Volker Roelcke, 'Psychiatrische Wissenschaft im Kontext nationalsozialistischer Politik
und "Euthanasie": Zur Rolle von Ernst Rüdin und der Deutschen Forschungsanstalt/
Kaiser-Wilhelm-Institut für Psychiatrie', in Doris Kaufmann (ed.), *Die Kaiser-Wilhelm-
Gesellschaft im Nationalsozialismus: Bestandsaufnahme und Perspektiven der Forschung,*
Göttingen: Wallstein, 2000, p. 137.

77 Jürgen Peiffer, 'Assessing neuropathological research carried out on victims of the
"Euthanasia" programme. With two lists of publications from the institutes in Berlin,
Munich and Hamburg', *Medizinhistorisches Journal,* 34 (1999), p. 350.

78 Paul Weindling, *Victims and Survivors of Nazi Human Experiments. Science and Suffering
in the Holocaust,* London: Bloomsbury, 2015, p. 35.

79 Ibid., p. 36.

80 Ibid.

81 Karl Heinz Roth, 'Psychosomatische Medizin und "Euthanasie": Der Fall Viktor
von Weizsäcker', in *Zeitschrift für Sozialgeschichte des 20. und 21. Jahrhunderts,* 1 (1986),
p. 86.

82 Wrocław, Archiwum Uniwersytetu Wrocławskiego, S 220 (Viktor von Weizsäcker
file), p.10.

83 In Carl Schneider's words "his attitude towards the movement was dispassionate but
absolutely loyal", see Jürgen Peiffer, *Hirnforschung in Deutschland 1849–1974. Briefe zur
Entwicklung von Psychiatrie und Neurowissenschaften sowie zum Einfluss des politischen
Umfelds auf Wissenschaftler,* Berlin and Heidelberg: Springer, 2004, quoted in Ernst Klee,
Euthanasie im Dritten Reich. Die "Vernichtung lebensunwerten Lebens", Frankfurt am Main:

Fischer Taschenbuch Verlag, 2010, p. 371. See also Wilhelm Rimpau, 'Viktor von Weizsäcker im Nationalsozialismus', in Gerrit Hohendorf and Achim Magull-Seltenreich (eds), *Von der Heilkunde zu Massentoetung. Medizin im Nationalsozialismus*, Heidelberg: Wunderhorn, 1990, pp. 113–130.

84 For a detailed account on the proceedings, see: Udo Benzenhöfer, 'Viktor von Weizsäcker und Breslau', *Jahrbuch der Schlesischen Friedrich Wilhelms Universität zu Breslau*, 26–27 (1995–96), pp. 454–465 and Udo Benzenhoefer, 'Die Berufung Viktor von Weizsäckers auf der Lehrstuhl für Neurologie in Breslau 1941', *Forschritte der Neurologie und Psychiatrie*, 61 (1994), pp. 438–444.

85 The University Archive does not hold his personal file, he is not even listed on the list of employees. The archivist explained it to me that at this point – 1942 – the archive was not systematically collecting documentation; besides the documents may have been destroyed during the last days of the war.

86 On Scherer's life and work see: Jürgen Peiffer, *Hirnforschung im Zwielicht. Beispiele verführbarer Wissenschaft aus der Zeit des Nationalsozialismus*, Husum: Mathiasen, 1997, pp. 56–70; Anonymous, 'Hans Joachim Scherer', Internet page of Institut Born-Bunge Universiteit Antwerpen (accessed 4 Sept 2013).

87 Peiffer reported after Zulch that Scherer had examined 350 brains of children; the existing documentation holds 217 autopsy reports signed by Scherer.

88 Viktor von Weizsäcker also declared that Scherer was forced to return to Germany because there was a lack of physicians there, see Marc Scherer, 'Letter to the editor: some comments on the paper "Hans Joachim Scherer (1906–45) – pioneer in glioma research"', *Brain Pathology*, 23 (2013), p. 485.

89 Udo Benzenhoefer and Wilhelm Rimpau, 'Introduction to Viktor von Weizsäcker: Euthanasia and experiments on human beings', in Karin Finsterbusch, Armin Lange and K.F. Diethard Römheld (eds), *Human Sacrifice in Jewish and Christian Tradition*, Leiden and Boston: Brill, 2007, p. 279; Benzenhöfer, 'Viktor von Weizsäcker und Breslau', pp. 464–465.

90 66 in 1942, 81 in 1943, 77 in 1944, see A.P. Katowice, J.P.K. Loben 763, passim.

91 FA, former assistant in the Institute, admitted that increasing frequency of shipments from Loben raised questions, see Rimpau, 'Viktor von Weizsäcker im Nationalsozialismus', p. 120.

92 Peiffer, *Hirnforschung im Zwielicht*, p. 71.

93 Benzenhöffer, *Arztphilosoph Viktor von Weizsäcker*, p. 160; idem, 'Viktor von Weizsäcker und Breslau', p. 465.

94 E. Hecker, 'Die Jugendpsychiatrische Klinik', *Archiv für Rasse u Gesselschaftsbiologie einschl. Rassen- u Gessleschaftshygiene*, 37 (1943/44), s. 183; quoted also in Klee, *Euthanasie im Dritten Reich*, p. 372.

95 Peiffer, 'Assessing neuropathological research', p. 350.

96 Idem, *Hirnforschung in Zwielicht*, p. 70.

97 Lutz Kaelber, 'Gedenken an die NS-"Kindereuthanasie" Verbrechen in Deutschland, Österreich, Tschechischen Republik und Polen', in idem and Raimond Reiter, *Kindermord und "Kinderfachabteilungen" im Nationalsozialismus. Gedenken und Forschung*, Frankfurt am Main: Peter Lang, 2011, p. 59

98 This number refers to those children whose names feature in the infamous luminal booklet. According to the author's calculation, the number of children who died at Loben amounts to 297; however, it remains unclear whether some of them died due to negligence and withdrawal of treatment or were poisoned with luminal.

99 Lutz Kaelber, 'Child Murder in Nazi Germany: The Memory of Nazi Medical Crimes and Commemoration of Children's Euthanasia Victims at Two Facilities (Eichberg, Kalmenhof)', *Societies*, 2 (2012), p. 179.

100 Ibid., p. 174.

101 A.P. Katowice, J.P.K. Loben 763, sygn. 13, p. 10.

Bibliography

Archival sources

Germany

Berlin, Bundesarchiv Berlin (BAB), R 96 I/Anhang

Poland

Katowice, Archiwum Państwowe w Katowicach (A.P. Katowice):
Jugendpsychiatrische Klinik Loben (JP.K. Loben) 763, sygn. 1–293
Oberschlesische Provinzial Verwaltung (O.P.V.) 118, sygn. 446–656; 5266–5816; dopływ sygn. 1/10–1/106
Opole, Archiwum Państwowe w Opolu, Rejencja Opolska I, sygn. 13 701
Wrocław, Archiwum Państwowe we Wrocławiu, Zbiór Wycinków Prasowych, sygn. 248
Wrocław, Archiwum Uniwersytetu Wrocławskiego, sygn. S 220

Literature

Benzenhöffer, Udo, 'Die Berufung Viktor von Weizsäckers auf der Lehrstuhl für Neurologie in Breslau 1941', *Forschritte der Neurologie und Psychiatrie*, 61 (1994), pp. 438–444
—— 'Viktor von Weizsäcker und Breslau', *Jahrbuch der Schlesischen Friedrich-Wilhelm Universitaet zu Breslau*, 26–27 (1995–96), pp. 454–465
—— *Der Arztphilosoph Viltor von Weizsäcker*, Göttingen: Vandenhoeck-Ruprecht, 2007
—— and Wilhelm Rimpau, 'Introduction to Viktor v Weizsaecker: Euthanasia and experiments on human beings', in Karin Finsterbusch, Armin Lange and K.F. Diethard Römheld (eds), *Human sacrifice in Jewish and Christian tradition*, Leiden and Boston: Brill, 2007, pp. 277–284
Czech, Herwig, 'Nazi Euthanasia Crimes in Second-World War Austria', *The Holocaust in History and Memory*, 5 (2012), pp. 51–73
Dahl, Matthias, 'Dr Elisabeth Hecker (1895–1986): Verdienste als Kinder- und Psychiaterin einerseits – Beteiligungan der Ausmerzung Behinderter andererseits', *Kinderpsychologie und Kinderpsychiatrie*, 52 (2003), pp. 98–108
Danforth, Scot, *The Incomplete Child. An Intellectual History of Learning Disabilities*, New York: Peter Lang, 2009
Friedlander, Henry, *The Origins of Nazi Genocide. From Euthanasia to the Final Solution*, Chapel Hill and London: The University of North Carolina Press, 1995
Haack, Kathleen, Frank Häßler and Ekkehardt Kumbier, 'Irgendeine angenehme Seite ist bei dem Jungen nicht zu entdecken. Aspekte der Kindereuthanasie in Schlesien', *Kinderpsychologie und Kinderpsychiatrie*, 62 (2013), pp. 391–404
Hecker, Elisabeth, 'Die Jugendpsychiatrische Klinik', *Archiv für Rassen- u Gesellschaftsbiologie einschl. Rassen- u Gesellschaftshygiene*, 37 (1943/44), pp. 180–184
Huck, Wilfried, 'Wunden der Errinerung. Eine künstlerische Annäherung an das Phänomenon Kindereuthanasie am Beispiel vom Elisabeth Hecker, erste Direktorin der Westphälischen Klinik für Jugendpsychiatrie, Gütersloh ab 1965 Hamm', *Mitteilungen des Landesjugendamtes*, 146 (2001), pp. 67–77

Jaroszewski, Zdzisław (ed.), *Pacjenci i pracownicy szpitali psychiatrycznych w Polsce zamordowani przez okupanta hitlerowskiego i los tych szpitali w latach 1939–1945*, Vol.1–2, Warsaw: PTP, 1989

—— *Zagłada chorych psychicznie w Polsce. Die Ermordung der Geisteskranken in Polen 1939–1945*, Warsaw: PWN, 1993

Kaelber, Lutz, 'Gedenken an die "NS-Kindereuthanasie", Verbrechen in Deutschland, Österreich, Tschechischen Republik und Polen"', in Lutz Kaelber and Raimond Reiter, *Kindermord und "Kinderfachabteilungen" im Nationalsozialismus. Gedenken und Forschung*, Frankfurt am M: Peter Lang, 2011, 33–67

—— 'Child Murder in Nazi Germany: The Memory of Nazi Medical Crimes and Commemoration of Child Euthanasia Victims at Two Facilities (Eichberg, Kalmenhof)', *Societies*, 2 (2012), pp. 157–194.

—— 'Jewish Children with Disabilities and Nazi Euthanasia Crimes', *The Bulletin of the Carolyn and Leonard Miller Center for Holocaust Studies*, 17 (2013), pp. 17–23

Klee, Ernst, *Euthanasie im Dritten Reich. Die "Vernichtung lebensunwerten Lebens"*, Frankfurt am Main: Fischer Taschenbuch Verlag, 2010

Kulesza, Witold, ' "Euthanasie" – Morde an polnischen Psychiatriepatient/innen während des zweiten Weltkriegs', in Maike Rotzoll, Gerrit Hohendorf, Petra Fuchs, Paul Richter, Christoph Mundt and Wolfgang U. Eckart (eds), *Die nationalsozialistische "Euthanasie" – Aktion "T4" und ihre Opfer. Geschichte und ethische Konsequenzen für die Gegenwart*, Paderborn: Ferdinand Schöningh, 2010, pp. 175–178

Lisiewicz, Paweł, ' "Casus Buchalik" jako zagadnienie unicestwiania dzieci w zakładzie psychiatrycznym na terenie Lublińca', in Andrzej Szefer (ed.), *Śląsk i Zagłębie Dąbrowskie w walce z okupantem hitlerowskim 1939–45*, Katowice: SIN, 1970, pp. 187–191

—— 'Zbrodnie na dzieciach i młodzieży popełnione w szpitalu psychiatrycznym w Lublińcu', in Czesław Pilichowski (ed.), *Zbrodnie i sprawcy. Ludobójstwo hitlerowskie przed sadem ludzkości i historii*, Warsaw: PWN, 1980, pp. 589–595

Marxen, Kazimiera and Hipolit Latyński, 'Dane ze sposobów leczenia dzieci upośledzonych umysłowo, na oddziale B przy Klinice Dziecięcej w Zakładzie Psychiatrycznym w Lublińcu, które to leczenie można traktować jako eutanazję', *Rocznik Psychiatryczny*, 1 (1949), pp. 113–116

Moska, Dionizy, 'Eksterminacja w zakładzie "Loben" ', *Przegląd Lekarski*, 1 (1975), pp. 112–114

Müller, Ulrich and Corina Wachsmann, 'Krankenakten als Lebensgeschichten', in Maike Rotzoll, Gerrit Hohendorf, Petra Fuchs, Paul Richter, Christoph Mundt and Wolfgang U. Eckart (eds), *Die nationalsozialistische "Euthanasie" – Aktion "T4" und ihre Opfer. Geschichte und ethische Konsequenzen für die Gegenwart*, Paderborn: Ferdinand Schöningh, 2010, pp. 190–199

Nasierowski, Tadeusz, *Zagłada osób z zaburzeniami psychicznymi w okupowanej Polsce. Początek ludobójstwa*, Warsaw: Neriton, 2008

—— 'Trzeba nieść tę noc . . . dlaczego i jak upamiętnić ofiary tanazji przewrotnie zwanej eutanazją', in Tadeusz Nasierowski, Grażyna Herczyńska and Dariusz Myszka (eds), *Zagłada chorych psychicznie. Pamięć i historia*, Warsaw: Eneteia, 2012, pp. 523–529

Peiffer, Jürgen, 'Assessing neuropathological research carried out on victims of the "Euthanasia" programme. With two lists of publications from the institutes in Berlin, Munich and Hamburg', *Medizinhistorisches Journal*, 34 (1999), pp. 339–335

—— *Hirnforschung im Zwielicht. Beispiele verführbarer Wissenschaft aus der Zeit des National-sozialismus*, Husum: Mathiasen, 1997

Rimpau, Wilhelm, 'Viktor von Weizsäcker im Nationalsozialismus', in Gerrit Hohendorf and Achim Magull-Seltenreich (eds), *Von der Heilkunde zu Massentoetung. Medizin im Nationalsozialismus*, Heidelberg: Wunderhorn, 1990, pp. 113–130

Roelcke, Volker, Gerrit Hohendorf and Maike Rotzoll, 'Psychiatric Research and "Euthanasia". The case of the Psychiatric Department at the University of Heidelberg, 1941–1945', *History of Psychiatry*, 5 (1994), pp. 517–532

—— 'Erbpsychologische Forschung im Kontext der "Euthanasie": neue Dokumente und Aspekte zu Carl Schneider, Julius Deussen und Ernst Rüdin', *Fortschrittte der Neurologie und Psychiatrie*, 66 (1998), pp. 331–336

Roth, Karl Heinz, 'Psychosomatische Medizin und "Euthanasie": Der Fall Viktor von Weizsäcker', *Zeitschrift für Sozialgeschichte des 20. und 21. Jahrhunderts*, 1 (1986), pp. 65–99

Scherer, Marc, 'Letter to the editor: some comments on the paper "Hans Joachim Scherer (1906–1945) – pioneer in glioma research"', *Brain Pathology*, 23 (2013), pp. 485–487

Schmuhl, Hans-Walther, *Hirnforschung und Krankenmord. Das Kaiser-Wilhelm- Institut für Hirnforschung 1937–1945. Vorabdrucke aus dem Forschungsprogramm Geschichte des KWG im NS, Ergebnisse 1*, Berlin: Impressum, 2000

—— 'Die Patientenmorde', in Angelika Ebbinghaus and Klaus Dörner (eds), *Vernichten und Heilen. Der Nürnberg Ärzteprozeß und seine Folgen*, Berlin: AtV, 2000, pp. 295–328

Schultze, Dietmar, 'Euthanasie Verbrechen in Oberschlesien', in Maike Rotzoll, Gerrit Hohendorf, Petra Fuchs, Paul Richter, Christoph Mundt and Wolfgang U. Eckart (eds), *Die nationalsozialistische "Euthanasie" – Aktion "T4" und ihre Opfer. Geschichte und ethische Konsequenzen für die Gegenwart*, Paderborn: Ferdinand Schöningh, 2010, pp. 179–183

Szwajca, Krzysztof, 'Eksterminacja dzieci w Szpitalu Psychiatrycznym w Lublińcu w latach 1942–1945', *Szkice Lublinieckie*, 5 (2000), pp. 24–30

Topp, Sascha, 'Der "Reichsausschuß zur wissenschaftlichen Erfassung erb- und anlagebedingter schwerer Leiden": Zur Organisation der Ermordung minderjähriger Kranker im Nationalsozialismus 1939–1945', in Thomas Beddies and Kristina Hübner (eds), *Kinder in NS Psychiatrie*, Berlin: Be.bra, 2004, pp. 17–55

Uzarczyk, Kamila, *Podstawy ideologiczne higieny ras i ich realizacja na przykładzie Śląska w latach 1924–1944*, Toruń: Marszałek, 2002

—— 'Rassenpolitik und "Erbgesundheit"', in Axel C. Hüntelmann, Johannes Vossen and Herwig Czech (eds), *Gesundheit und Staat. Studien zur Geschichte der Gesund-heitsämter in Deutschland, 1870–1950*, Husum: Matthiesen Verlag, 2006, pp. 221–236

—— 'Niechciane dzieci nazizmu: eugeniczna eutanazja w Dziecięcej Klinice Psychiatrycznej w Lublińcu (1942–44)', in Andrzej Furdal (ed.), *Problemy Współczesnej Tanatologii*, Wrocław: WTN, 2012, pp. 203–211

Weindling, Paul Julian, *Nazi Medicine and the Nuremberg Trials. From Medical War Crimes to Informed Consent*, Houndmills, Basingstoke: Palgrave Macmillan, 2004

—— *Victims and Survivors of Nazi Human Experiments. Science and Suffering in the Holocaust*, London: Bloomsbury, 2015

Part Three

Concentration camps

10 Children as victims of medical experiments in concentration camps

Astrid Ley

The news spread like wildfire through the Sachsenhausen Concentration Camp: Children had arrived. Not just juveniles, like those housed in the Youth Block, but real children – still of school age. This hadn't happened yet in the camp. They were now supposedly in the store. They put the youngest boy on the table there – he was so small. The old campmates who saw the children there were shaken and struck by the sight. Tears ran down the cheeks of one old campmate. That was how I got the first news of the arrival of these eleven Jewish children in the Sachsenhausen camp. . . . A deep unrest could be felt in the camp, because everybody sensed that the destiny of these eleven children would be a terrible one. What were these children doing here?[1]

The 11 young boys, whose arrival so shocked the prisoners of Sachsenhausen, had been earmarked for medical experiments to identify the pathogens of hepatitis (jaundice). There had been human experiments on prisoners in nearly all concentration camps since the beginning of the war. Some had been carried out on behalf of the SS or the *Wehrmacht* (German Army); some were the initiative of scientists themselves from civil research institutions in order to be able to test new vaccinations on camp prisoners.[2] In the experiments, the physicians basically treated their test subjects like animals, who, for research purposes, were infected with dangerous diseases or surgically mutilated. Furthermore, the medical researchers took the eventuality of lethal outcomes in the course of the testing into account. In some cases, the death of the subject was even a planned part of the experiment. Despite the brutal testing practices and their ethical reprehensibility, these experiments cannot be considered as senseless, pseudo-medical cruelty, as most of them corresponded in terms of their purposes and methods to the state of scientific practice at that time.[3]

Initially exclusively grown men were used as test subjects for such experiments, primarily Polish, Jewish, Soviet and German concentration camp inmates.[4] From the summer of 1942, the Nazis also used female prisoners, e.g. in the sulphonamide tests in Ravensbrück and the sterilisation experiments in Auschwitz. As the war persisted, even children were finally misused in concentration camps for medical experiments. The immunologist Dr Arnold Dohmen

(1906–80) undertook hepatitis experiments on the 11 Jewish boys mentioned above in Sachsenhausen from September 1944. In January 1945, the lung specialist Dr Kurt Heißmeyer (1905–67) deliberately infected 20 Jewish children in the Neuengamme Concentration Camp for test purposes with tuberculosis pathogens. The geneticist Dr Josef Mengele (1911–79), who was the camp physician in Auschwitz from May 1943, carried out genetic research on twin children there.

Why were experiments made on children in concentration camps?

Experiments with concentration camp prisoners began immediately after the beginning of the war in the autumn of 1939. That children were first involved as of mid-1943, i.e. relatively late, in such experiments, allows the presumption that the concentration camp experiments on children were the apex of morally uninhibited research in the "Third Reich", in which children, particularly Jewish children, were "considered as a type of 'subhuman' species".[5] Yet the selection of the groups of persons misused for experiments in the individual phases of the war did not follow any linear development leading from men to women to children. Even in the later years of the war, a significant portion of experiments was conducted on men. To trace the reasons for the experiments on children, it is therefore worthwhile to investigate how the test subjects were selected and what interests were affected. To do so, it is indispensable to consider things, at least in part, from the perspective of the perpetrators.

For physicians who wanted to use the special possibilities of the concentration camp for ethically uninhibited research, there were three ways to request prisoners as test subjects for scientific projects: via the SS *Ahnenerbe* Association that carried out from 1942 human experiments that were "important for the war effort", via "SS Reich Physician" Dr Ernst Grawitz (1899–1945), whose scope of responsibilities included medical tests in concentration camps, or via Heinrich Himmler (1900–45) himself, if the relevant researcher had personal access to him. Himmler was responsible for deciding about such requests. Grawitz presented Himmler recommendations, often together with the opinion of a high-ranking Nazi doctor, such as Professor Dr Karl Brandt (1904–48), Hitler's Commissioner for Sanitation and Health.[6] When approving the experiments, Himmler also determined the prisoner groups from which the test subjects to be used should come.

Officially Himmler thus decided in each case what types of prisoners were to be used for experiments. In fact, however, the participants executing the experiments had a certain degree of leeway, as can be shown by the example of the experiments on the 11 boys in Sachsenhausen.[7] The immunologist and Medical Corps' Captain Arnold Dohmen, whose experiments will be discussed below, had carried out experimental studies since the start of 1942 as an employee of the Academy for Military Doctors of Berlin in order to identify the pathogen causing hepatitis, which was still unknown at that time. He had succeeded in culturing a germ that produced symptoms of jaundice in animal experiments. Dohmen then wanted to clarify by experiments on humans whether he, in fact, had succeeded in isolating the hepatitis pathogen. Once Karl Brandt advocated the experiments, Grawitz requested Himmler on 1 June 1943 "obediently for a decision" whether Dohmen could carry out the planned experiments "in the prisoners' infirmary of the Sachsenhausen Concentration Camp".[8] Himmler approved this, stating in writing, "that eight criminals under the sentence to death in Auschwitz (eight Jews sentenced to death from the Polish resistance) were to be used for the tests".[9]

Nearly two weeks later, however, Dohmen selected 12 boys in Auschwitz for his experiments, of which 11 were later transferred to Sachsenhausen.[10] As Himmler required, these were Jews from Poland, but they definitively were not resistance members who had been sentenced to death. Dohmen's actions point towards a certain amount of leeway with respect to the selection of test subjects.

When determining test subjects for a research project, the interests of two parties were affected: those of the experimenting physicians and those of the concentration camp command on site. The physicians were interested in obtaining healthy prisoners in a sound state of nutrition, so that their test results would not be influenced by sickness or weaknesses. Moreover, the subject group had to be comparable in terms of gender and age.[11] For infection tests, prisoners without respective prior disease were sought if possible so as to rule out immunities against the relevant pathogen. The different concentration camp commands met these requirements until 1942 by providing suitable male inmates. After this time, however, physically strong and healthy prisoners, who were thus capable of working, were needed for other purposes. After the failure of the "*Blitzkrieg* Strategy" in the winter of 1941/42 in front of Moscow, the function of the concentration camps changed. To assure weapons production, the Nazis used a much higher quantity of concentration camp prisoners as forced labourers. The camps became a "labour reserve" for the German war industry.[12] In this situation, further groups of prisoners came into the focus of the aforementioned parties: in addition to women also children, who were now being handed over in greater numbers to the SS in the concentration camps since the start of the mass deportations in the course of the "Final Solution".

While the children deported with their families to Auschwitz were uninteresting for the concentration camp command as labourers, they generally did meet the physicians' requirements. Based on their young age and the resulting low probability of prior diseases, children were obviously deliberately chosen by the physicians for infection experiments. As Saul Oren-Hornfeld (born 1929), one of Dohmen's test victims, later recounted, the immunologist selected his young subjects in Auschwitz himself from an arriving transport. On the ramp, he asked them: "Children, were you sick? Did you have jaundice?" When the children failed to understand, he pointed to the yellow star on their clothes. "That", Oren said, "we understood".[13]

As with Dohmen's experiments, the test subjects were deliberately infected with disease germs in Kurt Heißmeyer's TB experiments in Neuengamme Concentration Camp. In this case, too, children who had just arrived at Auschwitz without any detrimental histories of internment and who were relatively unlikely to have immunity against the pathogen were selected for testing. Likewise in this case, logical test-related reasons were likely decisive in selecting children as test subjects. And even with Mengele's camp studies on twins, the selection of the subjects resulted from the question being studied. In the experiments, pairs of twins deported to Auschwitz were examined and autopsied in comparative terms. In contrast to child twins, adult twins rarely arrived at the camp together.

In the following, the experiments of the three physicians on children will be shortly depicted, with main emphasis on Dohmen's experiments in Sachsenhausen.

Hepatitis experiments on Jewish boys in Sachsenhausen

As explained in the report cited at the outset from the former medical orderly Bruno Meyer, 11 Jewish boys arrived at the Sachsenhausen Concentration Camp in August 1943. The youngest was eight, the oldest 23 years old. Most were between 12 and 16. Two months before, the boys had been transported with their families from the city of Będzin (Upper Silesia), whose Jewish population was almost completely exterminated by the Nazis, to Auschwitz. Every one of them lost relatives in Auschwitz, most their entire families.

For unknown reasons, Dohmen only began to experiment on the boys in September 1944. The tests were to prove that hepatitis, which was still largely unresearched at the time, was an infectious disease.[14] As explained, Dohmen had isolated a pathogen that came into consideration as a cause in earlier laboratory experiments on animals. He infected some of the boys in Sachsenhausen with this and undertook a biopsy of the liver. Because the medical orderly Bruno Meyer later reported on the experiments in detail, we are well informed about their course. In addition, Meyer's report impressively shows the suffering and fear experienced by the test victims:

> Dr Dohmen wore the grey-green uniform of the Nazi *Wehrmacht*. He was not very tall, stocky and a seemingly strong man of about 40 years. His face was a little flushed, the cheeks round and full. Upon his strong, curved nose, he wore glasses with big, round lenses. That made him look a bit like an owl. His hair was ash-blonde, straight and sat solidly on his head. His limbs were short and powerful. With solid steps and stocky legs, he followed me down the narrow corridor of the infirmary to the room where the children were locked up. I opened the door. He entered without hesitation or words. No greeting, nothing. The children stood motionless with pale faces, pressed together in front of the window and starred, terrified, at the strange man in uniform, who came towards them in there. . . .

Dohmen then ordered the children to uncover their upper bodies. Then he took each one and examined them routinely, but very thoroughly. The examination was carried out almost without words. He dealt with the children as if it was an inspection. Everything was carried out with complete prudence and with an accustomed flick of the wrist, he felt the boys' bodies. In this setting, it seemed almost unreal. It was completely inconceivable to me how a man, a doctor, could have absolutely no feeling for the terrible situation in which these helpless and abandoned children found themselves. . . . Finally, he completed the examination of the last boy. . . . [He] turned to me and ordered: strict isolation, strict quarantine, daily check of the early morning urine, blood sedimentation and blood count every three days, measure fever twice daily, morning, evening. Then he put his stethoscope back in his briefcase and left the room, without a word or a farewell, just as he had come in.

He wanted to come back in approximately two weeks. Nevertheless almost three weeks past before he appeared again. . . . He brought a small, suitcase-like leather bag with him. Inside, he kept four or five glass ampoules packed in ice. . . . Dr Dohmen selected four children. Once again, they had to undress their upper-bodies. Then he took a couple of syringes, which he had brought with him, out of his briefcase and filled them with the contents of the mysterious ampoule. . . . Then the doctor injected approximately 10 cc of the prepared fluid into the deltoid muscle of each selected boys' upper arm. . . .

Soon after the injection a raised area about the size of a five mark piece, which felt very solid and only began to slowly recede after several days, developed on the place where the injections had been made on the four boys. A slight fever was already detectable on the first evening. After several days, Dr Dohmen returned.

This time the Medical Corps' Captain brought two big ampoules carefully wrapped in paper in his briefcase. As he unpacked them, I saw that they contained a reddish-brown, gel-like substance. I recognised that from the laboratory! Those were bacteria cultures! A heat sensation shot through my body from head to toe and I felt as if my hands began to moisten. Did this man want to. . .? My God! The children – his victims – also stood crowded together with pale faces and stared at the hands of the Medical Corps' Captain with frightened, wide-open eyes, which now took some glass syringes and rubber hoses – those were duodenum probes! – out of the bag. He carefully placed these obviously sterilised things on top of a white cloth, with which he had already covered the small table beforehand. Then he selected two of the boys. They were Saul Hornfeld and Wölfchen Silberglett – our youngest!

They both had to undress completely. Naked, they stood full of fear before their torturer. He examined them both again thoroughly. Then a duodenum probe was inserted into each of them by the doctor. When the children had choked down the tubes far enough, they had to sit on a wooden stool. The Medical Corps' Captain put on rubber gloves, opened the ampoule with a small steel saw, and extracted its contents into a 20 cc syringe. Only with difficulty did the gel glide into the needle of the glass syringe. Then he placed the end of the rubber tube that hung out of Wölfchen's mouth on the tip of the syringe and began to pump the gel into the tube. It was even more difficult to force the viscous content out of the syringe and through the little one's thin tube in order to inject him in the intestines. Then Saul was next. . . . Once he had finished his horrific "work", he strictly ordered both of the young ones to stay in bed.

. . .

Dr Dohmen came almost eight days later to examine Saul and Wölfchen. . . . Saul had to then undress his upper body and climb onto the operation table. . . . Dr Dohmen took a diagonally-cut probing tube with a needle sticking out of it out of his bag of instruments, stepped behind Saul, felt up his back with his fingers, positioned the tube and thrust it deeply through the back muscles into the child's body cavity. Saul screamed and bit his little fists in pain. I quickly jumped close in front of him and implored him in a pressed, heated whisper to stay brave. Blind with tears, he looked at me without seeing me. The tears streamed over his pale cheeks. Then the Medical Corps' Captain thrust for the second time. I threw a worried look to [inmate doctor] Sven Oftedal. "Liver Puncture", he whispered.

Then I saw how Dr Dohmen took the long needle out of the probing tube and quickly held a test tube under the opening of the probe. Thick, dark blood dropped into the test tube. Also some pieces of tissue, ripped completely out of the liver by the needle, floated in the glass. Now the Medical Corps' Captain again took the probe out of the boy's back, threw it in a kidney dish, and quickly pressed a swab on the wound. Then he stuck one or two wide elasticated plaster strips on top. The torture was over.

We lifted Saul from the operation table and brought him back, back to his comrades and laid him on top of his straw sack. There this small person was lying. Facing the boarded wall; he cried and whimpered quietly to himself. Again and again his slight body twitched under the heartbreaking sobs of this boy's mistreated soul.[15]

Meyer's report ends at this point. Due to the course of the war, Dohmen had to abort his experiments at the start of 1945. The boys were to be murdered a short while later as the camp was being evacuated. It was only thanks to the courageous intervention of the Norwegian prisoners that the 11 test victims survived. In May 1945 they were freed by Allied troops.

Tuberculosis tests on 20 Jewish children in Neuengamme

From mid-1944, the lung doctor Kurt Heißmeyer experimented on the prisoners of the Neuengamme Concentration Camp. His tests initially concerned the question of whether tuberculosis in the lungs could be favourably influenced by deliberately placing a further tuberculosis herd on the skin, i.e. the testing of a therapeutic procedure. In addition, Heißmeyer was also interested in a potential connection between "race" and TB susceptibility. The experiments thus touched on questions from "race research" and hereditary pathology.[16]

For the tests, Heißmeyer initially infected probably more than 100 adult Russian and Serbian prisoners with TB pathogens.[17] At least a part of the men – who had been mostly deported to Germany as civilian forced labourers – already suffered from different forms of tuberculosis. They, therefore, presumably were considered unfit for work, which surely formed an important reason for their being chosen as "test subjects". After many of these adults had died under the experiments, Oswald Pohl, the head of the SS Economic and Administrative Office, who – as of 1942 – was also in charge of the concentration camps, provided 20 Jewish children aged between five and 12 years for further tests.[18]

From January 1945, Heißmeyer infected the children with TB pathogens. In order to test the effect of his therapeutic procedure, he took lymph nodes from the children for histological testing. The scars from the operations were then carefully documented by photographs. As the Allied troops approached shortly thereafter, Heißmeyer buried the pictures and other test documents in order to be able to use the material for scientific purposes at a later date.[19]

The victims of the experiments, 10 girls and 10 boys, most from Poland, were hung on 20 April 1945 in the basement of the Hamburg School in Bullenhuser Damm, which was used as a subsidiary camp, in order to remove any traces. Most of the adult prisoners initially used for the testing had died during the experiments or were murdered after they were concluded.

Heredity research on twin children in Auschwitz

The name "Josef Mengele" has become synonymous with the crimes of German physicians during the Nazi period. From May 1943 *Dr. phil. et med.* Mengele was the camp physician at the Auschwitz concentration and extermination camp. He participated there in the murder of hundreds of thousands of mostly Jewish people. Like no other, he also used the extra-legal space of the concentration camp for medical research.

Mengele was a student of Otmar Freiherr von Verschuer (1896–1969), one of Europe's leading geneticists, and in 1938 submitted a dissertation on hereditary medicine that was highly regarded in professional circles. Having served in the *Waffen-SS* since 1940, the researcher presumably viewed the position at Auschwitz as a chance to reinitiate his scientific activity, which had been suspended since the start of the war. His work there focused on genetic research conducted on twins.[20] The beginning of Mengele's experiments on Jewish twins was recently dated at mid-1944.[21]

Before the discovery of the gene, the phenomenon of heredity could only be studied based on external features. One of the key methods of "classic genetics" at the end of the 1930s was comparative research of twins. Pairs of identical twins were precisely measured and studied in order to determine conformity and variation in their physical and mental development. Geneticists in this way sought indications as to the features and diseases of human beings that were genetically conditioned and those that were acquired through the external circumstances of life.

Being the largest concentration and extermination camp in the German sphere of influence, Auschwitz offered special opportunities for hereditary research. Among the nearly 1.3 million persons deported there, a corresponding percentage was twins, so that a significant number of identical twin children could be investigated there more broadly and intensively than was conceivable outside a concentration camp.

According to the statements of former prisoners, Mengele often came onto the ramp in order to select twins from arriving transports. His subjects were accommodated in a special section, where relatively good living conditions prevailed. This was to prevent test results from being influenced by hunger or disease. Several hundred pairs of twins lived in Mengele's section for some time.

Mengele's experiments had two phases. The first phase encompassed research "on the living object". Exact measurements of the skull and other extremities were made. The twins were X-rayed, photographed and examined physically and psychiatrically. Comprehensive data material thus arose, which Mengele planned to evaluate at a later time. Furthermore, he conducted cruel experiments, such as experimental operations without anaesthesia, possibly in order to compare the sensitivity of twins to pain. Other children received blood transfusions or were injected with disease pathogens, because Mengele wanted to study the blood serum reactions of pairs of twins.

The second investigatory phase consisted in autopsies. In order to be able to compare the internal organs of twins, Mengele killed the children at the same time by injecting chloroform into their hearts. To carry out the post-mortem examinations, Mengele had a modern autopsy room set up in the camp. There, the Hungarian pathologist Dr Miklós Nyiszli, who was deported to Auschwitz in 1944, had to perform the dissections.[22]

The total number of twins Mengele misused for his research, as Paul Weindling pointed out on the basis of testimonies by former Auschwitz inmate doctors and anthropologists, was around 730, a considerable number of whom survived.[23] Some of these were among the Auschwitz inmates liberated and photographed by the Soviets in January 1945. The picture of the children behind barbed wire has become a photographic icon in international visual memory.

Conclusions

Experiments on human subjects were carried out in all of the large concentration camps from the beginning of the Second World War. The doctors who misused camp inmates as "test subjects" came from the ranks of the SS, the *Wehrmacht* and respectable research centres and universities. Their experiments had a variety of aims. By far the larger part of them belonged to applied military research and army medicine, aimed at testing therapies and vaccines for treating war-related injuries, illnesses and epidemics. Other groups were related to the planned settlement and population policy in occupied Eastern Europe or consisted of attempts to provide scientific legitimation to racist Nazi ideology such as Mengele's twin research in Auschwitz.

Initially exclusively adult men were used as test subjects for such experiments, as up to early 1942 the vast majority of the concentration camp inmates were male. From the summer of 1942, also female prisoners and later even children were used in concentration camps for medical experiments, who – since the start of the mass deportations in the course of the "Final Solution" – were now being handed over in greater numbers to the SS in the concentration camps. Besides the principal availability of women and children as "test subjects", another factor was relevant. After the failure of the "*Blitzkrieg* Strategy", the concentration camps began to be seen as a reservoir of labour for the German armaments industry. To support the German war effort, the SS from mid-1942 massively increased the degree of forced labour in the camps. As a consequence, only inmates who could not be used as forced labourers were provided for medical experiments by the concentration camp commands.

Therefore, after the start of the mass deportations associated with the "Final Solution" and due to the increased use of the labour of adult prisoners as of 1942, children became potential objects for medical experiments in concentration camps. As the examples outlined above show, children were used as test subjects when this was advantageous in terms of the logic of the experiment, i.e. when children were, according to the opinion of the medical perpetrator, the best suited subjects for the test purpose or, in the case of Mengele's research on twins, the only possible subjects.

Notes

1 Eyewitness report of the former medical orderly Bruno Meyer, *Bericht über die Hepatitis-Versuche im KZ Sachsenhausen*, unpublished typescript, 1960, in Oranienburg, Sachsenhausen Archive: P3 Bruno Meyer, Vol. I, p. 1.

2 For overviews of the different kinds of human experiments in Nazi concentration camps and the medical research areas behind it, see: Rolf Winau, 'Medizinische Experimente in den Konzentrationslagern', in Wolfgang Benz and Barbara Distel (eds), *Der Ort des Terrors. Geschichte der nationalsozialistischen Konzentrationslager*, Vol. 1, Munich: C.H. Beck, 2005, pp. 165–178; and, with more differentiated categories: Volker Roelcke, 'Humanexperimente während der Zeit des Nationalsozialismus', in Ralf Forsbach (ed.), *Medizin im "Dritten Reich". Humanexperimente, "Euthanasie" und die Debatten der Gegenwart*, Berlin: LIT Verlag, 2006, pp. 99–134.

3 For the epistemological and ethical dimension of human experimentation in concentration camps, see: Volker Roelcke, 'Die Sulfonamid-Experimente in nationalsozialistischen Konzentrationslagern: Eine kritische Neubewertung der epistemologischen und ethischen Dimension', *Medizinhistorisches Journal*, 44 (2009), pp. 42–60.

4 On the victims of the experiments, among others in relation to nationality and sex: Paul Weindling, 'Die Opfer von Humanexperimenten im Nationalsozialismus. Ergebnisse eines Forschungsprojekts', in Insa Eschebach and Astrid Ley (eds), *Geschlecht und "Rasse" in der NS-Medizin*, Berlin: Metropol, 2012, pp. 81–99.

5 Paul Weindling, 'Genetik und Menschenversuche in Deutschland, 1940–1950, Hans Nachtsheim, die Kaninchen von Dahlem und die Kinder vom Bullenhuser Damm', in Hans-Walter Schmuhl (ed.), *Rassenforschung an Kaiser-Wilhelm-Instituten vor und nach 1933*, Göttingen: Wallstein, 2003, pp. 247–248. Further reasons for experimenting on children: Weindling, 'Die Opfer von Humanexperimenten im Nationalsozialismus', pp. 90–91.

6 Judith Hahn, *Grawitz, Genzken, Gebhardt. Drei Karrieren im Sanitätsdienst der SS*, Münster: Klemm & Oelschläger, 2008, pp. 401–407.

7 See: Astrid Ley and Günter Morsch, *Medical Care and Crime. The Infirmary at Sachsenhausen Concentration Camp 1936–1945*, Berlin: Metropol, 2007, pp. 338–361.

8 'Ernst Grawitz to Heinrich Himmler, 1 June 1943: Evidence Document NO-010', in Klaus Dörner et al. (eds), *Der Nürnberger Ärzteprozeß 1946/47. Wortprotokolle, Anklage- und Verteidigungsmaterial, Quellen zum Umfeld*, Micorfiche ed., Munich: K.G. Saur, 1999, (MF) 3/1229–1230.

9 'Heinrich Himmler to Ernst Grawitz, 16 June 1943: Evidence Document NO-011', in Dörner et al., *Der Nürnberger Ärzteprozess 1946/47*, (MF) 3/1231.

10 On Dohmen's official trip to Auschwitz: Ley and Morsch, *Medical Care and Crime*, pp. 342–343.

11 Volker Roelcke, 'Fortschritt ohne Rücksicht. Menschen als Versuchskaninchen bei den Sulfonamid-Experimenten im Konzentrationslager Ravensbrück', in Eschebach and Ley, *Geschlecht und "Rasse"*, pp. 101–114; Weindling, 'Die Opfer von Humanexperimenten im Nationalsozialismus', pp. 89–90.

12 Jan Erik Schulte, *Zwangsarbeit und Vernichtung. Das Wirtschaftsimperium der SS. Oswald Pohl und das SS-Wirtschafts-Verwaltungshauptamt 1933–1945*, Paderborn: Schöningh, 2001.

13 Oranienburg, Sachsenhausen Archive: Video interview of Saul Oren-Hornfeld, in 'Jedesmal musste es ein Wunder sein', Filmhochschule Potsdam, 1996.

14 On Dohmen's hepatitis experiments: Brigitte Leyendecker and Burghard F. Klapp, 'Deutsche Hepatitisforschung im Zweiten Weltkrieg', in Christian Pross und Götz Aly (eds), *Der Wert des Menschen. Medizin in Deutschland 1918–1945*, Berlin: Edition Hentrich, 1989, pp. 261–293; Ley and Morsch, *Medical Care and Crime*, pp. 338–337.

15 Eyewitness report of Bruno Meyer, pp. 9–15.

16 See: Weindling, 'Genetik und Menschenversuche in Deutschland'; on Heißmann's victims: Günther Schwarberg, *Der SS-Arzt und die Kinder. Bericht über den Mord vom Bullenhuser Damm*, Hamburg: Gruner & Jahr, 1979.

17 On the adult victims, who found only little interest in historical research for a long time, fundamentally: chapter by Anna von Villiez in this volume.

18 Iris Groschek and Kristina Vagt, ". . . *dass du weißt, was hier passiert ist*". *Medizinische Experimente im KZ Neuengamme und die Morde am Bullenhuser Damm*, Bremen: Edition Temmen, 2012, pp. 28–33.

19 Herbert Diercks, 'Gesucht wird: Dr. Kurt Heißmeyer', *Beiträge zur Geschichte der nationalsozialistischen Verfolgung in Norddeutschland*, 9 (2005), pp. 102–115.

20 On Mengele's research on twins in Auschwitz: Benoît Massin, 'Mengele, die Zwillingsforschung und die "Auschwitz-Dahlem Connection"', in Carola Sachse (ed.), *Die Verbindung nach Auschwitz. Biowissenschaften und Menschenversuche an Kaiser-Wilhelm-Instituten*, Göttingen: Wallstein, 2003, pp. 201–254.

21 Paul Weindling, *Victims and Survivors of Nazi Human Experiments. Science and Suffering in the Holocaust*, London: Bloomsbury, 2015, pp. 157–265.

22 See eyewitness report of Miklós Nyiszli, *Im Jenseits der Menschlichkeit: Ein Gerichtsmediziner in Auschwitz*, Berlin: Dietz, 1992.

23 Weindling, *Victims and Survivors of Nazi Human Experiments*, pp. 157–265. Massin, 'Mengele', p. 236, estimated a higher number of test persons and victims.

Bibliography

Archival sources

Germany

Oranienburg, Sachsenhausen Archive:
P3 Bruno Meyer
Video interview of Saul Oren-Hornfeld

Literature

Diercks, Herbert, 'Gesucht wird: Dr. Kurt Heißmeyer', *Beiträge zur Geschichte der nationalsozialistischen Verfolgung in Norddeutschland*, 9 (2005), pp. 102–115

Dörner, Klaus, Angelika Ebbinghaus and Karsten Linne (eds), in cooperation with Karl Heinz Roth and Paul Weindling, on behalf of the Stiftung für Sozialgeschichte des 20. Jahrhunderts, *Der Nürnberger Ärzteprozeß 1946/47. Wortprotokolle, Anklage- und Verteidigungsmaterial, Quellen zum Umfeld*, Micorfiche ed., Munich: K.G. Saur, 1999

Groschek, Iris and Kristina Vagt, *". . . dass du weißt, was hier passiert ist". Medizinische Experimente im KZ Neuengamme und die Morde am Bullenhuser Damm*, Bremen: Edition Temmen, 2012

Hahn, Judith, *Grawitz, Genzken, Gebhardt. Drei Karrieren im Sanitätsdienst der SS*, Münster: Klemm & Oelschläger, 2008

Ley, Astrid and Günter Morsch, *Medical Care and Crime. The Infirmary at Sachsenhausen Concentration Camp 1936–1945*, Berlin: Metropol, 2007

Leyendecker, Brigitte and Burghard F. Klapp, 'Deutsche Hepatitisforschung im Zweiten Weltkrieg', in Christian Pross and Götz Aly (eds), *Der Wert des Menschen. Medizin in Deutschland 1918–1945*, Berlin: Edition Hentrich, 1989, pp. 261–293

Massin, Benoît, 'Mengele, die Zwillingsforschung und die "Auschwitz-Dahlem Connection"', in Carola Sachse (ed.), *Die Verbindung nach Auschwitz. Biowissenschaften und Menschenversuche an Kaiser-Wilhelm-Instituten*, Göttingen: Wallstein, 2003, pp. 201–254

Nyiszli, Miklós, *Im Jenseits der Menschlichkeit: Ein Gerichtsmediziner in Auschwitz*, Berlin: Dietz, 1992

Roelcke, Volker, 'Humanexperimente während der Zeit des Nationalsozialismus', in Ralf Forsbach (ed.), *Medizin im "Dritten Reich". Humanexperimente, "Euthanasie" und die Debatten der Gegenwart*, Berlin: LIT Verlag, 2006, pp. 99–134

—— 'Die Sulfonamid-Experimente in nationalsozialistischen Konzentrationslagern: Eine kritische Neubewertung der epistemologischen und ethischen Dimension', *Medizinhistorisches Journal*, 44 (2009), pp. 42–60

—— 'Fortschritt ohne Rücksicht. Menschen als Versuchskaninchen bei den Sulfonamid-Experimenten im Konzentrationslager Ravensbrück', in Insa Eschebach and Astrid Ley (eds), *Geschlecht und "Rasse" in der NS-Medizin*, Berlin: Metropol, 2012, pp. 101–114

Schulte, Jan Erik, *Zwangsarbeit und Vernichtung. Das Wirtschaftsimperium der SS. Oswald Pohl und das SS-Wirtschafts-Verwaltungshauptamt 1933–1945*, Paderborn: Schöningh, 2001

Schwarberg, Günther, *Der SS-Arzt und die Kinder. Bericht über den Mord vom Bullenhuser Damm*, Hamburg: Gruner & Jahr, 1979

Weindling, Paul, 'Genetik und Menschenversuche in Deutschland, 1940–1950, Hans Nachtsheim, die Kaninchen von Dahlem und die Kinder vom Bullenhuser Damm', in Hans-Walter Schmuhl (ed.), *Rassenforschung an Kaiser-Wilhelm-Instituten vor und nach 1933*, Göttingen: Wallstein, 2003, pp. 245–274

—— 'Die Opfer von Humanexperimenten im Nationalsozialismus. Ergebnisse eines Forschungsprojekts', in Insa Eschebach and Astrid Ley (eds), *Geschlecht und "Rasse" in der NS-Medizin*, Berlin: Metropol, 2012, pp. 81–99

—— *Victims and Survivors of Nazi Human Experiments. Science and Suffering in the Holocaust*, London: Bloomsbury, 2015

Winau, Rolf, 'Medizinische Experimente in den Konzentrationslagern', in Wolfgang Benz and Barbara Distel (eds), *Der Ort des Terrors. Geschichte der nationalsozialistischen Konzentrationslager*, Vol. 1, Munich: C.H. Beck, 2005, pp. 165–178

11 The story of how the Ravensbrück "Rabbits" were captured in photos[1]

Aleksandra Loewenau

Introduction

The story of the Polish women who were subjected to experimental treatment of war wounds at the female concentration camp of Ravensbrück has been presented in many publications. We therefore know: what the purpose of this research was; how many women were operated on; how many of them died at the camp; who was involved in performing these operations and what were the side effects of these procedures. Yet, the Ravensbrück sulphonamide experiments theme has gone through a considerable transformation over time. The first person to give a very detailed medical description of the procedures involved was a former Polish prisoner and herself a physician – Zofia Mączka, who witnessed several operations.[2] Soon after this topic was analysed within the broader aspect of the Nuremberg Medical Trial by Alexander Mitscherlich and Fred Mielke, who quoted a great deal of original trial documents.[3] More recent historiography re-evaluates the importance of the post-war trials and, at least to some extent, includes the victims' position as presented by Paul Weindling in his two remarkable monographs *Nazi Medicine and the Nuremberg Trials: From Medical War Crimes to Informed Consent* [4] and *Victims and Survivors of Nazi Human Experiments: Science and Suffering in the Holocaust.*[5] Moreover, Volker Roelcke in his recent articles "Sulfonamide Experiments on Prisoners in Nazi Concentration Camps: Coherent Scientific Rationality Combined with Complete Disregard of Humanity"[6] and "Die Sulfonamid-Experimente in nationalsozialistischen Konzentrationslagern: Eine kritische Neubewertung der epistemologischen und ethischen Dimension" focused on critical analysis of the sulphonamide experiments performed in Nazi concentration camps.[7] Furthermore, two German authors, Freya Klier and Loreta Waltz, presented horrifying experiences of the "Rabbits" in Ravensbrück.[8] In addition, victims' written collective and individual memoirs had already been published in the 1960s.[9] In general, the historiography to this date was based either on interrogation reports or witness testimonies collected after the war ended. Scholars in their analysis of historical sources have ignored photo images.

This chapter presents the story of the "Rabbits" captured in photos. In other words, I will analyse photo images of the "Rabbits", which were taken during and after war, as evidence of crime and torment at Ravensbrück.

Who were the "Rabbits"

In July 1942, over 100 Polish political prisoners incarcerated at Ravensbrück were gathered on the roll call square for an informal medical examination.[10] On 24 July, 74 randomly selected Polish women were called to the camp office where they were met by Commandant Koegel and the camp doctors: Schiedlausky, Rosenthal and Oberheuser.[11] The women who became known as the "Rabbits", *Kaninchen*, *Lapins*, or *króliki*,[12] came to the camp in two groups. The first arrived on 23 September 1941 and the second on 31 May 1942.[13] Approximately 80 per cent of Polish female inmates at Ravensbrück were classified as political prisoners. Moreover, according to post-war testimonies, a certain number of Polish women came to the camp under sentence of death.[14] The vast majority of them had experienced brutal interrogation in Gestapo offices and in prisons before they were sent to Ravensbrück. For instance, 68 of the "Rabbits" were transported from Lublin, where they had spent months being questioned and beaten in a prison located inside Lublin Castle[15] and in the Gestapo head office called *Więzienie pod Zegarem*[16] (the Prison under the Clock). The remaining six "Rabbits" were transported to Ravensbrück from Warsaw where they had undergone interrogation at Pawiak prison. Zofia Kiecol

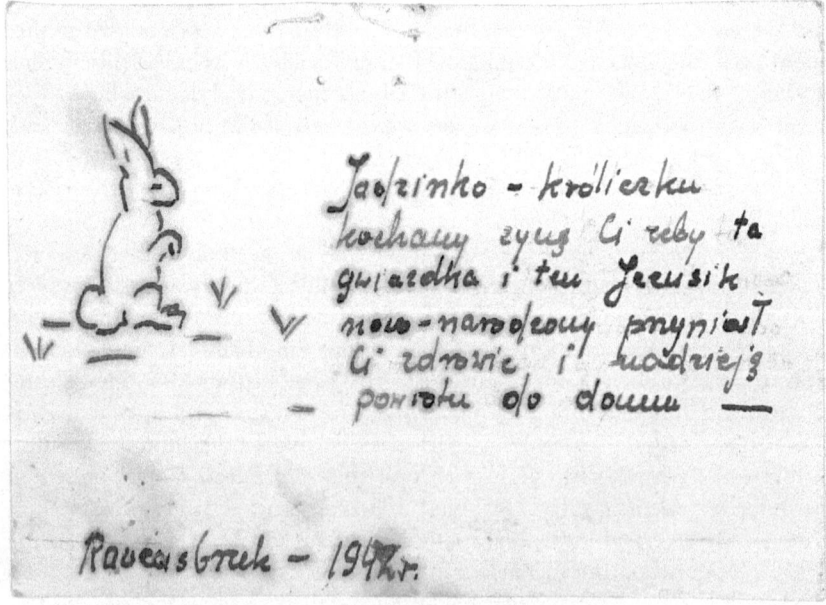

Figure 11.1 Christmas card given to Jadwiga Dzido by another inmate in which Dzido is referred to as a "Rabbit", Ravensbrück, 25 December 1942

Source: Washington, DC, United States Holocaust Memorial Museum (hereafter USHMM) Photo Archives, No. 63555

and Helena Piasecka were heavily pregnant at the time of their arrest and delivered their babies at Lublin Castle prison. The new-borns died.[17]

During the examination each prisoner's personal data were recorded, and then their health history was checked. Particular interest was given to the state of the skin on their legs.[18] Although most of them had spent almost a year at the camp, their health was still in good condition. After doctors had collected the desired information, they sent the women back to their block. During the next few days the women were gathered several times during the roll call without receiving any explanation. On 28 July 1942, the first group from among the 74 selected Polish women was taken to the *Revier* (the camp clinic), where they were undressed, bathed and had their legs shaved. On 1 August 1942, the first experimental operations on six of the "Rabbits" began.[19]

Existing secondary literature commonly suggests that Polish women became victims of two types of experiments at Ravensbrück: a) research with the use of sulphonamides, and b) experimental operations on the regeneration of bones, muscles and nerves. In turn, the sulphonamide tests can be divided into three stages, each of which was performed in several series.[20] The first phase involved an incision into a calf and the introduction of bacterial cultures into the wounds. The second stage featured the introduction of other materials (e.g. pieces of wood) into the wound in addition to the bacteria cultures. The final phase of the infection experiments utilised specific cultures of gangrene-inducing bacteria. The second type of experiment involved: fractures, transplants and bone grafting, along with the excision of parts of muscles and nerves. All experimental operations were performed with the use of a general anaesthetic – either Evipan or Ether.[21]

The "Rabbits" – 74 Polish women – experienced suffering and were left with horrendous scars and damaged health. Many of them were operated on several times, particularly the victims of bone regeneration experiments. Forty-six such procedures were conducted on a group of 22 prisoners. In addition, 17 muscle regeneration operations were performed on four "Rabbits".

Overall, 116 operations were performed. Władysława Karolewska under-went six operations. Barbara Pietrzyk, who practised gymnastics before the war in the hope of fulfilling her dream of becoming a ballerina, ended up as a cripple from five bone regeneration operations. Leonarda Bień-Dymska was also operated on five times. When the war began, 47 of the "Rabbits" were in their 20s, and 16 were still in school. The youngest victim was 16 at the time of her first operation, and the oldest was 45. Out of the 74, 63 survived the war. Six "Rabbits" were executed after their operations were performed, and five died as a result of experimental procedures.

Crippled "Rabbits" fight for their lives

The relationship between the "Rabbits" went beyond friendship. The common experience of pain and the feelings of injustice and violation that they shared resulted in powerful bonds based upon mutual understanding, compassion and assistance in the provision of care. Among the "Rabbits" were university-educated women, who came from eminent families, as well as those less privileged with limited schooling. However, for the "Rabbits" boundaries, such as education, background or age, did not exist. They looked after each other by feeding those who were too weak to eat by themselves or changing bandages. This solidarity applied particularly to the "Rabbits" who were in the first group of victims, as they did not receive any medical help from either the Nazi doctors or the German nurses.[22]

The unique relationship among the "Rabbits" had a great influence in developing mental strength, courage and determination, qualities which enabled them to establish fundamental aims, such as surviving the camp and informing the outside world about the crimes committed at Ravensbrück.

At first, the "Rabbits" felt intimidated by the Nazi physicians and the SS. The situation changed on 11 February 1943, when they discovered that two "Rabbits" had been executed. These two killings were not unprecedented, as the execution of political prisoners at Ravensbrück began in 1941/1942.[23] At that point, they realised that they had nothing to lose and had to fight for their survival. Thus, in early March 1943, over 60 crippled victims of medical experiments – many on crutches or being carried by fellow prisoners – organised a march to the camp commandant.[24] Their aim was to promote awareness among the other prisoners that the "Rabbits" had not agreed to any experimental operations, regardless of what the SS claimed. According to post-war recollections, the following day, the "Rabbits" sent a letter to the commandant inquiring as to whether the experimental operations were part of their death sentences.[25] They did not receive any answer.[26]

In September 1943, 10 "Rabbits" were ordered to go the hospital. The message was clear; they were to undergo more operations. As a further sign of protest, the "Rabbits", supported by other women at their block, refused to go to the infirmary. Sensing the rising tension, camp doctors told the "Rabbits" that they were being sent to work at a factory. The 10 women requested written confirmation. When they realised that it was just a deceptive pretext, they avoided the transport by hiding among other prisoners.[27] However, this desperate attempt was not effective, as they were captured and dragged by force to the *Bunker*, where they were operated on. In her testimony at the Ravensbrück trial, Helena Piasecka recalled that she resisted and was thrown on a bed and "without taking any precautions, [or] any measurement . . . some amount of ether was poured on [her] face".[28] She also reported that none of the selected women were bathed or undressed before the operation. The collective display of defiance brought negative consequences for the 500 women who participated in hiding the "Rabbits". As a punishment, they were locked in Block 24 for three days with very limited supplies of water and food.[29]

The strong conviction of injustice and the awareness that their chances of surviving the camp were very small caused the "Rabbits" to undertake a mission to disseminate information about the crimes committed by the Nazis at Ravensbrück. The increase in the number of executions of Polish political prisoners in the camp in 1943 catalysed this action.[30] According to Kiedrzyńska, prisoners established several ways of contacting the world outside of the camp. First of all, they passed information to French POWs who worked near the SS sanatorium of Hohenlychen, and who managed to inform the French underground about the situation at the camp.[31] Additional contacts were Polish forced labour workers and Polish officers who worked in Neustrelitz, 28 kilometres from Ravensbrück. The information provided was very precise and included details about operations, including the number performed and the number of subsequent deaths, as well as information regarding executions. In the "Rabbits' " opinion, it was absolutely crucial for those letters to be preserved in their original format as testimonies so they could be used as evidence in case none of them survived.[32]

The "Rabbits" also found another way to inform members of their families about the true conditions at the camp. In general, the inmates' correspondence was strictly censored; however, the "Rabbits" managed to pass on details regarding the experimental operations performed on them in letters written using "funny ink" – a euphemism for urine.[33] Moreover, it is believed that an American-Polish prisoner Aka Kołodziejczyk, who was released from the camp in late 1942, took with her a list of experimental victims, which she later handed over to the Polish government-in-exile.[34] The publicity around the "Rabbits" resulted in the cessation of further executions of "human guinea pigs" at Ravensbrück.

In late September 1944, another opportunity to gather evidence of the Nazi crimes committed in Ravensbrück arose when one of the women transported from Warsaw traded her camera for a piece of bread. Joanna Szydłowska, also a victim, agreed to take photos of three of the "Rabbits" – Maria Kuśmierczuk, Bogumiła Bąbińska and Barbara Pietrzyk. In sum, five photos of the "Rabbits" were taken on Sunday, 1 October 1944.[35]

The photo images presented below contain very important information with regard to the conditions of the "Rabbits" at Ravensbrück. A good place to begin the analysis of these images is with the circumstances under which they were taken. Namely, the victims were hiding at the back of the block, imbuing the photos with a clandestine character. The absence of crutches indicates that the women's wounds had healed well and no longer significantly impaired their ability to walk. An analysis of the women's appearance yields several insights into aspects of camp life. For example, the victims had long hair, which communicates that the position of the Polish prisoners was higher than that of the Jews, whose heads were completely shaved upon arrival. The fact that they were not dressed in camp uniforms could come across as rather odd. One may think that they dressed up for the occasion; however, it would have drawn attention to the women and thus jeopardise the mission. In reality, there was a shortage of camp uniforms; therefore, inmates were allowed to wear civilian clothes that were marked with a cross on the back and also had their prisoner number sewn on to their coats. The first photo of the series below might be confusing to the reader, as Pietrzyk smiled for the camera; therefore, the scars on her legs may be overlooked. Pietrzyk was one of the youngest of the victims. She died of TB shortly after the war at the age of 22.[36]

The next two images, on the other hand, clearly achieve their purpose – drawing attention to the women's wounds. Bąbińska (Figure 11.3), not only refrained from smiling, but also lifted her skirt up to show scars on her legs caused by experimental operations. Similarly, Kuśmierczuk (Figure 11.4), who can be seen in previous photos in the top-left corner waiting for her turn, also exposed her right leg without looking directly into the camera.

By the end of 1944 it seemed that the "Rabbits" had achieved the desired goal – their safety in the camp. The experiments were concluded and the

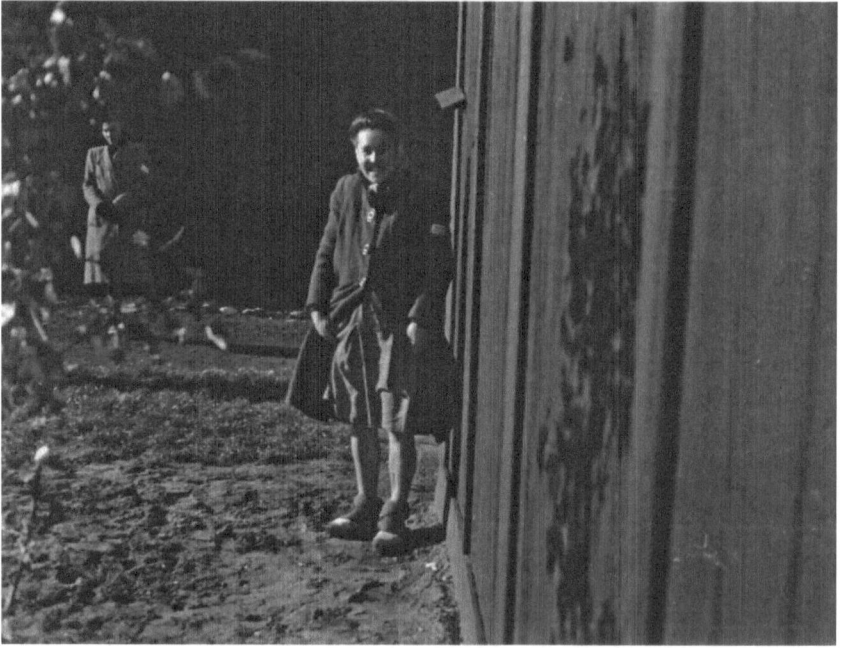

Figure 11.2 Clandestine photograph of a Polish political prisoner and medical experimentation victim in the Ravensbrück concentration camp. Pictured is Barbara Pietrzyk. Her prisoner number patch is visible on the sleeve of her coat. Maria Kuśmierczuk is standing in the background. Photo was taken by Joanna Szydłowska on 1 October 1944

Source: USHMM Photo Archives, No. 69342. The negative was kept by the "Rabbits" at Ravensbrück until April 1945 and then was given to the French prisoner Germaine Tillion, who sent it back to the "Rabbits" in Poland after the liberation. Władysława Karolewska was then in possession of the negatives, until she gave them to Anna Jarosky, who deposited it at the USHMM, see USHMM Photo Archive, Nos. 69339, 69340, 69341, 69342, 69343; Germaine Tillion, 'A la recherche de la vérité', in *Ravensbrück*, Neuchâtel: Cahiers du Rhône, 1946

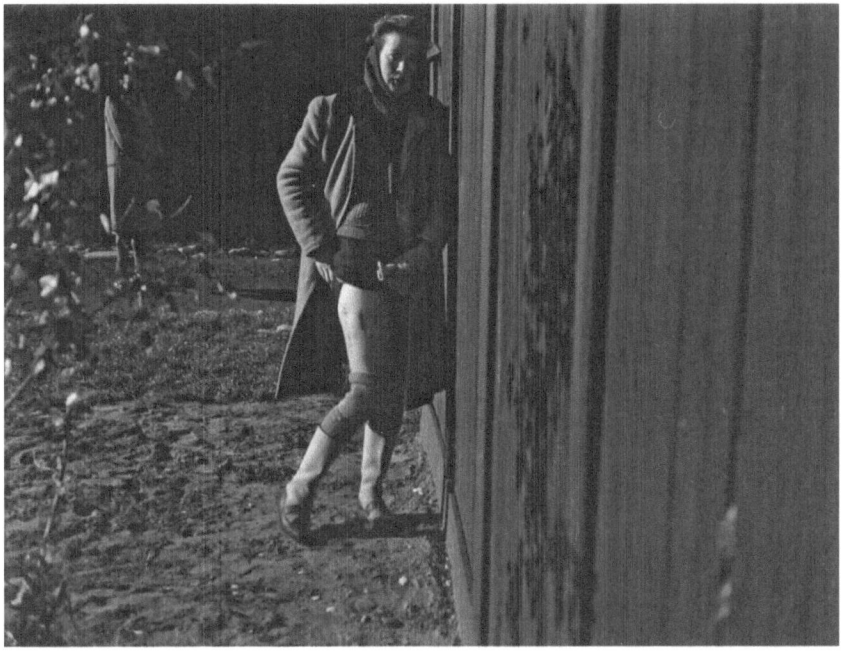

Figure 11.3 Clandestine photograph of a Polish political prisoner and medical
experimentation victim in the Ravensbrück concentration camp.
Pictured is Bogumiła Bąbińska (Jasiuk). Photo was taken by Joanna
Szydłowska on 1 October 1944

Source: USHMM Photo Archives, No. 69343

executions of the "Rabbits" were stopped. However, shortly before the
liberation the SS attempted to cover up their crimes. Thus, the "Rabbits" once
again found themselves in great danger. On 2 February 1945, the information
that the "Rabbits" would be liquidated was spread among the prisoners. On
4 February, all 63 surviving experimental victims were ordered to stay in their
block after the morning roll call. After long deliberation the "Rabbits" decided
that they would not give up and would try to escape and hide. It was an
extremely difficult task because many of them could barely walk, and their
prisoner numbers began from 7,000; therefore, they were easily recognisable
among other inmates. This time, however, saving the lives of the "Rabbits"
became a joint action of prisoners of various nationalities. When the Gestapo
surrounded their block, the Soviet prisoners who worked in the electrician
commando turned the power off; as a result, several "Rabbits" were able to
jump out of the window.[37] When the remaining women were gathered in
front of Block 24, suddenly a group of Sinti and Roma prisoners deliberately
began shouting and running around creating confusion, which provided an
opportunity for the rest of the "Rabbits" to escape. On many occasions while

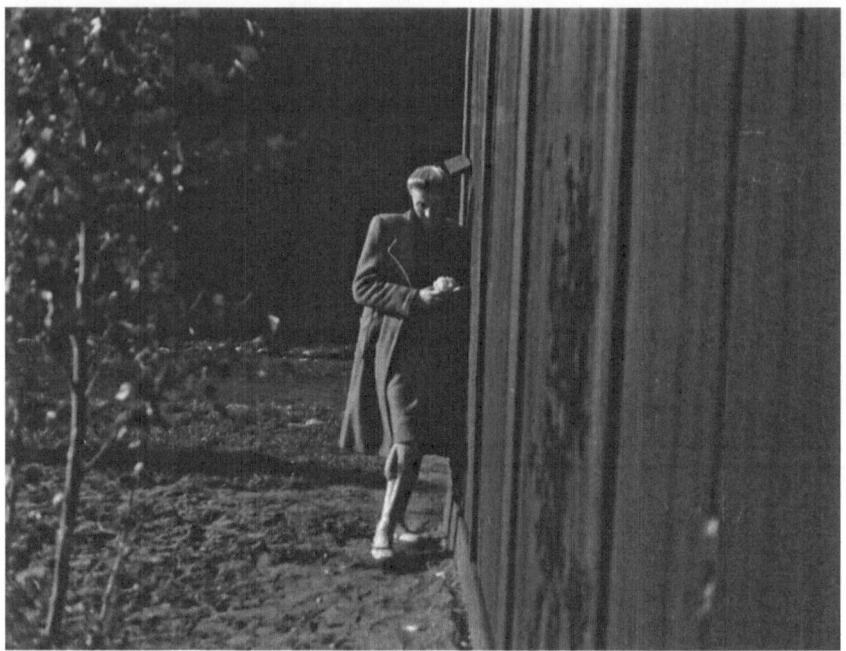

Figure 11.4 Clandestine photograph of a Polish political prisoner and medical
           experimentation victim in the Ravensbrück concentration camp.
           Pictured is Maria Kuśmierczuk. Photo was taken by Joanna Szydłowska
           on 1 October 1944

Source: USHMM Photo Archives, No. 69341

the search for the "Rabbits" was in progress, some prisoners of other nationalities
offered their coats, so the "Rabbits" could cover their camp numbers. Despite
the inherent danger, inmates offered to hide them in their blocks.[38] Thus, some
of the "Rabbits" were hidden in the typhus block, whereas others found a
place in the *Revier* among the ill and dying.[39] However, a number of women
whose scars were too visible could not be hidden. As Wanda Półtawska
described, they "took a spade and dug themselves in underneath the block,
armed with stolen blankets and a little food. For seven days and seven nights
they stayed buried in that cold, dark hole".[40]

Even when the situation of the "Rabbits" was at its most dramatic, the
women still managed to inform their families and the Polish underground about
their struggle. As a result, details about experiments performed on them once
again reached the Polish government-in-exile in London. Subsequently, on 6
March 1944, the government-in-exile issued a report describing the situation
in various camps, including Ravensbrück, in order to alert the Allies.[41] As the
unethical treatment of the "Rabbits"/political prisoners had already been
exposed, the SS were forced to change their tactics.[42] They tried to convince

several women to sign documents, which stated that the scars on their legs were effects of accidents at work.[43] The more gentle approach of the camp commandant towards the "Rabbits" was an evident sign that the Nazis were aware that information in regard to the experiments conducted at the camp had become known abroad; thus the "Rabbits", being slightly more confident, categorically rejected the Nazis' "reconciling gesture". Moreover, their action brought an improvement regarding the hunger issue, as the "Rabbits", in addition to other prisoners, began receiving food parcels that were sent by the International Committee of the Red Cross.[44]

As described above, the publicity action of the "Rabbits" was successful and resulted in various advantages. First, fellow prisoners were willing to help the "Rabbits" who found themselves in great danger on several occasions. Second, the information regarding the experiments reached abroad, which meant that the scale of Nazi crimes at Ravensbrück was to a large extent revealed, and could not be covered up even by killing all the victims. This process of publicising the experiments was continued after the war along with the "Rabbits'" demand for punishing those who were responsible for damaging their health.

Liberation

The condition in which they were freed varied from the relatively safe to the highly disturbing. The process of releasing prisoners had begun before the Red Army entered the camp thanks to the efforts of the Director of the Swedish Red Cross, Folke Bernadotte, who negotiated with Heinrich Himmler for a gradual release of women incarcerated at Ravensbrück.[45]

In late February, Himmler met Folke Bernadotte, who – aware of the "Rabbits'" situation at the camp – requested their release. Himmler, although not keen on the request, said that he would think about it.[46] Meanwhile, the "Rabbits" were still in hiding while seeking to escape the camp. The Swedish Red Cross's efforts began to be effective after a second meeting with Himmler in early April, during which he agreed for Norwegian and Danish prisoners to be evacuated from Ravensbrück.[47] On 21 April 1945, the third meeting between Himmler and Bernadotte took place. Also present during discussions were the representative of Swedish Jewry – Norbert Masur, and Himmler's healer – Felix Kersten. This time Bernadotte negotiated the rescuing of inmates of other nationalities including Polish Jews and gentiles.[48] As a consequence of the Swedish Red Cross engagement, on 5 April 1945, the first inmates were evacuated from Ravensbrück to Switzerland. These included 299 French inmates and a Polish woman, Karolina Lanckorońska who shortly after her release deposited a complete list of the "Rabbits" to the Red Cross (see below).[49]

On 22 April 1945 the white buses of the Swedish Red Cross rescued 2,873 Ravensbrück prisoners, among them 954 Polish females.[50] In the end, however, the large-scale action of rescuing women from Ravensbrück did not include the "Rabbits" and only Alicja Jurkowska, Janina Marczewska and Zofia

NO.	NAME	PRISONER NO.	NO.	NAME	PRISONER NO.
1.	Wojtasik Wanda	7709	48.	Backiel Irena	7890
2.	Gnaś Stefania	7883	49.	Bień Leokadia	7861
3.	Zielonka Maria	7771	50.	Bąbińska Bogumiła	7693
4.	Gutek Rozalia	7871	51.	Cabaj Maria	11306
5.	Okoniewska Aniela	7873	52.	Czajkowska Stanisława	7864
6.	Kulczyk Wanda	---	53.	Grabowska Maria	7674
7.	Kamińska Jadwiga	7783	54.	Hegier Helena	7896
8.	Kormańska Zofia	7884	55.	Plater-Broel Maria	7911
9.	Kawińska Zofia	7935	56.	Bielska Jadwiga	7922
10.	Karolewska Władysława	7928	57.	Czyż Krystyna	7708
11.	Jurkowska Alicja	7716	58.	Andrzejak Wacława	7718
12.	Karczmarz Maria	7912	59.	Sienkiewicz Anna	---
13.	Karwacka Urszula	7920	60.	Buraczyńska Wojciecha	7926
14.	Iwańska Krystyna	7710	61.	Gisges Jadwiga	7889
15.	Iwańska Janina	7711	62.	Mann Eugenia	7873
16.	Mitura Janina	7932	63.	Mikluska Genowefa	7897
17.	Sobolewska Aniela	7678	64.	Dzido Jadwiga	7860
18.	Sokulska Zofia	7919	65.	Michalik Pelagia	7918
19.	Dąbska Krystyna	7650	66.	Marczewska Janina	7763
20.	Stefaniak Zofia	7697	67.	Marczewska Władysława	7892
21.	Łotocka Stefania	7707	68.	Marciniak Janina	7910
22.	Młodkowska Stanisława	7880	69.	Michalik Stanisława	7907
23.	Pietrzak Maria	7909	70.	Piotrowska Halina	7923
24.	Prus Alfreda	7657	71.	Modrowska Zofia	7681
25.	Hoszowska Zofia	7095	72.	Szydłowska Joanna	7914
26.	Kraska Weronika	7672	73.	Piasecka Helena	7927
27.	Nowakowska Maria	8651	74.	Sieklucka Stefania	---
28.	Rakowska Maria	7728			
29.	Szuksztul Weronika	7829			
30.	Pajączkowska Maria	---			
31.	Kuśmierczuk Maria	7888			
32.	Kostecka Czesława	7688			
33.	Maćkowska Pelagia	7886			
34.	Kwiecińska Leokadia	7682			
35.	Lefanowicz Aniela	7719			
36.	Kurowska Kazimiera	7670			
37.	Kiecol Zofia	7866			
38.	Kluczek Genowefa	11326			
39.	Łuszcz Jadwiga	11275			
40.	Krawczyk Irena	11329			
41.	Jabłońska Stanisława	11319			
42.	Kapłon Maria	11322			
43.	Pietrzyk Barbara	---			
44.	Śladziejowska Stanisława	7712			
45.	Pytlewska Barbara	7899			
46.	Rek Izabella	11286			
47.	Baj Zofia	7685			

Figure 11.5 List of "Rabbits" submitted to the International Committee of the Red Cross by Karolina Lanckoronska

Source: USHMM, ITS Digital Collection, KL Ravensbrück, Folder 54. Several spelling errors on the original list have been corrected

Sokulska managed, under false names, to join the Red Cross transport to Sweden, which left on 25 April with approximately 4,000 Polish prisoners.[51] The rest of the "Rabbits" were not released. Jadwiga Dzido recalled after the war that she tried to get onto the transport list but was unsuccessful because her injuries were too serious.[52] The camp commandant compiled the lists of prisoners to be rescued. The Polish victims of medical experiments were excluded. Bernadotte's influence was not strong enough to help the "Rabbits".[53]

Meanwhile, the three "Rabbits" who managed to falsify their numbers and that way joined the other women selected by the Swedish Red Cross, were loaded onto a train to Sweden where they were provided with medical help and general support. Despite the fact that the journey took several days, they could consider themselves free persons as soon as they left the camp. Following a few days of travelling in crowded freight wagons, they arrived in Denmark where they were greeted by a Polish priest and Danish Red Cross medical staff. The rest of the trip to Malmö was spent on a comfortable train and a ferry. On 1 May, they arrived in Lund where they were able to rest and receive medical assistance from the local physicians. Similarly to other rescued women, the three "Rabbits" were given various employment opportunities and the option to settle in Sweden. Janina Marczewska, chose to return, leaving Lund on 6 October 1945 with the first transport to Poland.[54] The two remaining "Rabbits", on the other hand, never returned to Poland. Zofia Sokulska lived

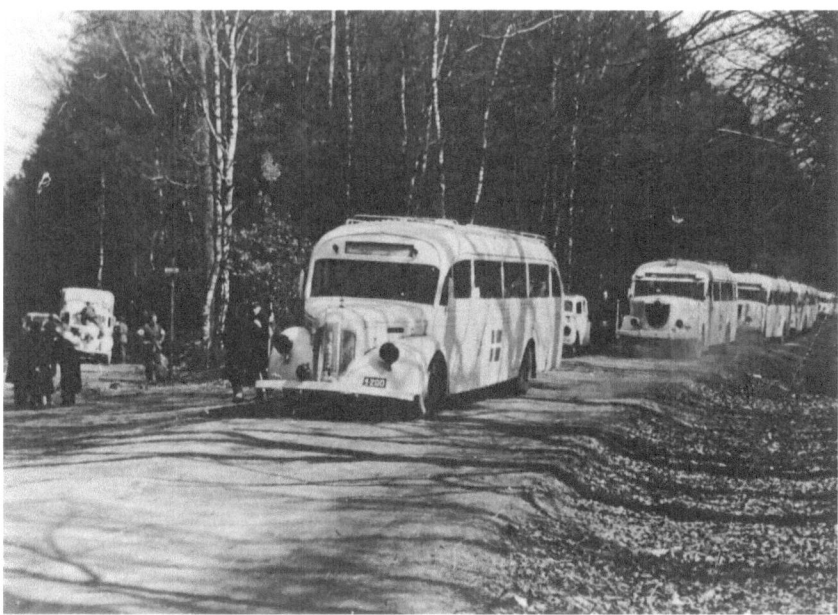

Figure 11.6 Red Cross white buses
Source: USHMM Photo Archives, No. 45696

in Sweden for several years and then immigrated to the United Kingdom where she met her future husband Ryszard Kaczmarski. Alicja Jurkowska also left Sweden for the UK. She later moved to Argentina with her husband.[55]

Meanwhile, for the vast majority of the "Rabbits" the last days of incarceration and their journey back to Poland proved to be exhausting and traumatic. After the last transport to Sweden left Ravensbrück, there were still several thousand prisoners remaining at the camp. The final order was to evacuate the camp leaving behind only the severely ill. Thus, inmates were forced to march to other concentration camps. The last group to be evacuated left Ravensbrück on 28 April 1945.[56] Among them were approximately 40 "Rabbits".[57] They composed just a small proportion of the approximately 2,000 hungry and exhausted women who were herded along narrow roads with civilians trying to escape the Soviets.[58] The chaos and uncertainty resulted in growing anxiety and tensions between inmates. In addition, the promised parcels delivered by the Swedish Red Cross were never distributed to prisoners. Women were given barely any food and were therefore forced to feed themselves with anything they were able to find or catch along the way. After hours of walking they were ordered to sleep on the bare ground. The constant bombing raids and ensuring panic created opportunities to run away. The women, who could not see the end of their marching and believed that separating from the SS-guarded columns was a better solution, organised themselves into groups. When the opportunity arose they either joined columns of escaping civilians or ran into nearby forest.[59] On 29 April, a group of "Rabbits" guarded by SS officers separated themselves from the evacuation column. On 3 May in Parchim, the crippled women were handed over to the British. Because there was a great deficiency of food supplies in Germany a small group of the liberated "Rabbits" decided to make their way to Poland after three days. Their journey was long and exhausting but relatively safe as they had the company of several men for protection.[60]

For the 18 "Rabbits" who managed to leave Ravensbrück with transport to the Neustadt-Glewe and Bergen-Belsen camps in February 1945 the suffering continued. Although they were not frightened of being shot by the execution commando, they were still forced to fight for survival. Their position within the camp as newcomers was extremely difficult. They did not know other prisoners and thus did not receive any help. Półtawska recalled after the war that all food distribution in Bergen-Belsen resulted in physical and verbal violence between inmates.[61] The "Rabbits" had great difficulty in adapting to the new reality since they were "not used to fight for food".[62] In addition, the horrendous accommodation conditions, which resulted in deteriorating camp hygiene, caused epidemics of typhus and other contagious diseases killing thousands of prisoners during the months before the end of the war.[63] On 15 April 1945, the British Army entered the Bergen-Belsen concentration camp.[64] The conditions in the camp were severely disturbing. Approximately 10,000 corpses were found in decomposed stages lying around the campsite. The death rates were increasing due to malnutrition and various diseases.[65]

Two "Rabbits" – Maria Cabaj and Stanisława Michalik – suffered from typhus.[66] In June 1945, after quarantine and primary medical assistance provided by the British, they were sent by the Swedish Red Cross to Sweden to recover. After several months, they were reunited with their families in Poland. On 2 May 1945, the Red Army liberated the sub-camp of Ravensbrück, Neustadt-Glewe. The severely ill prisoners were taken to the nearby hospitals and the rest were gradually repatriated to their native countries.[67] Wanda Wojtasik, Zofia Kawińska, Zofia Modrowska, Halina Piotrowska and Krystyna Czyż were not willing to wait for transport to Poland and they made their way on their own, unaware of any impending danger. Many of the Soviet soldiers had not interacted with women for a long time. Therefore, being in a position of power, a number of them took advantage of civilians, as well as female inmates liberated from concentration camps.

Post-war trials

During the war the "Rabbits" were determined to stay alive and to inform their families in regard to the crimes that were committed by the Nazi doctors at Ravensbrück. When the war was over, they focused on seeking justice and on informing the world about their experiences at the camp. Thanks to the "Rabbits'" efforts, particularly those of the released inmate, Aka Kołodziejczyk, the Allies already had in their possession the list of victims of medical experiments along with a detailed description of experiments before the liberation of Ravensbrück. As soon as the war ended, a number of the victims of Nazi medical experiments, including the "Rabbits", were seeking judicial prosecution and punishment for their tormentors. The process of putting the Nazi criminals on trial, however, was very complex and time-consuming.

The British military at Bergen-Belsen began to receive survivor reports on the experiments with a deposition by Maria Cabajowa on 25 June 1945.[68] The scale of the medical atrocities committed at Ravensbrück was to some extent revealed by the early autumn of 1945, after nearly all members of the "Hohenlychen group", who had operated on the "Rabbits", had been captured and interrogated by British investigators. The situation was further complicated when French and Polish governments demanded extradition of captured criminals. Each country, however, had different motives. The French government argued that a substantial quantity of French prisoners had died at the camp; thus, their concern was that the British would marginalise this issue. The Polish Provisional Government of National Unity made their demand, on the other hand, based on the fact that the majority of the victims of medical experiments performed by the "Hohenlychen group" were of Polish nationality.[69] The British argued that in fact the nationality of prisoners was irrelevant since their focus was on crimes against human beings in general that took place at Ravensbrück regardless of prisoners' origin.[70] Three sides, i.e. the US, the UK and Poland, collected evidence for potential trial independently.

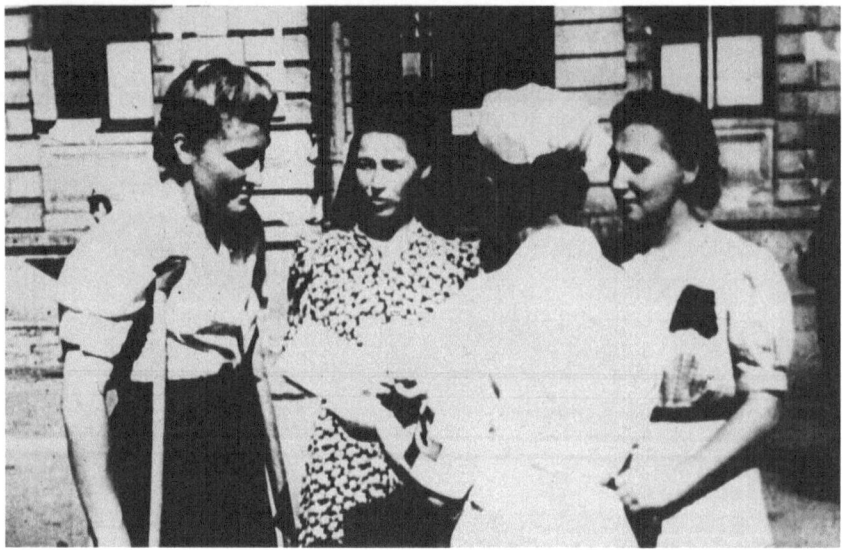

Figure 11.7 Maria Kuśmierczuk (on crutches), Władysława Karolewska and Jadwiga
    Dzido in Warsaw, 1945

Source: USHMM Photo Archives, No. 63553

By November 1945 the Polish government had contacted 54 of the
"Rabbits" who were invited to Gdańsk Medical Academy to undergo an
extensive medical examination. 49 of them were well enough to participate
in this process. Dr Kornel Michejda – Polish specialist in surgery – took photos
and X-rays of their legs and evaluated the damage to their health caused by
the Nazi medical experiments.

Although the "Rabbits" received relatively good medical care upon their
return, their physical health was far from ideal as shown on a photo above
that represents Maria Kuśmierczuk, Władysława Karolewska and Jadwiga
Dzido chatting to a nurse in 1945 in Warsaw. The eyewitness account by Zofia
Mączka, a former prisoner-anaesthetist at Ravensbrück camp hospital, was an
integral part of the report compiled by the Polish Commission to Investigate
German Crimes against Poles.[71] The materials collected by the Polish authorities
were very impersonal as they present only injured limbs; however, they contain
valuable information regarding side effects of these experiments.

Krystyna Iwańska was a victim of sulphonamide experiments. She was
operated on on 14 August 1942. She was one of the women who had additional
material inserted into the wound. The Nazis put her leg into a plaster cast
instead of applying stitches. She recollected that after several days the object
was taken out of the wound and she was operated on again three months later
by a single incision in the same place. No stitches were applied; therefore, the
scar was quite wide and the process of re-cutting and long-lasting healing caused
minor damage to the muscle tissue.[72]

The injuries of Leonarda Bień and Janina Marczewska were more severe. Both were victims of bone experiments, which were conducted by the Berlin surgeon Ludwik Stumpfegger. Leonarda Bień, who was 28 at the time of her first experimental procedure, was subjected to a total of 5 operations on both legs. As a result, bones of both legs were deformed. The victim experienced problems with walking since her ankle joint (*articulatio talocruralis*) was affected by the experiment. Similarly Marczewska, who was experimented upon on 3 December 1942, also on both legs.[73]

The damaged tissue of the right calf that is visible in the photo below may give the impression that Kuśmierczuk was a victim of the muscle experiments. In fact, she was infected with tetanus – a form of the infection produced by very aggressive bacteria, which caused the death of five of the "Rabbits". Weronika Kraska was infected with tetanus on 7 October 1942. She died within a few days. Kazimiera Kurowska died in the middle of October the same year from infection caused by gas bacilli. Aniela Lefanowicz, Zofia Kiecol and Alfreda Prus died within a week after being infected with malignant oedema.[74] Kuśmierczuk testified after the war that it took a year and a half for her wounds to heal. The result of the experiment was considerable damage of the muscle tissue (Figure 11.8); thus, she experienced problems with walking for the rest of her life.[75]

Despite very strong evidence and a large number of witnesses willing to testify, the Polish government was unsuccessful in its efforts to extradite the Ravensbrück perpetrators. Meanwhile, both the Americans and the British competed with each other for the right to put the Rabbits' oppressors on trial. However, as a result of complicated political relations, the British were forced to give up Herta Oberheuser, Fritz Fischer and Karl Gebhardt who all stood trial in Nuremberg led by the American prosecutors; whereas, Rolf Rosenthal and Gerhard Schidlausky were put on trial before the British judges in Hamburg.[76] The participation of the "Rabbits" in the post-war trials of war criminals in Hamburg and in Nuremberg had a double meaning. First of all, they continued the mission of informing the world in regard to the crimes that Nazis conducted on them at Ravensbrück. Second, they aimed for the perpetrators to be punished. Both proceedings overlapped during the first few months. The person who worked on the "Rabbits" case most extensively was a British pathologist for the War Crimes Group, Keith Mant. He spent months preparing the case travelling to Sweden, Belgium and Paris to interview several of the "Rabbits", and document their injuries.[77] Overall, he interviewed more than 100 witnesses. The Soviet authorities created several obstacles for Mant, for example, they repeatedly denied him access to the crime scene – Ravensbrück camp. On 5 December 1946, the British Military tribunal began its proceedings. The trial was held at the Curiohaus in Hamburg and lasted two months. Mant managed to call two "Rabbits" as witnesses. Helena Piasecka came from Paris and Zofia Sokulska arrived from Sweden.[78] The questions they were asked mainly concerned the issues of their death sentence and the forcible participation in the experiments. The "Rabbits" described their brave attempt in protesting against further experiments with astonishing precision.[79] The trial was concluded on

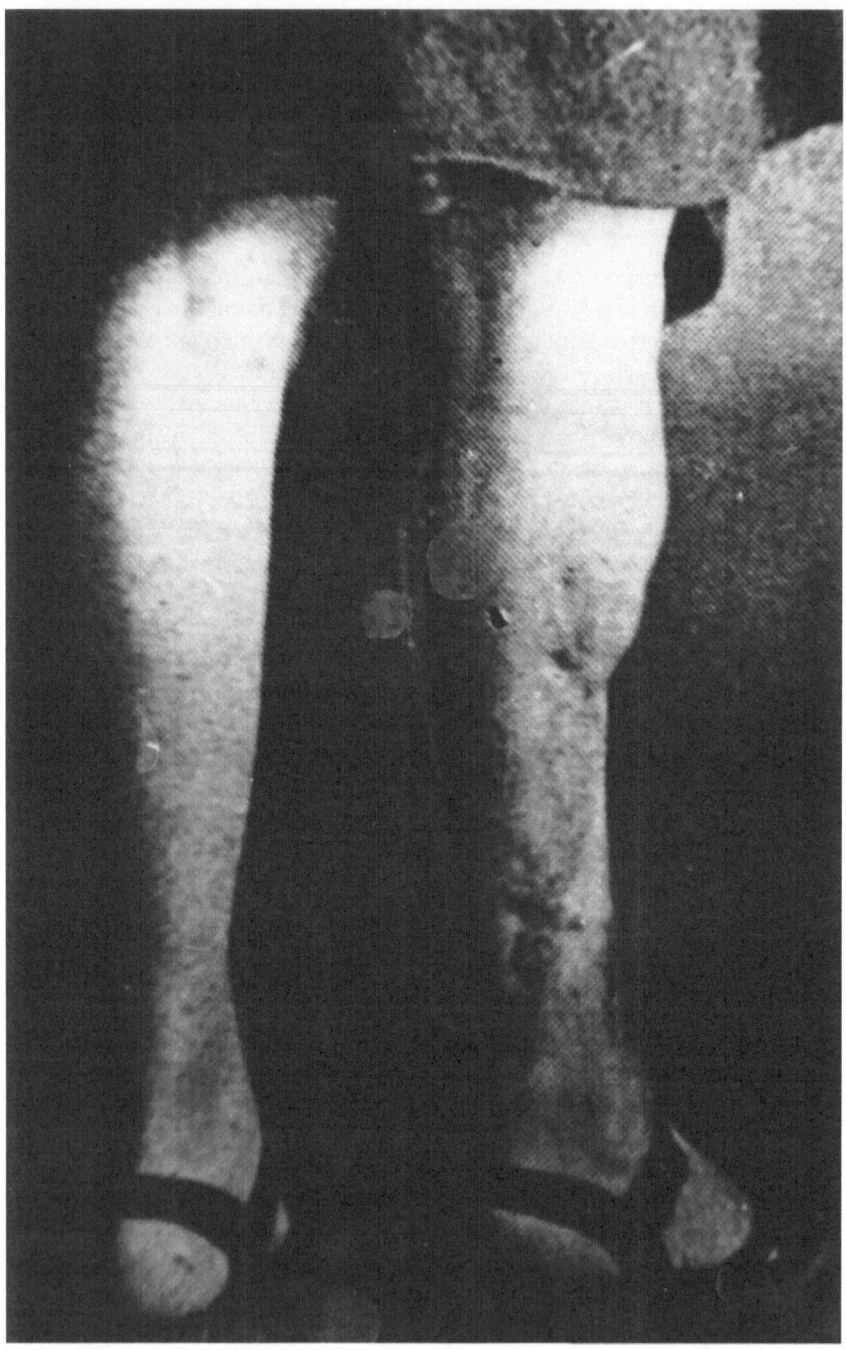

Figure 11.8 Maria Kuśmierczuk
Source: USHMM Photo Archives, No. 63562

3 February 1947. Schidlausky, Rosenthal and Treite, who were involved in sterilisation experiments on Sinti and Roma, were all condemned to death.[80]

Mant had to accept the decision by the British for Gebhardt, Fischer and Oberheuser to be tried at Nuremberg. He went to Nuremberg to brief the medical adviser to the prosecution, Leo Alexander and the prosecutor McHaney, and to conduct further interrogations.[81] The investigator comprehensively involved in preparation to the Nuremberg Medical Trial was the Expert Consultant to the Secretary of War, the neurologist Leo Alexander, who was more successful in bringing witnesses into the courtroom. As a result, Władysława Karolewska, Jadwiga Dzido, Maria Kuśmierczuk and Maria Broel-Plater, came to Nuremberg from Poland to tell their horrific stories, and to show their scars.[82] Leo Alexander greeted them upon their arrival at the Nuremberg train station on 15 December 1946 (see photo below). From that point, the image of these victims was established as they were seen as fashionably dressed, sophisticated and well educated women.

The trial began on 9 December 1946.[83] It has been known as the Nuremberg Medical Trial, and it was the first out of 12 Nuremberg trials. Despite the fact that reports from proceedings of the trial held by the British in Hamburg

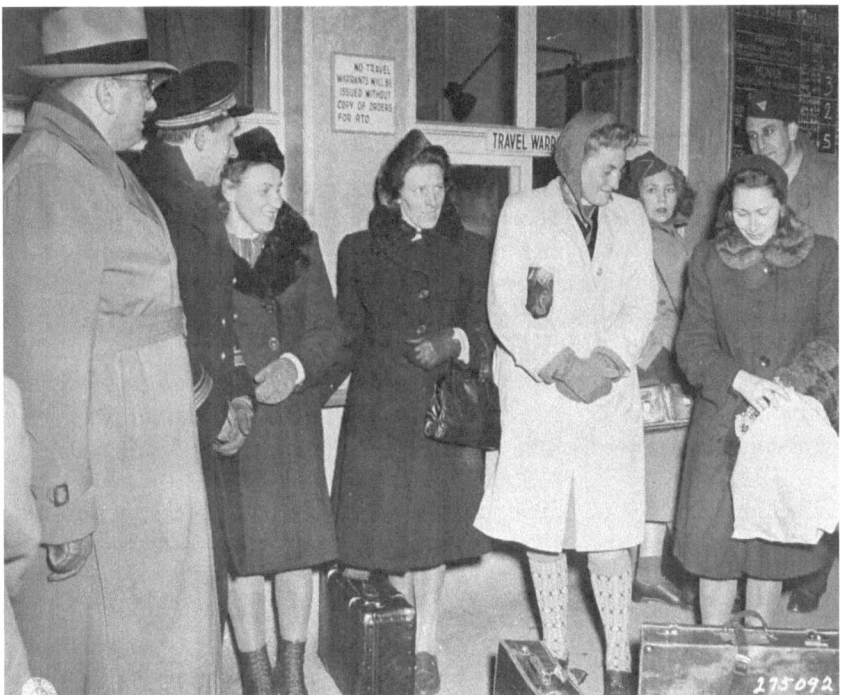

Figure 11.9 From left: Leo Alexander greeting, Jadwiga Dzido, Maria Broel-Plater, Maria Kuśmierczuk and Władysława Karolewska in Berlin

Source: USHMM Photo Archives, No. 43033

regularly appeared in the press in the UK, the publicity given to the trial in Nuremberg by the Americans was without question more substantial.

While the British relied on cross-examination in court (with some success), the Americans under Chief Prosecutor Telford Taylor took a different approach in gathering materials for the trial. These included documents, such as witnesses' statements and photo images of the victims of the Nazi medical crimes, which were later used as evidence in the courtroom.[84] Unlike the image materials collected by the Polish authorities that, one can presume, focused only on scarred limbs, the Americans immortalised the four "Rabbits" in photographs in a rather humanised if not in personal way. In other words, the "Rabbits" were facing the camera regardless of whether it was a front or a profile photo, which could be understood as giving the victims the face and the voice rather than presenting them as nameless statistics (see photos below). Moreover, the fact that they were dressed only in white sheets, which covered just the private parts of their body, gives these images a gender character. Details, such as long hair, jewellery and slightly shy smile (see Figure 11.10) gave the "Rabbits" a more feminine and innocent look. Strictly speaking, the "Rabbits" were not only presented as victims and witnesses but also as attractive, young and physically fragile women, whose awfully scarred legs proved beyond any doubt that they were experimented upon.

Moreover, the presence of the "Rabbits" in the courtroom as witnesses, and the content of their testimonies gave the prosecuting team an additional weapon against the defendants. The experiences related to the incarceration and forcible medical experiments described by the victims made an unforgettable impression. However, what had an even greater impact was the fact that the "Rabbits" could be identified with American women who were present during proceedings. The goal of the prosecutors was not presenting their witnesses as emotionally unstable but rather the opposite. For instance, Karolewska, who appears in the photo below, through her outfit and body posture, indicated her relatively high social background and good manners.

In addition, the sophisticated behaviour in conjunction with the eloquent way of communicating, presented the four "Rabbits" as extremely reliable witnesses who did not look for sympathy or compassion but for justice.[85]

Despite the horrifying stories told by the "Rabbits" in the courtroom, the prosecutors managed to gain a satisfying verdict only for Gebhardt who was sentenced to death and executed on 2 June 1948.[86] Oberheuser based her defence on the fact that she did not perform any surgery but was only responsible for post-operative care of victims.[87] Fischer, on the other hand, was the only doctor who showed repentance.[88] In addition, the fact that he lost his arm in combat, as he claimed he was sent to the Front for refusing to participate in further experiments, most likely had an impact on the final verdict of the court.[89] The judges treated both Fischer and Oberheuser rather gently. Fischer was sentenced to life in prison. Oberheuser was given a sentence of 25 years in prison.[90] In the end, they were freed after only five years.[91]

The Hamburg and the Nuremberg Trials received considerable press coverage both in Poland and abroad. The Polish newspaper *Dziennik Polski i Dziennik Żołnierza* published several short articles informing Polish refugees in London about the proceedings in both courts. The news from the Hamburg Trial appeared several times a week presenting topics beyond simply the testimonies of the "Rabbits", whereas articles with reference to the proceedings in Nuremberg were concerned mainly with the suffering of Polish inmates at Ravensbrück.[92] In Poland, on the other hand, the press was controlled to a huge extent by the Communist regime and paid a great deal of attention to the Nuremberg Medical Trial. However, the motive of support given by the Polish government to the "Rabbits" case, despite how it was presented in the press, was mainly ideological. In other words, highlighting the crimes of the Nazis was a larger concern than seeking justice for Polish victims of medical experiments. The fact that the four "Rabbits" had to cover their travel expenses from Poland to Nuremberg and did not receive help regarding accommodation and food supplies in Berlin before they arrived in Nuremberg proves that they were not a priority for the Polish Military Mission in Berlin.[93] Unlike the French who complained about the verdict of the Hamburg Trial, the Polish observers had no objections.[94] The Polish press in Great Britain did not mention the verdicts of either of the trials. However, the "Rabbits'" actions were successful to a certain extent. Thanks to their determination the Ravensbrück perpetrators were either executed or placed behind bars.

The American help in the fight for compensation

In July 1951, the German cabinet of Chancellor Adenauer issued a decree according to which victims of medical experiments were entitled to compensation. Provided, however, that there were political relations between the Federal Republic of Germany and the country of origin of the applicant.[95] In 1956, the compensation law was revised; as a result, only a small number of victims were qualified to receive compensation. In addition, victims who were imprisoned as political prisoners, and members of the Resistance, were omitted.[96] Thus, Polish victims who resided in Poland were excluded, and consequently the claims submitted by the "Rabbits" were rejected on the same grounds.[97]

Neither the British nor American governments took a stand in regard to the issue of financial compensation for the victims of the Nazi medical crimes who settled in their countries, thus the victims sought support from elsewhere. The Catholic Women's League, for example, provided financial assistance in addition to moral support for several victims including the only "Rabbit" who settled in the UK long term, Zofia Sokulska-Kaczmarska.[98]

In the US, however, the traumatic story of the "Rabbits", who as victims of extremely brutal medical experiments were deprived of the compensation, moved a lot of people abroad. Therefore, in 1958 three individuals, Caroline Ferriday,[99] Benjamin Ferencz and Norman Cousins established the

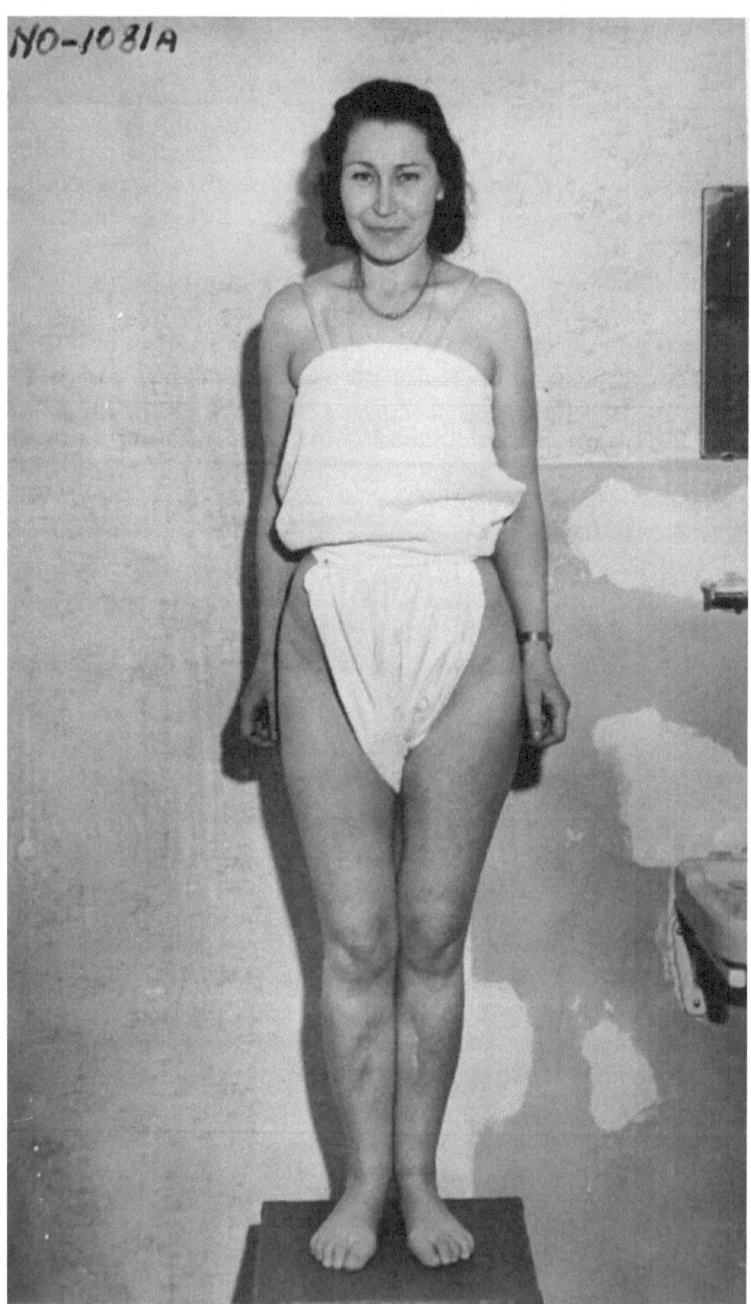

Figures 11.10 and 11.11 Władysława Karolewska and Jadwiga Dzido

Source: USHMM Photo Archives, No. 78599 and 78600. These are copies of the original photo images that are held at the National Archives and Records Administration in College Park in Maryland, USA

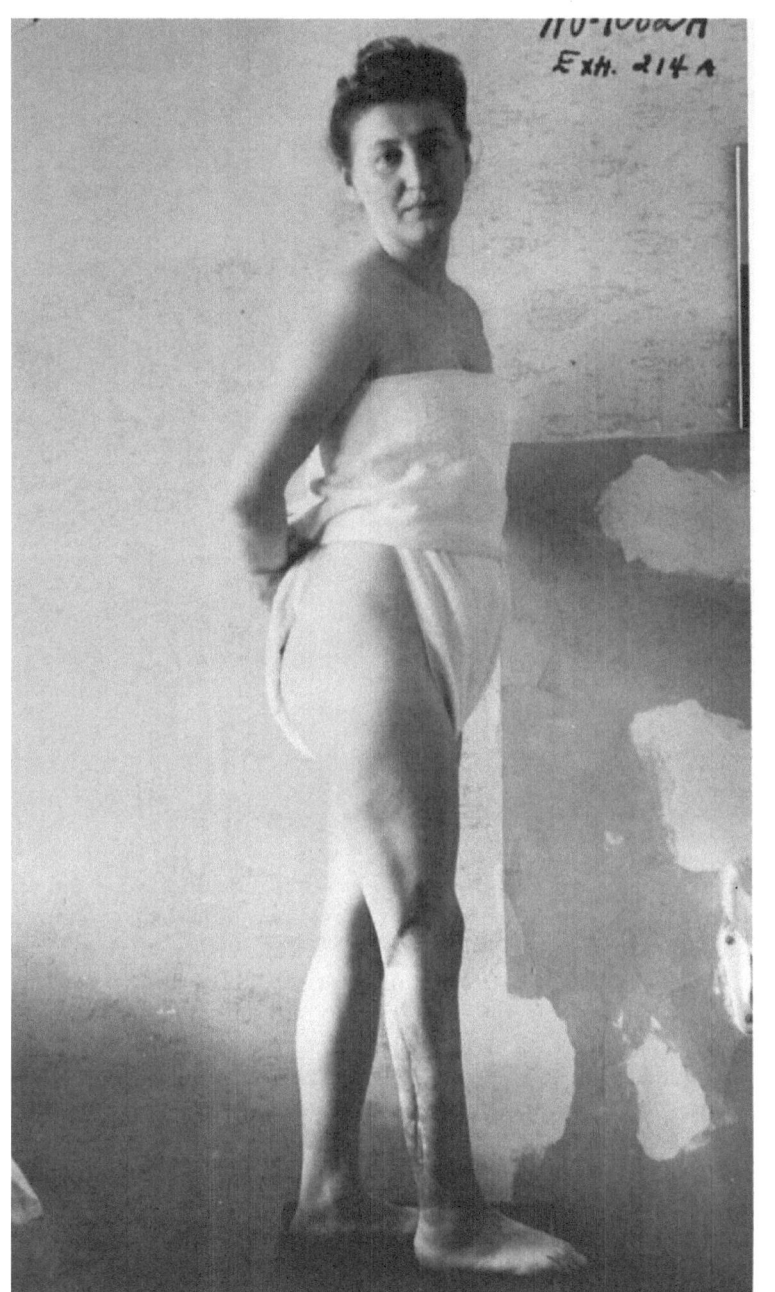

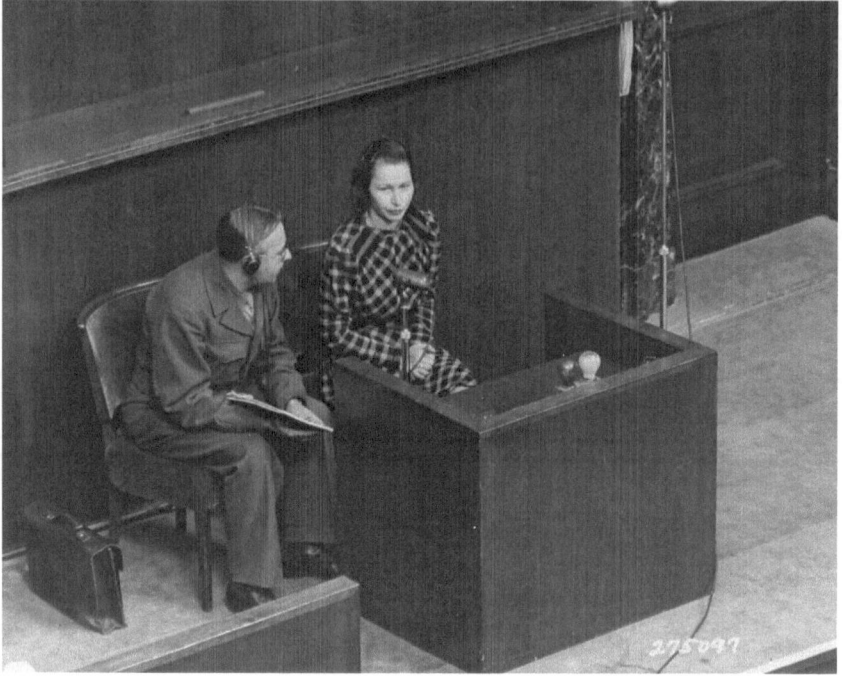

Figure 11.12 Władysława Karolewska in courtroom
Source: USHMM Photo Archives, No. 43019

"Ravensbrück Lapins Project", which was devoted to fighting for justice on behalf of the "Rabbits". Ferriday, who had broad contacts in Europe and was very familiar with the issue of compensation, acted on behalf of all victims of the Nazi medical experiments. Ferencz, as a solicitor, was responsible for the legal side of the issue, such as negotiating with the UN, with the *Bundestag* and with the Polish Ambassador in the US. Cousins, on the other hand, as a well-known journalist kept the public well informed. Yet, the project's initiative came from Ferriday. In 1957, Caroline Ferriday met Piasecka, one of the "Rabbits" who after the war left Poland. Piasecka illustrated the dramatic situation of the "Rabbits" in Poland who at that time were still waiting for compensation.[100] Ferriday heard about Norman Cousins' "Hiroshima Maidens Project" thanks to which a group of 24 Japanese women were brought to the US to undergo free of charge plastic surgery to minimise skin defects caused by the atomic bomb.[101] Therefore, soon after she contacted Cousins via the medical consultant of the "Hiroshima Maidens Project", William Hitzig. In the middle of 1958, the first meeting between Cousins and Ferriday took place, during which she presented all gathered documentation in regard to medical experiments, post-war trials, personal profiles of the "Rabbits" and their medical files. During that meeting the "Ravensbrück Lapins Project" was established.[102] The next step to be taken was organising a medical commission to examine the "Rabbits" in order to choose how many of them were well enough to travel to the US and what kind of medicines were urgently needed in Poland. The American specialists in Warsaw made the final selection of t he participants for the treatment supported by the "Ravensbrück Lapins Project".[103]

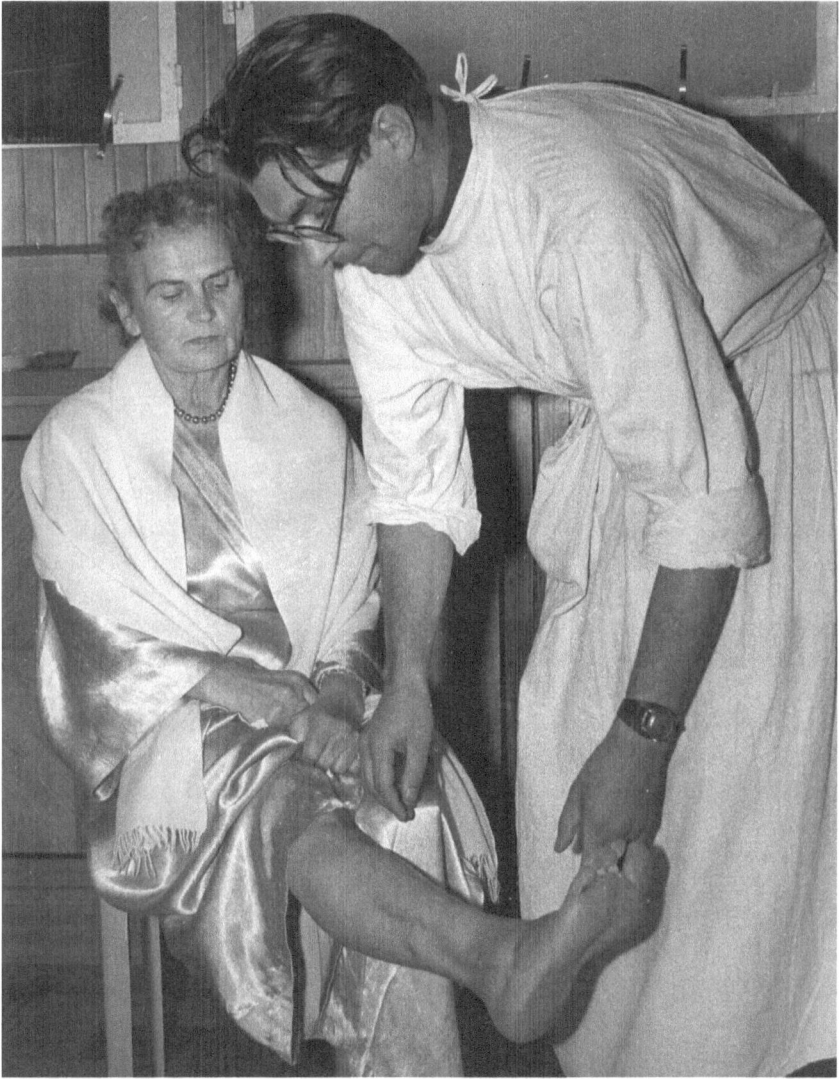

Figure 11.13 Dr William Hitzig examines Pelagia Maćkowska
Source: USHMM Photo Archives, No. 54906

As can be seen in the above photo of Pelagia Maćkowska,[104] who was being examined by Hitzig, the concerns of Piasecka were not exaggerated. After the Nuremberg Medical Trial was concluded and the Cold War became apparent, victims of the Nazi medical experiments who resided in Poland were abandoned and forgotten.[105] However, the very warm and positive attitude of the "Ravensbrück Lapins Project" staff towards the "Rabbits" restored their hope for a better future.

On 18 December 1958, after months of negotiations with the Polish government, 27 Polish victims of medical experiments arrived in New York. The additional eight "Rabbits" flew to the US in March 1959.[106] Not all of them were able to take advantage of that opportunity. Health issues and family problems prevented several of the "Rabbits" from leaving Poland. The "Ravensbrück Lapins Project" was a great success. Several of the "Rabbits" were operated on, and others received optical or dental treatment. In addition, while travelling across the US, they were also able to highlight their struggle for compensation before several American politicians.[107] Meanwhile, the American public opinion followed the "Rabbits'" steps in the US. Several photos of smiling, glamorous, healthy and happy looking Polish ladies appeared in *The Saturday Review*. It was a reward and assurance to all those who contributed to this mission that this trip was essential.

For the "Rabbits", however, this visit was more than an adventure. Stefania Łotocka said after her return to Poland: "Many people with whom we lived, or had contact with showed us countless signs of friendship, which will remain in my heart forever. I've regained my faith in people".[108]

Several months later, the pressure of the "Ravensbrück Lapins Project" forced the German politicians to reconsider their standpoint regarding the "Rabbits'" compensation request. On 13 July 1960, the Vice-President of the *Bundestag*, Carlo Schmidt, sent a letter to Ferencz in which he expressed that the German government was aware of the urgent need to solve the "Rabbits'" problem.[109] On 22 June 1961, during a discussion between members of the German government, finally the decision was made to compensate victims of the Nazi medical experiments who lived in countries with which the Federal Republic had no official political relations.[110] The Federal Finance Ministry agreed to distribute to the victims DM 5,000,000 in a form of single instalments, which each was not supposed to exceed DM 25,000.[111] The vast majority of the "Rabbits" received the "financial support" in early 1961.[112]

The compensation claims process took place between 1961 and 1971. The "urgent" applications of the "Rabbits" and the Polish Catholic priests from Dachau were considered mainly because of the publicity around them, but also because of the fact that they did not require much work since they were very well documented and, more importantly, already completed. All the "Rabbits" who lived in Poland were compensated in 1962, and the vast majority of them received their payments in early January.[113] The money was sent to the individual accounts of *Polska Kasa Opieki Spółka Akcyjna* (The Polish

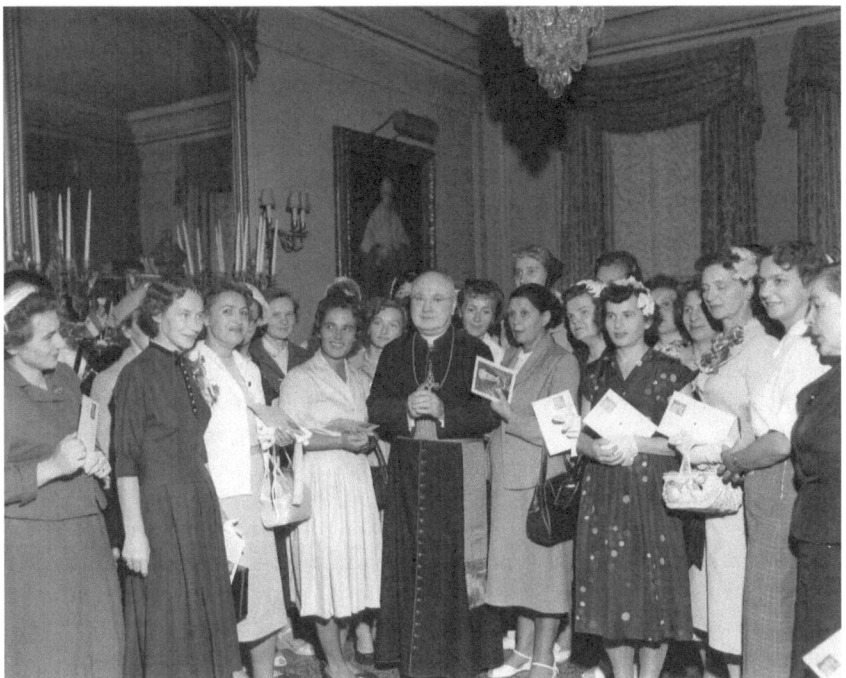

Figure 11.14 Cardinal Spellman grants a private audience to a delegation of
"Rabbits" in the USA, 1959

Source: USHMM Photo Archives, No. 54908

PEKAO SA Bank). Moreover, the amount was processed in American
Dollars. The sum varied from $ 7,500.63 up to $ 10,000.85 according to the
health damage caused by the experiment.[114] Those "Rabbits" who were
victims of the sulphonamide experiments with use of gangrenous cultures such
as *streptococci* and *staphylococci*, and women who were operated on by Ludwig
Stumpfegger received the highest amount of money. Each of the "Rabbits"
upon receiving the money had to declare that it was financial assistance rather
than compensation as stated: "[The] sum was put at my disposal to help victims
of the title of pseudo-medical experiences in German concentration camps
under the National Socialist regime".[115]

In early 1972, the first discussion to establish relations between Poland and
the Federal Republic of Germany took place. The prime ground for discussion
was security in Europe. On 27 May 1972, the Polish government ratified the
pact with West Germany. Official political relations between the two countries
were established in the middle of September 1972.[116] Meanwhile, corresponding
negotiations took place in the name of the remaining victims of the Nazi medical
experiments whose number was estimated at 6,000 and who were waiting to
be compensated. As a result, on 16 November 1972, an agreement was signed

between the Federal German Finance Ministry and the Polish Ministry of Health and Public Care under which Poland was granted DM 103 million towards further compensation.[117] Those negotiations did not meet the expectations of the "Rabbits". First of all, the word "compensation" was replaced by "financial help" for Polish victims of medical experiments, wherein the Federal German government thereby washed its hands from taking any responsibility for medical crimes committed by the Nazis. Second, the Polish government was put in charge of distributing the money instead of the Polish Red Cross; thus, the risk of abuses increased. Finally, the sum of DM 103 million was to be the final act in the compensation issue, which meant that the topic of lifelong pensions for the "Rabbits" was abandoned, and they were excluded from further support since they had already received compensation in 1962.[118]

The "Rabbits" have been identified as a group of extraordinary women – victims of medical experiments who survived the Ravensbrück concentration camp thanks to their determination and bravery. The photo images presented in this chapter confirm their heroic behaviour. However, in addition to evidence of the Nazi medical crimes in the form of scars that were visible on several photos, one can also read emotions, captured at a particular moment. Jadwiga Dzido-Hassa's face, for instance, shows signs of concern, pain and hopelessness. Whereas, Władysława Karolewska, despite her suffering, represented feminine innocence, kindness and trust in a positive future. The diverse state of mind of the "Rabbits" expressed in these photo images reveals that behind this icon of the brave heroic victims were ordinary women who had moments of fear, physical pain, anxiety, as well as hope and happiness.

Notes

1 This chapter is an extended version of a paper published in German in 2012, see Aleksandra Loewenau, 'Die Kaninchen von Ravensbrück: Eine Fotogeschichte', in Insa Eschebach and Astrid Ley (ed.), *Geschlecht und "Rasse" in der NS-Medizin*, Berlin: Metropol Verlag, 2012, pp. 115–139.

2 Zofia Mączka, 'Operacje doświadczalne przeprowadzone w obozie koncentracyjnym Ravensbrück', *Biuletyn Głównej Komisji Badania Zbrodni Niemieckich w Polsce*, 2 (1947), pp. 123–133.

3 Alexander Mitscherlich and Fred Mielke, *Doctors of Infamy: The Story of the Nazi Medical Crimes*, New York: Henry Schuman, 1949.

4 Paul Julian Weindling, *Nazi Medicine and the Nuremberg Trials: From Medical War Crimes to Informed Consent*, Houndmills, Basingstoke: Palgrave Macmillan, 2004. For information related to the British investigation regarding the medical crimes committed in Ravensbrück, see idem, 'Auf der Spur von Medizinverbrechen: Keith Mant (1919–2000) und sein Debut als forensischer Pathologe', *1999. Zeitschrift für Sozialgeschichte des 20. und 21. Jahrhunderts*, 16 (2001), pp. 129–139; Ulf Schmidt, '"The Scars of Ravensbrück": Medical Experiments and British War Policy, 1945–1950', *German History*, 23 (2005), pp. 20–49.

5 Paul Weindling, *Victims and Survivors of Nazi Human Experiments: Science and Suffering in the Holocaust*, London: Bloomsbury, 2015.

6 Volker Roelcke, 'Sulfonamide Experiments on Prisoners in Nazi Concentration Camps: Coherent Scientific Rationality Combined with Complete Disregard of

Humanity', in Sheldon Rubenfeld and Susan Benedict (eds), *Human Subjects Research after the Holocaust*, New York: Springer, 2014, pp. 51–66.

7 Idem,'Die Sulfonamid-Experimente in nationalsozialistischen Konzentrationslagern: Eine kritische Neubewertung der epistemologischen und ethischen Dimension', *Medizinhistorisches Journal*, 44 (2009), pp. 42–60.

8 Klier did not present the depth of the issue as she included too comprehensive analysis of the perpetrators; therefore, it is hard to get what is her argument, see: Freya Klier, *Die Kanninchen von Ravensbrück: Medizinische Versuche an Frauen in der NS-Zeit*, Munich: Knaur, 1994. Waltz, on the other hand, managed to interview several of the "Rabbits" presenting their perspective, see: Loretta Walz, *"Und dann kommst du dahin an einem schönen Sommertag": Die Frauen von Ravensbrück*, Munich: Kunstmann, 2005.

9 Wanda Półtawska, *And I Am Afraid of My Dreams*, London: Hodder & Stoughton, 1964; Helena Klimek (ed.), *Ponad ludzka miarę*, Warsaw: Książka i Wiedza, 1972; Urszula Wińska, *Więzi: Losy wieźniarek z Ravensbrück*, Gdańsk: Wydawnictwo "Marpress", 1992.

10 Mączka, 'Operacje doświadczalne', p. 124.

11 Alexander Mitscherlich and Fred Mielke, *Medizin ohne Menschlichkeit: Dokumente des Nürnberger Ärzteprozesses*, Frankfurt am Main: Fischer Taschenbuch Verlag, 1981, p. 141. Also Kew, The National Archives (hereafter TNA), WO 235/306: Judge Advocate General's Office: War Crimes Case Files, Second World War, Ravensbrück Case, Testimony by Helena Piasecka, 30 Dec 1946.

12 *Kaninchen* – Rabbits in German; *Lapins* – in French as well as so referred to in American English; *króliki* – in Polish. In this chapter I will use the term "Rabbits".

13 Wanda Szymonowicz, *Beyond Human Endurance*, Warsaw: Interpress Publishers, 1970, pp. 8–9.

14 Helena Piasecka, testifying at the Hamburg Ravensbrück Trial, said that personally she never saw the written order for a death sentence. However, her mother had informed her that the Gestapo had confirmed that her daughter had received a death sentence. TNA, WO 235/306, Witness Testimony, Helena Piasecka, 30 Dec 1946.

15 Lublin Castle was built in the 1820s as a prison on the grounds of a destroyed castle that dated from the twelfth century. The Nazis took it over in 1939. Approximately 40,000 people were interrogated in this prison that, next to Pawiak in Warsaw, Montelupich in Cracow, and Fort VII in Posen, was one of the biggest prisons in occupied Poland. Thousands of inmates were executed or died as a result of torture, or were sent to Nazi camps. On 22 July 1944, the Nazis murdered 300 prisoners in the massacre at Lublin Castle. In Aug 1944, the Castle was transformed into a prison for opponents of the Communist regime. It held approximately 35,000 Poles, 333 were executed. In 1957, the Castle became a location for a state museum. For other information, see Zygmunt Mannkowski and Róża Bieluszko-Świechowa (eds), *Hitlerowskie Więzienie na Zamku w Lublinie 1939–1944*, Lublin: Wydawnictwo Lubelskie, 1988.

16 *Więzienie pod Zegarem* was built between 1928 and 1930 as the main building for the Land Office. Between 1940 and 1944 it was a prison. Thousands of Poles and Jews, mainly political opponents and members of the resistance movement, were interrogated and tortured there. It was called "the Prison under the Clock" because there is a clock above the main entrance to the building. See http://zamek-lublin.pl (Accessed on 12 Jan 2015).

17 Helena Piasecka delivered twins. See http://jtajchert.w.interia.pl/zyciorysykrolikow. htm (Accessed on 12 Jan 2015).

18 Szymonowicz, *Beyond Human Endurance*, p. 88; also see Jack G. Morrison, *Ravensbrück: Everyday Life in a Women's Concentration Camp, 1939–1945*, London: Eurospan Group, 2000, p. 246.

19 The number of the "Rabbits" who were exposed to each series of experiments has been differently estimated by scholars. The difficulty comes from contradictory figures being given by defendants at the Nuremberg Medical Trial. Estimates given in this article are based on testimony of Zofia Mączka and her medical report, 'Operacje doświadczalne w obozie koncentracyjnym Ravensbrück', published in 1946.

20 For division according to applied drugs see Volker Roelcke, 'Tiermodell und Menschenbild; Konfigurationen der epistemologischen und ethischen Mensch-Tier-Grenzziehung in der Humanmedizin zwischen 1880 und 1945', in Birgit Griesecke, Markus Krause, Nicolas Pethes and Katja Sabisch (eds), *Kulturgeschichte des Menschenversuchs im 20. Jahrhundert*, Frankfurt am Main: Suhrkamp, 2009, p. 33.

21 Mączka, 'Operacje doświadczalne', p. 124.

22 The prisoner nurses did not assist during the experimental operations but were also not allowed to help any of the "Rabbits". See Karolina Lanckorońska, *Michelangelo in Ravensbrück: One Woman's War Against the Nazis*, Boston: Da Capo, 2008, p. 205.

23 The first executed Polish prisoner was Wanda Maciejewska on 1 Feb 1941. However, starting from 1942 several prisoners at a time were taken. The last execution of Poles took place in 1945. For more information on that matter, see Wanda Kiedrzyńska, Irena Pannenkowa and Eliza Sulińska, *Ravensbrück*, Warsaw: Książka i Wiedza, 1961, pp. 163–186.

24 Based on testimonies by Leokadia Kwiecińska, Pelagia Maćkowska and Eugenia Mikulska-Turowska. For detailed descriptions, see Szymonowicz, *Beyond Human Endurance*, pp. 91–92, 123 and 133.

25 Ibid.

26 Urszula Wińska, *Zwyciężyły wartości: wspomnienia z Ravensbrück*, Gdańsk: Wydawncitwo Morskie, 1985, pp. 304–305; also Kiedrzyńska et al., *Ravensbrück*, p. 211.

27 Walz, *Und dann kommst*, pp. 301–303.

28 TNA, WO 235/306, Testimony by Helena Piasecka, 30 Dec 1946.

29 Wińska, *Zwyciężyły wartości*, pp. 306–307.

30 On 28 September 1943, Rosalia Gutek, Maria Zielonka, Stanisława Śledziowska and Apolonia Rakowska were shot. For additional information see Jarek Górecki's website: http://individual.utoronto.ca/jarekg/Ravensbruck/Photographsofvictims.html (Accessed on 15 Nov 2015)

31 Kiedrzyńska based her observation on Agnieszka Glinczanka who translated many of those letters into French. See Kiedrzyńska et al., *Ravensbrück*, p. 276.

32 Washington DC, United States Holocaust Memorial Museum (hereafter USHMM), International Tracing Service, 1.1.35.1 List Material Ravensbrück, Briefe an Häftlinge des Männer Lagers über die Untergrundtätigkeit im Lager, medizinische Versuche und Exekutionen 1942/43. There is an error in the description of the folder. These are letters written by Polish women in Ravensbrück. Several of those letters were published. See Kazimierz Smoleń (ed.), *Aby świat sie dowiedział . . . : nielegalne dokumenty z obozu Ravensbrück*, Oświęcim: Wydawn. Państwowego Muzeum w Oświęcimiu, 1980, pp. 66–109.

33 Weindling, *Victims and Survivors*, p. 91. Families on the other hand hid replies in food parcels that were sent to the camp starting from December 1942. Smoleń, *Aby świat sie dowiedział*, p. 53. Several of those letters have been displayed at the Lublin Museum "Under the Clock".

34 Kiedrzyńska et al., *Ravensbrück*, p. 212.

35 Apart from the five photos of the "Rabbits" the negative film also contained two pictures of Polish women who were transported to Ravensbrück after the failure of the Warsaw Uprising. See USHMM Photo Archives, Nos. 69337 and 69338.

36 http://jtajchert.w.interia.pl/zyciorysykrolikow.htm (Accessed on 10 Jan 2015).

37 Lanckorońska, *Michelangelo in Ravensbrück*, p. 273.

38 Wińska, *Zwyciężyły wartości*, pp. 311–313.

39 Szymonowicz, *Beyond Human Endurance*, p. 54.
40 Półtawska, *And I Am Afraid*, p. 151.
41 London, "Studium Polski Pozdziemnej" (The Polish Underground Movement Trust), Delegatura Rządu Sprawozdania-Raporty, Raport dotyczący obozu w Majdanku i innych obozów w Rzeszy, 6 Mar 1944.
42 Henryk Świebodzki (ed.), *London Has Been Informed: Reports by Auschwitz Escapees*, Oświęcim: The Auschwitz-Birkenau State Museum, 1997, p. 97. For information about what was known about atrocities committed at Ravensbrück before the war ended see Paul Weindling, 'Was wussten die Allierten während des Krieges und unmittelbar danach über die Menschenversuche in deutschen Konzentrationslagern?', in Astrid Ley and Marion Maria Ruisinger (eds), *Gewissenlos Gewissenhaft: Menschenversuche im Konzentratonslager*, Erlangen: Specht, 2001, pp. 54–58.
43 Półtawska, *And I Am Afraid*, p. 151.
44 The International Committee of the Red Cross (ICRC) was informed about the situation of the "Rabbits" by the Liaison Committee of Women's International Organisation already in October 1944. In December, the first food parcels were sent to the "Rabbits". See Geneva, Archives du Comité international de la Croix-Rouge, Microfilm G 44/01, 44/13–11 otages, détenus politiques. Allemagne. Corréspondance générale avec Croix-Rouge 1.12.1943–30.05.1945, Resolution of the Liaison Committee of Women's international Organisations signed Elsie Zimmern, 23 Oct 1944. Also see Jean-Claude Favez, *The Red Cross and the Holocaust*, Cambridge: Cambridge University Press, 1999, p. 43. In addition, for a detailed description of the standpoint of the ICRC towards the "Rabbits'" issue see Weindling, *Nazi Medicine*, pp. 15–20.
45 Folke Bernadotte was born on 2 Jan 1895 in Stockholm to Prince Oscar Bernadotte Count of Wisborg. His grandfather was King Oscar II of Sweden. From an early age he attended military school and in 1915 he took his officer's exam. In 1943 Bernadotte was appointed the vice chairman of the Swedish Red Cross, which opened opportunities to negotiate between the Allies and the Axis for prisoner exchanges and further for their release. Thanks to his "white buses" action, which rescued concentration camp prisoners under protection of the Red Cross approximately 31,000 inmates left concentration camps before their liquidation. His contribution was recognised and in 1948 he was appointed as the first UN mediator in Palestine. Unfortunately, on 17 Sept 1948, Bernadotte was assassinated by a Jewish terrorist Zionist group and as a result he died on the same day. See Ralph Hewins, *Count Folke Bernadotte: His Life and Work*, London: Hutchinson & Co., 1948; Sarah Helm, *If this is a Woman: Inside Ravensbrück Hitler's Concentration Camp for Women*, London: Little Brown, 2015.
46 Hewins, *Count Folke Bernadotte*, p. 123.
47 Ibid., pp. 115 and 122–125.
48 For more information in regard to help that Bernadotte provided to inmates of the Nazi concentration camp, see article written by a witness: Zygmunt Łakociński, 'Folke Bernadotte i akcja Szwedzkiego Czerwonego Krzyża', *Przegląd Lekarski*, 1 (1968), pp. 145–152. Also see Peter Padfield, *Himmler Reichs Führer-SS*, London: Cassell & Co., 2001, pp. 590–591.
49 Kiedrzyńska *et al.*, *Ravensbrück*, p. 242.
50 Hewins, *Count Folke Bernadotte*, pp. 154–155.
51 Irith Dublon-Knebel (ed.), *A Holocaust Crossroads: Jewish Women and Children in Ravensbrück*, London: Vallentine Mitchell, 2010, pp. 228–229.
52 http://jtajchert.w.interia.pl/zyciorysykrolikow.htm (Accessed on 12 Jan 2015).
53 For more information in reference to rescue actions of Poles see Hewins, *Count Folke Bernadotte*, pp. 154–155.
54 Wińska, *Więzi*, pp. 90–91.
55 http://jtajchert.w.interia.pl/zyciorysykrolikow.htm (Accessed on 10 Jan 2015).
56 Wińska, *Więzi*, p. 45.

57 Ibid., p. 54.
58 Kiedrzyńska *et al.*, *Ravensbrück*, p. 245.
59 Wińska, *Więzi*, p. 62.
60 Ibid., pp. 64–65.
61 Półtawska, *And I Am Afraid*, p. 155.
62 Wińska, *Więzi*, p. 80.
63 About the conditions at Neustadt-Glewe, see Morrison, *Ravensbrück*, pp. 215–217.
64 Hagit Lavsky, *New Beginnings: Holocaust Survivors in Bergen-Belsen and the British Zone in Germany, 1945–1950*, Detroit: Wayne State University Press, 2002, p. 37.
65 Joanne Reilly, *Belsen: The Liberation of a Camp*, London: Routledge, 1998, p. 25. More in regard to the British medical efforts at Bergen-Belsen after the liberation, see Susanne Bardgett and David Cesarani (eds), *Belsen 1945: New Historical Perspective*, London: Vallentine Mitchell, 2006, pp. 31–51. Bardgett and Cesarani favoured the way the British handled the liberation; however, issues such as the incorrect handling of malnutrition and infectious diseases were ignored. Weindling, on the other hand, emphasised both problems related to immediate health and hygiene problems and immigration of survivors to other European countries, see Paul Weindling, ' "Belsenitis": Liberating Belsen, Its Hospitals, UNRRA, and Selection for Re-emigration, 1945–1948', *Science in Context*, 19 (2006), pp. 401–418.
66 A third person to be liberated from Bergen-Belsen was Hanna Sienkiewicz who returned to Poland relatively soon after the war. She studied art in Cracow and in Warsaw and died in 1986. Go to http://jtajchert.w.interia.pl/zyciorysykrolikow.htm (Accessed on 10 Jan 2015).
67 Rochelle G. Saidel, *The Jewish Women of Ravensbrück Concentration Camp*, Madison: University of Wisconsin Press, 2004, p. 158.
68 TNA, WO 309/1697, Deposition of Maria Cabajowa, 25 June 1945. Also TNA, WO 209/3944A, 'In the Matter of War Crimes and Operations at Ravensbrück', 26 June 1945.
69 Schmidt, 'The Scars of Ravensbrück', p. 24; Weindling, *Nazi Medicine*, p. 107.
70 TNA, WO 309/468.
71 Mączka, 'Operacje doświadczalne', pp. 123–175.
72 Ibid., p. 137.
73 Ibid., p. 160–161.
74 Mitscherlich and Mielke, *Doctors of Infamy*, p. 56.
75 For more information regarding her health state shortly after the war, see Mączka, 'Operacje doświadczalne', pp. 146–147; Ulf Schmidt, *Justice at Nuremberg: Leo Alexander and the Nazi Doctors' Trial*, New York: Palgrave Macmillan, 2006, p. 188–189.
76 Fischer was in the beginning held by the British who interrogated him; however, later he was hand over to the Americans.
77 Zofia Sokulska testified before Mant on 11 July 1946 in Lund 3/713; Zofia Baj testified on 12 Aug 1946 in Brussels 3/718; Janina Iwańka testified in Paris 3/724; Helena Piasecka was questioned on 28 June in Paris 3/733, see A.K. Mant, 'The Medical Services in the Concentration Camp of Ravensbruck', *The Medico-Legal Journal*, 17 (1949), pp. 99–118.
78 Mant on the British side faced problems in calling witnesses who lived in Poland; therefore, only the "Rabbits" who lived abroad were able to testify.
79 For testimonies of Sokulska and Piasecka see TNA, WO 235/306, 31 Dec 1946.
80 Ibid.
81 On Mant's investigations of Ravensbrück and the International Scientific Commission, see Paul Weindling, *John W. Thompson, Psychiatrist in the Shadow of the Holocaust*, Rochester, NY: Rochester University Press, 2010, pp. 116–121.
82 Schmidt, *Justice at Nuremberg*, p. 180.

83 For lists of documents selected for the Nuremberg Medical Trial including exhibits, defendants' interrogation, as well as witness testimonies, see Klaus Dörner *et al.* (eds), *The Nuremberg Medical Trial 1946/1947. Transcripts, Material of the Prosecution and Defense. Related Documents. Guide to the Microfiche-Edition*, Munich: Saur, 2001.

84 Paul Weindling, 'Victims, Witnesses and the Ethical Legacy of the Nuremberg Medical Trial', in Kim Priemel and Alexa Stiller (eds), *Reassessing The Nuremberg Military Tribunals: Transitional Justice, Trial Narratives, and Historiography*, New York: Berghahn, 2014, pp. 74–103.

85 All four women had a relatively high social background. Broel-Plater, Kuśmierczuk and Dzido were university students when the war began see http://jtajchert.w.interia.pl/zyciorysykrolikow.htm. Moreover, for information regarding the social division and the impact of higher education in the pre-war Poland see: Alicja Iwańska, *Polish Intelligentsia in Nazi Concentration Camps and American Exile: A Study of Values in Crises Situations*, Lewiston: Edwin Mellen Press, 1998.

86 There are several photos that depict Gebhardt's execution, see College Park, MD, National Archives and Records Administration (hereafter NARA), RG 238, Box 4; Mitscherlich and Mielke, *Medizin ohne Menschlichkeit*, p. 281.

87 NARA, 1019/50, Testimony of Herta Oberheuser, 25 Sept 1945; TNA, WO 309/469, 55799, Report on Herta Oberheuser.

88 Jarosław Gajewski, 'Odzyskana wiara w ludzi: Sprawa ofiar niemieckich eksperymentów medycznych w KL Ravensbrück', *Glaukopis*, 9 (2007), p. 105.

89 Fischer's correspondence with his wife during the war and while being imprisoned by the British, in which he confidently and positively spoke about his future as his action were justified to some extent, was also used in his defence.

90 Mitscherlich and Mielke, *Medizin ohne Menschlichkeit*, pp. 281–282.

91 According to Landsberg officers Fischer, who worked as doctor at the prisons hospital, was a model inmate, which in fact led to his rather early release, see NARA, RG 238, Report written by Capt. M. Love, 23 June 1950.

92 Examples of articles include: 'Zeznania Polki więźniarki z Ravensbrück', *Dziennik Polski i Dziennik Żołnierza*, 291.7 (10 Dec 1946), p. 1; 'Egzekucje w Ravensbrück', ibid., 293.7 (12 Dec 1946), p. 4; 'Ofiara nieludzkich eksperymentów', ibid., 301.7 (21 Dec 1946), p. 1.

93 'Więźniarki z Ravensbrück jadą do Norymbergi', ibid., 21.8 (21 Feb 1947), p. 4.

94 For the reaction of the French to the Hamburg Trial, see Weindling, *Nazi Medicine*, p. 108.

95 Krzysztof Ruchniewicz, *Polskie zabiegi o odszkodowania niemieckie w latach 1944/45–1975*, Wrocław: Wydawnictwo Universytetu Wrocławskiego, 2007, p. 100.

96 USHMM, Benjamin Ferencz Collection, R.G.12.012.02–01, Chronological Outline of Steps Taken by the Ravensbrueck Lapins and Groups Acting on Their Behalf to Obtain Indemnification from the Federal Republic of Germany, Mar 1960.

97 The precise explanation for this decision was the fact that because of lack of diplomatic representation it was impossible to verify the evidences collected by the Polish side.

98 Geneva, United Nations Archive, UNOG/SO 262/2, Part A, Letter of Sokulska to Ferriday, 3 Nov 1957. Another organisation involved in fighting for compensation for the victims of Nazi medicine both in Europe and in the US since the early 1950s was the Friends of the *Association Nationale des Anciennes Déportées et Internées de la Résistance* (National Federation of Resistance Fighters Imprisoned and Deported and Patriots, ADIR). ADIR was founded on 4 Nov 1945 by former French resistance fighter who suffered during the war. The prime aim of this organisation was supporting members of resistance in need and their widow red partners if necessary. After the compensation decree of the German Federal government became valid ADIR sought for compensation application French victims of Nazi medical experiments to be submitted before the Human Rights Division of the UN. Later due to small number of applicants' victims

from other countries also received ADIR's support, which meant financial payment to hundreds of victims worldwide including the US and UK. As a result, in 1950s Caroline Ferriday created Friends of the ADIR, which aimed to help victims in the US. Later this organisation was involved in the fight for compensation for the "Rabbits" in Poland. For more information see USHMM, Benjamin Ferencz and Caroline Ferriday Collections; also on organisation and achievements of the ADIR, see Anne-Marie Pavillard, 'Les archives de l'Association des anciennes déportées at internées de la Résistance (ADIR) à la BDIC', Histoire@Politique. Politique, culture, société, 2.5 (2008), pp. 1–5.

99   Caroline Ferriday was an American philanthropist. In her early years, she was an actress. During the war, she actively supported the French Resistance. She was a member of "France Forever". In addition, she was awarded the Legion of Honour. She died in New York, where she lived almost all her life, aged 87. See 'Carolyn Ferriday, Philanthropist, 87, Who Aided Poles', *The New York Times* (27 Apr 1990).

100   Norman Cousins, 'Dialogue in Warsaw', *The Saturday Review* (28 June 1958).

101   For more information on that matter see: Donald Reid, 'America so far from Ravensbrück', *Histoire@ Politique. Politique, culture, société,* 2.5 (2008), p. 11; also Gajewski, 'Odzyskana wiara w ludzi', pp. 95–96.

102   Ibid., p. 96 and pp. 106–107.

103   Ibid.

104   Jadwiga Dzido got married to Józef Hassa after the war hence the name change.

105   Gajewski, 'Odzyskana wiara w ludzi', p. 112.

106   Reid, 'America so far', p. 8.

107   Gajewski, 'Odzyskana wiara w ludzi', pp. 125–126.

108   Ibid.

109   USHMM, Benjamin Ferencz Collection, RG.12.012.02–01, Carlo Schmidt to Benjamin Ferencz, 13 July 1960.

110   Ruchniewicz, *Polskie zabiegi*, p. 126; Reid, 'America so far', p. 8.

111   Ruchniewicz, *Polskie zabiegi,* p. 128.

112   Each of the "Rabbits" when receiving money had to declare that it was a financial help rather than compensation as quoted: "[The] sum was put at my disposal to help victims of the title of pseudo-medical experiences in German concentration camps under the National Socialist regime". As an example file, see Koblenz, Bundesarchiv Koblenz (hereafter BAK), Politisches Archiv des Auswärtigen Amts (hereafter PAAA), B 126/27578, Teil 1, Irena Bakiel: Pokwitowanie, 3 Jan 1962.

113   Stefania Łotocka received her compensation in November 1962, see BAK, PAAA, B 126/27580, Human Experiments Poland 30–40, Stefania Łotocka: Pokwitowanie, 30 Nov 1962.

114   The entire documentation in regard to compensation for the "Rabbits" is held at the Archives of the Polish Red Cross in Warsaw and in the *Bundesarchiv* in Koblenz. The files deposited at the archives of the Polish Red Cross are not accessible because of the Data Protection Act. However, files can be viewed at the *Bundesarchiv*. Subject to special access criteria negotiated for the project "Victims of Human Experiments and Coercive Research under National Socialism". For details of all 1,357 victims compensated between 1961 and 1971, see a collection BAK PAAA, B 126.

115   As an example file, see BAK, PAAA, B 126/27578, Teil 1, Irena Bakiel: Pokwitowanie, 3 Jan 1962.

116   'Uchwała Rady Państwa o ratyfikacji układu między Polską a NRF, Warszawa, 26.05.1972', in Tadeusz Walichnowski (ed.), *Układy Związku Radzieckiego i Polski z Niemiecką Republiką Federalną na drodze do pokojowej i bezpiecznej Europy. Dokumenty, przemówienia, wywiady, komentarz,* Warsaw: Książka i Wiedza, 1972, p. 68.

117   Gajewski, 'Odzyskana wiara w ludzi', p. 129.

118   Ruchniewicz, *Polskie zabiegi*, pp. 205–207.

Bibliography

Archival sources

Germany

Koblenz, Bundesarchiv Koblenz (BAK), Politisches Archiv des Auswärtigen Amts (PAAA), B 126

Poland

Lublin, Państwowe Muzeum "Pod Zegarem", photo of "Rabbits" in the USA, 1959
Warsaw, Instytut Pamięci Narodowej (IPN), photos of Krystyna Iwańska, Leonarda Bień, Janina Marczewska and Maria Kuśmierczuk

Switzerland

Geneva, Archives du Comité international de la Croix-Rouge, Microfilm G 44/01 and 13–11
Geneva, United Nations Archive, UNOG/SO 262/2, Part A

United Kingdom

Kew, The National Archives (TNA):
WO 209/3944A
WO 235/305–306
WO 309/468–469 and 1697
London, "Studium Polski Pozdziemnej" (The Polish Underground Movement Trust), Delegatura Rządu Sprawozdania-Raporty

USA

College Park, MD, National Archives and Records Administration (NARA), RG 238 Box 4; 1019/50
Washington DC, United States Holocaust Memorial Museum (USHMM):
Benjamin Ferencz Collection, R.G.12.012.02–01
International Tracing Service, 1.1.35.1 List Material Ravensbrück
International Tracing Service Digital Collection, KL Ravensbrück, Folder 54
USHMM Photo Archives: Nos. 43019, 43033, 45696, 54906, 63553, 63555, 69337–69343 and 78599–78600

Literature

Bardgett, Susanne and David Cesarani (eds), *Belsen 1945: New Historical Perspective*, London: Vallentine Mitchell, 2006
Dörner, Klaus, Angelika Ebbinghaus and Karsten Linne (eds), in cooperation with Karl Heinz Roth and Paul Weindling, on behalf of the Stiftung für Sozialgeschte des 20. Jahrhunderts, *The Nuremberg Medical Trial 1946/1947. Transcripts, Material of*

the Prosecution and Defense. Related Documents. Guide to the Microfiche-Edition, Munich: Saur, 2001

Dublon-Knebel, Irith (ed.), *A Holocaust Crossroads: Jewish Women and Children in Ravensbrück*, London: Vallentine Mitchell, 2010

Favez, Jean-Claude, *The Red Cross and the Holocaust*, Cambridge: Cambridge University Press, 1999

Gajewski, Jarosław, 'Odzyskana wiara w ludzi: Sprawa ofiar niemieckich eksperymentów medycznych w KL Ravensbrück', *Glaukopis*, 9 (2007), pp. 94–138.

Helm, Sarah, *If This is a Woman: Inside Ravensbrück Hitler's Concentration Camp for Women*, London: Little Brown, 2015

Hewins, Ralph, *Count Folke Bernadotte: His Life and Work*, London: Hutchinson & Co., 1948

Iwańska, Alicja, *Polish Intelligentsia in Nazi Concentration Camps and American Exile: A Study of Values in Crises Situations*, Lewiston: Edwin Mellen Press, 1998

Kiedrzyńska, Wanda, Irena Pannenkowa and Eliza Sulińska, *Ravensbrück*, Warsaw: Książka i Wiedza, 1961

Klier, Freya, *Die Kanninchen von Ravensbrück: Medizinische Versuche an Frauen in der NS-Zeit*, Munich: Knaur, 1994

Klimek, Helena (ed.), *Ponad ludzka miarę*, Warsaw: Książka i Wiedza, 1972

Łakociński, Zygmunt, 'Folke Bernadotte i akcja Szwedzkiego Czerwonego Krzyża', *Przegląd Lekarski*, 1 (1968), pp. 145–152

Lanckorońska, Karolina, *Michelangelo in Ravensbrück: One Woman's War Against the Nazis*, Boston: Da Capo, 2008

Lavsky, Hagit, *New Beginnings: Holocaust Survivors in Bergen-Belsen and the British Zone in Germany, 1945–1950*, Detroit: Wayne State University Press, 2002

Loewenau, Aleksandra, 'Die Kaninchen von Ravensbrück: Eine Fotogeschichte', in Insa Eschebach and Astrid Ley (ed.), *Geschlecht und "Rasse" in der NS-Medizin*, Berlin: Metropol Verlag, 2012, pp. 115–139

Mączka, Zofia, 'Operacje doświadczalne przeprowadzone w obozie koncentracyjnym Ravensbrück', *Biuletyn Głównej Komisji Badania Zbrodni Niemieckich w Polsce*, 2 (1947), pp. 123–133

Mańkowski, Zygmunt, and Róża Bieluszko-Świechowa (eds), *Hitlerowskie Więzienie na Zamku w Lublinie 1939–1944*, Lublin: Wydawnictwo Lubelskie, 1988

Mant, A.K., 'The Medical Services in the Concentration Camp of Ravensbruck', *The Medico-Legal Journal*, 17 (1949), pp. 99–118

Mitscherlich, Alexander and Fred Mielke, *Doctors of Infamy: The Story of the Nazi Medical Crimes*, New York: Henry Schuman, 1949

—— *Medizin ohne Menschlichkeit: Dokumente des Nürnberger Ärzteprozesses*, Frankfurt am Main: Fischer Taschenbuch Verlag, 1981

Morrison, Jack G., *Ravensbrück: Everyday Life in a Women's Concentration Camp, 1939–1945*, London: Eurospan Group, 2000

Padfield, Peter, *Himmler Reichs Führer-SS*, London: Cassell & Co., 2001

Pavillard, Anne-Marie, 'Les archives de l'Association des anciennes déportées at internées de la Résistance (ADIR) à la BDIC', *Histoire@Politique. Politique, culture, société*, 2.5 (2008), pp. 1–5

Półtawska, Wanda, *And I Am Afraid of My Dreams*, London: Hodder & Stoughton, 1964

Reilly, Joanne, *Belsen: The Liberation of a Camp*, London: Routledge, 1998

Reid, Donald, 'America so far from Ravensbrück', *Histoire@ Politique. Politique, culture, société*, 2.5 (2008), p. 11

Roelcke, Volker, 'Die Sulfonamid-Experimente in nationalsozialistischen Konzentrationslagern: Eine kritische Neubewertung der epistemologischen und ethischen Dimension', *Medizinhistorisches Journal*, 44 (2009), pp. 42–60

—— 'Tiermodell und Menschenbild; Konfigurationen der epistemologischen und ethischen Mensch-Tier-Grenzziehung in der Humanmedizin zwischen 1880 und 1945', in Birgit Griesecke, Markus Krause, Nicolas Pethes and Katja Sabisch (eds), *Kulturgeschichte des Menschenversuchs im 20. Jahrhundert*, Frankfurt am Main: Suhrkamp, 2009, pp. 16–47

—— 'Sulfonamide Experiments on Prisoners in Nazi Concentration Camps: Coherent Scientific Rationality Combined with Complete Disregard of Humanity', in Sheldon Rubenfeld and Susan Benedict (eds), *Human Subjects Research after the Holocaust*, New York: Springer, 2014, pp. 51–66

Ruchniewicz, Krzysztof, *Polskie zabiegi o odszkodowania niemieckie w latach 1944/45–1975*, Wrocław: Wydawnictwo Uniwersytetu Wrocławskiego, 2007

Saidel, Rochelle G., *The Jewish Women of Ravensbrück Concentration Camp*, Madison: University of Wisconsin Press, 2004

Schmidt, Ulf, ' "The Scars of Ravensbrück": Medical Experiments and British War Policy, 1945–1950', *German History*, 23 (2005), pp. 20–49

—— *Justice at Nuremberg: Leo Alexander and the Nazi Doctors' Trial*, New York: Palgrave Macmillan, 2006

Smoleń, Kazimierz (ed.), *Aby świat sie dowiedział . . .: nielegalne dokumenty z obozu Ravensbrück*, Oświęcim: Wydawn. Państwowego Muzeum w Oświęcimiu, 1980

Świebodzki, Henryk (ed.), *London Has Been Informed: Reports by Auschwitz Escapees*, Oświęcim: The Auschwitz-Birkenau State Museum, 1997

Szymonowicz, Wanda, *Beyond Human Endurance*, Warsaw: Interpress Publishers, 1970

Tillion, Germaine, 'A la recherche de la vérité', in *Ravensbrück*, Neuchâtel: Cahiers du Rhône, 1946

'Uchwała Rady Państwa o ratyfikacji układu między Polską a NRF, Warszawa, 26.05.1972', in Tadeusz Walichnowski (ed.), *Układy Związku Radzieckiego i Polski z Niemiecką Republiką Federalną na drodze do pokojowej i bezpiecznej Europy. Dokumenty, przemówienia, wywiady, komentarz*, Warsaw: Książka i Wiedza, 1972, p. 68

Walz, Loretta, *"Und dann kommst du dahin an einem schönen Sommertag": Die Frauen von Ravensbrück*, Munich: Kunstmann, 2005

Weindling, Paul, 'Auf der Spur von Medizinverbrechen: Keith Mant (1919–2000) und sein Debut als forensischer Pathologe', *1999. Zeitschrift für Sozialgeschichte des 20. und 21. Jahrhunderts*, 16 (2001), pp. 129–139

—— 'Was wussten die Alliierten während des Krieges und unmittelbar danach über die Menschenversuche in deutschen Konzentrationslagern?', in Astrid Ley and Marion Maria Ruisinger (eds), *Gewissenlos Gewissenhaft: Menschenversuche im Konzentratonslager*, Erlangen: Specht, 2001, pp. 54–58

—— *Nazi Medicine and the Nuremberg Trials: From Medical War Crimes to Informed Consent*, Houndmills, Basingstoke: Palgrave Macmillan, 2004

—— ' "Belsenitis": Liberating Belsen, Its Hospitals, UNRRA, and Selection for Re-emigration, 1945–1948', *Science in Context*, 19 (2006), pp. 401–418

—— *John W. Thompson, Psychiatrist in the Shadow of the Holocaust*, Rochester, NY: Rochester University Press, 2010

—— 'Victims, Witnesses and the Ethical Legacy of the Nuremberg Medical Trial', in Kim Priemel and Alexa Stiller (eds), *Reassessing The Nuremberg Military Tribunals: Transitional Justice, Trial Narratives, and Historiography*, New York: Berghahn, 2014, pp. 74–103

—— *Victims and Survivors of Nazi Human Experiments: Science and Suffering in the Holocaust*, London: Bloomsbury, 2015

Wińska, Urszula, *Zwyciężyły wartości: wspomnienia z Ravensbrück*, Gdańsk: Wydawncitwo Morskie, 1985

—— *Więzi: Losy wieźniarek z Ravensbrück*, Gdańsk: Wydawnictwo "Marpress", 1992

12 Rascher and the "Russians"

Human experimentation on Soviet prisoners in Dachau – a new perspective

Nichola Farron

On either 9 or 10 June 1945, Wassilij Kowaltschuk, formerly of the USSR, died in Dachau concentration camp and was buried under grave marking G/2/1048 by the liberating authorities. The cause of death is listed as tuberculosis. Like so many victims of Nazism, the details of Kowaltschuk's life are lost to history; we cannot discern the personal details of the man he was beyond the biographical details recorded by the concentration camp system. Surviving camp records tell us he was born in the USSR on 24 March 1918 and had the occupation of a baker. We can also ascertain that he was given the prisoner number 34885. The paper trail for this prisoner also contains another document; one that sets him apart from the vast majority who suffered the concentration camp experience. He experienced something particular in the spectrum of Nazi atrocities: Kowaltschuk was a victim of human experimentation during his incarceration in Dachau, Nazi documents have him listed as one of six prisoners included in the research being undertaken by Dr Sigmund Rascher.[1] The record of his death after the camp liberation, by which time Rascher was already dead, is testament to the fact that he survived this experiment. He was buried in-between two other prisoners by the liberating forces, one of thousands who had lived to see the end of Nazism, only to die because of its lasting effects. The story of Wassilij Kowaltschuk, even in its limited form, is one where developments in archival access and the study of surviving documentation have afforded a rare insight into the experience of a Soviet prisoner subjected to the Nazi human experimentation programme. Kowaltschuk emerges as a face among the anonymous mass of Soviet victims of this particular subset of Nazi atrocities. His story tells us something about the history of the use of Soviet prisoners in Nazi human experimentation and forced research at Dachau. As a recognised racial and military enemy, regarded with contempt and hatred by the Nazi social and political hierarchy, Soviet prisoners were susceptible to selection for experiments that it was understood were likely to be fatal.

Following the prompt provided by the discovery of Kowaltschuk's history as a test subject, this chapter will offer a focused "micro-study" approach, framing the experience of Kowaltschuk and his companions through the parameters of experimentation undertaken by Sigmund Rascher. Rascher, it will be demonstrated, was prolific and unceasing in his choice of Soviet prisoners for his experiment series: Kowaltschuk was one of many who ended up in the medical dominion he managed to establish at Dachau. Assessing motivations and personalities, and examining the experiments that were undertaken, this chapter will offer an insight into the story of the use of Soviet prisoners in human experimentation in the setting of Dachau Concentration camp, and under the specific research control of Dr Sigmund Rascher. As a victim group who suffered from the human experimentation and coerced research programmes, there is scant research devoted to Soviet prisoners, so there are benefits to breaking down various components of the broader history of medical testing in Dachau and refining the focus to singular elements. For this chapter, there will be a concentration on the stories of the use of Soviet prisoners in Dachau. The camp itself is selected as an example from the vast concentration and penal system of Nazis where the interaction between a Nazi doctor and this victim group was particularly pronounced. Refining the study further, Sigmund Rascher emerges from the hundreds of culpable doctors and medical professionals involved in the moral bankruptcy of medicine under Hitler to take central scrutiny. Wassilij Kowaltschuk was just one among the many Soviet prisoners who would fall under Rascher's control.

The story of Soviet victims is an important part of the history of Nazi medicine, but it is a chapter that has long been given only cursory treatment, if at all. Wassilij Kowaltschuk was one of thousands of Soviet prisoners who would be selected to undergo unethical treatment across the extended Reich. As a Soviet, his life was not regarded as having any worth beyond the utility that could be extracted from him. It was the use he could provide as a test subject for medical experiments prompted by the desperation that his country's military resurgence ignited in his captors. Kowaltschuk represents the possibilities we now have to expand our understanding of the Soviet prisoner experience in Nazi human experimentation at Dachau and beyond, to retrieve some of the status denied to him by the Nazi regime.

Historiographical problems

Unlike other victim groups of the Nazi human experimentation programmes,[2] Soviet prisoners have hitherto not received an individual exploration of their specific story in the historiography of Nazi medicine. Following the surrender of Germany, discoveries of the true extent of the complicity of some of the medical profession in the worst abuses of the Holocaust and war crimes came into the public consciousness, coalescing first of all in the Nuremberg Medical Trial of 1946. A historiography then developed over the following decades, beginning with the initial observational, empirical publications that strove to report the revelations of the experimentation programmes and the role of the medical profession in the "euthanasia" killings. Mitscherlich and Mielke's

Doctors of Infamy,[3] was quickly established as the keystone of the field. Over the years, the historiography developed to include more nuanced treatments, with key publications emerging that remain the foundation of the field.[4] What characterised these treatments of the history of Nazi medicine however, was the reliance on perpetrator-created source material to convey the whole history: often the voice of the victim was silent. As Weindling has noted:

> The problem with research on Nazi medicine, and indeed more broadly with research on human experimental abuses, is that these are perpetrator oriented. The victims are generally seen as incidental figures, as episodic evidence, rather than as having identity. Their life histories are passed over in silence, even though their lives were brutally terminated by the experiments or they had to live with the physical and psychological consequences of the atrocity. This has unfortunate consequences for the understanding of the atrocities, as well as for post-war responses to such crimes.[5]

More recent efforts to redress this imbalance have seen a greater focus on the victims themselves;[6] but the experience of Soviet victims has been absent from the literature at any stage in the development of scholarship. This stems from a number of combining factors (which certainly constitute a separate consideration beyond the remits of this chapter). Broadly speaking, the treatment of the Holocaust in the post-war Soviet era was stunted and problematic; indigenous scholarship in no way reflected the vast and unheralded destruction and brutality experienced by millions of citizens. This has well-explored roots in the post-War Soviet attitude of applying a universalism to wartime experience without acknowledging the realities of specified racially based treatment towards the Jews. Specificity of suffering was regarded as the antithesis to the Communist system of government, and also ran parallel to very real and entrenched anti-Semitism that prevailed in the Soviet Union. Instead, focus remained on the heroism and military successes of the Soviet forces: that is not to downplay the very real and huge sacrifices made by the Soviet military and home population, but the reality was that Soviet citizens experienced the war in different ways according to whether they were Jewish or not. Also contributing to the absence of a more lateral historical treatment was a culture that did not foster an environment for surviving victims to share their stories of trauma in any meaningful or public way. Accusations of collusion were a very real threat for returning survivors; the ability to survive the concentration camp system was attributed to some kind of traitorous behaviour. As Rees has commented, for liberated Soviet prisoners, the reality was that their individual stories:

> ... so conspicuously lack the redemptive quality that many in the West have come to expect from the history of World War II. For generations of British and Americans, this war has attained a near mythic quality of a fight of "good" against "evil". . . . But the history of the aftermath is not as simplistic as the popular myth would have us believe. There were

certainly few "happy endings" for the Soviet prisoners liberated by the Red Army . . .[7]

Further obstacles come from the fact that physical access to material in Soviet archives was blocked to the West for decades. In addition, concerns about the veracity of Soviet-produced documentation and evidence meant that it was only with the collapse of the Soviet regime that a more consistent and complex tackling of the history of the Holocaust began. The Soviet experience of Nazi medicine remained an obscure element in a largely clandestine history of Nazi occupation and of the Holocaust in the Soviet Union, and in the narrative of the Soviet prisoner.

Defining the starting point for an investigation into the history of the use of Soviet prisoners is more problematic than for other victim groups, in particular those groups who were given post-war opportunities to tell their story and identify with other survivors who had experienced similar abuses. For this chapter, the main source material originates from perpetrator created documentation that was subsequently investigated and presented as part of the Nuremberg Medical Trial. But crucially, it is now possible to consult materials from the collection of the International Tracing Service,[8] for years inaccessible to researchers and it is from the ITS that we find the records pertaining to Kowaltschuk. From a name and recorded prisoner number on a Dachau file, the ITS records can add more biographical details to the prisoner and help a victim like Kowaltschuk emerge from the opacity of history. An approach that marries together perpetrator source materials with the post-war investigative efforts allows researchers to have a more in-depth view than ever before.

It is important to acknowledge a caution here concerning the difficulties that arise with the Nazi practice of universally describing Soviet prisoners as "Russian" without distinction. Frequently, perpetrator-created documentation, from concentration camp administrations and beyond, describe prisoners as "Russian" when the reality may be that the prisoner was from a completely different country of the Soviet Union. The harsh realities of racial ignorance, as well as the speedy and often chaotic intake processes at camps and prisons meant that there was often some error in the recording of nationality and other biographical details. One of the major issues in studying the demographics and biographies of the Soviet victims of human experimentation was the Nazi propensity to group all Soviet people under a catch-all description of "Russian" without distinction. This is an issue that has been highlighted by Berkhoff, who draws attention to this practice and the ramifications it had for those in the camps. In Nazi-controlled locations, an unfavourable and incorrect national designation could result in dire consequences, namely the cruelty exhibited toward this prisoner group:

> . . . that callousness resulted to a large degree from racist orders from German policy-makers who thought of the multi-ethnic Soviet prisoners as "Russians", and who tried to eliminate most of these "Russians" . . .[9]

These practices were to have direct consequences on the prisoners themselves; to be labelled as one of the lowest strata on the Nazi racial hierarchy was to be at a massive disadvantage in camps and prisons, and could be the designation that led to extermination:

> Russifying the prisoners in this way is no small matter. During the years 1941 and 1942 . . . the very imposition of a Russian identity upon the multi-ethnic multitudes of Soviet POWs was crucially important in shaping their fate.[10]

And, as this chapter will demonstrate, to be a "Russian" within the sphere of Rascher's influence was particularly dangerous as experiments with their roots in issues associated in the Eastern Campaign began to gain importance. For the purposes of this chapter, the term "Russian" has been used as designated in the source material; but the author advises caution and recognition of this issue when investigating this particular victim group.

The experiments

Much of the source material that helps gain an understanding of these experimental procedures emerges from the statements and correspondence of the key players. We have the words of Rascher himself, recorded in his numerous letters and communications with Himmler and his superiors. His death at the end of the war (executed by the SS, the very group that he hoped to ascend and in which he had placed so much esteem) meant he was never called to account in the courtroom. But he left a substantial "paper-trail"; keen to continue to foster the favour of Himmler, his detailed letters are full of insight into his cross-departmental and organisational manoeuvrings, and the extent of his research work at Dachau. They reveal key details of his attitude towards his Soviet experimental subjects. In parallel to Rascher's personal correspondence, the testimony of Walter Neff, his prisoner-assistant, provides a crucial insight into the experimental work undertaken at Dachau. In fact, much of what we know about the realities of Rascher's experiments comes from Neff who stood as witness to countless testing rounds: his testimony is crucial, and he was extensively questioned by the US prosecution. Neff himself is a complicated figure: he was taken on as a prisoner assistant and came to be regarded as indispensable by Rascher; in fact, he continued in this role even after his official release:

> Rascher found an apparently dependable assistant in Walter Neff, who had been imprisoned in 1937. . . . He was released on 15 September 1942, but stayed on to assist Rascher, keeping records and statistics of Rascher's experiments. . . . Himmler considered that Neff should be retained for the rest of the war, because he could work effectively with the prisoners.[11]

As witness for the prosecution in the Nuremberg Medical Trial, Neff left a lasting record of the realities of Dachau's experimental blocks, and of the cruel fate of those unfortunate enough to be used as test subjects.

From the hundreds of physicians and other professionals who can be implicated in the medical crimes carried out in the name of Nazi ideals, Sigmund Rascher has emerged as one with a certain degree of notoriety, both in scholarly research and in the broader public consciousness. He used the prisoner population of Dachau for experiments in high altitude recovery, wet and dry freezing and also for trials with blood coagulants. His experimental work at Dachau was a manifestation of ruthless personal ambition, and the result of fortuitous personal connections. In 1937, he passed his medical exams at age 28 and accepted a post at the Schwabinger Krankenhaus in Munich. Associating on a daily basis with more distinguished practitioners and professors inspired the young doctor to aim for greater career heights, and his call-up to the *Luftwaffe*'s Munich-based Medical Research Centre in 1939 was a key step along the way. Perhaps even more important to his career was the turn his personal life took when he met and subsequently married Nini Diehls, slightly older than him, but crucially a member of Himmler's inner circle. From this privileged position, Rascher was able to move into an arrangement with Himmler that allowed personal letters and appeals, as well as sentiments of familiarity that would facilitate his research ambitions. This favour with the *Reichsführer SS* was to prove crucial in advancing his research ideas, and in gaining the support to requisition equipment and test subjects. His experiments would affect hundreds of prisoners, and were marked by numerous fatalities. It is important to recognise that a number of nationalities and prisoner groups were used, and it is not the intention of the author to lead to the misconception that Soviet prisoners were used exclusively. However, for the purposes of this focused investigation, the experience of Rascher's work will be looked at through the lens of their experience, especially in view of the historiographical absence of any dedicated investigation.

It was German misfortune in the war that would provide the impetus for all of Rascher's experimental series. Recognising the opportunities afforded by *Luftwaffe* struggles in the air war with Great Britain in 1940–41 Rascher reached out to Himmler, who would increasingly offer protection from rivals, to seek authorisation to begin experimentation on high altitude. With the RAF successfully reaching higher altitudes, there was a pressing need to help the *Luftwaffe* counter their rival's superiority. Unexperienced in the internal power play of the SS, and surrounded by colleagues who questioned his ability, Rascher was shrewd in cultivating his relationship with Himmler. In the *Reichsführer SS* he had an ally that could sanction all of his experimental ambitions with one flick of the pen. With the *Luftwaffe* falling behind, Rascher saw an opening to place himself as a valuable researcher. An altitude and pressure experiment was devised where prisoners would be placed in a pressure chamber and subjected to increasing force. The contents of a letter to Himmler of 15 May 1941 set in motion the use of prisoners as test subjects, and illustrate the over-arching Nazi world-view that under-pinned all the medical abuses that transpired during Hitler's Chancellorship:

> . . . is there any possibility that two or three professional criminals can be made available for these experiments? . . . The experiments, in which the experimental subject may of course die, would take place with my collaboration.[12]

Some lives were considered expendable: the very crux of National Socialist theory. Himmler's return correspondence indicated that any condemned prisoner who undertook the experiment would see their sentence pardoned;[13] Rascher's contempt for Soviet prisoners would become apparent when he was concerned that the offers of a pay-off for "voluntary" participation would be applied to them. A written enquiry of 20 October 1942 indicates that it was thus far Poles and Russians who had been used in the high altitude tests, with Rascher wanting clarification that they were exempt from any judicial or punitive leniency. His fears were alleviated when a terse telegram from Rudolf Brandt to his superior succinctly summarised the Nazi position to their Soviet and Polish prisoner population:

> Please inform SS Untersturmfuhrer Dr. Rascher with regard to his teletype enquiry that the instruction given some time ago by the Reich Leader SS concerning amnesty of test persons does not apply to Poles and Russians.[14]

With such entrenched attitudes prevailing throughout the medical and SS worlds, the fate of Soviet prisoners in Rascher's Dachau-based experiments was determined: there was no obstacle to their unrestricted use in human experiments.

Testimony concerning the high-altitude experiments is crucial to understanding the role Russians played as test subjects. Walter Neff provided the prosecuting authorities at Nuremberg with an insight into the processes of experimentation. For the high-altitude tests he detailed how a group of Russian prisoners were selected from the prisoner population and exclusively used in a round of testing:

> One day . . . Rascher told me . . . he was going to make a serious experiment and that he would need 16 Russians who had been condemned to death, and he received these Russians . . .[15]

On further questioning from the American prosecution about the nationalities of test subjects, Neff confirms that certainly, subjects were selected from across the groups interned in the camp, and that those selected as "prisoners of war" were Russians.[16] Neff estimates that between 180 and 200 inmates were used in the altitude testing, with approximately 70 to 80 fatalities. Of these 70 to 80, he relayed to the court there were approximately 40 who had in fact, not been condemned to death, in contravention of the original agreement between Rascher and Himmler.[17] We can safely conjecture that a number of those fatalities would likely have been Soviet prisoners. More recent research has put a total figure of prisoners used for the pressure experiments at 540.[18] The prisoner of war status that excluded them from the pardon Himmler and Rascher offered meant Soviets were easily available test subjects, already categorised as dangerous enemies to be eradicated for the sake of the Reich.

Accounts of the use of Soviet prisoners in other experimental cycles emerged post-war, testifying to their continued use and selection by Rascher; in particular, the "freezing" experimentation he undertook through the submersion of prisoner subjects in a specially constructed basin. The impetus for the experimentation was counter-acting the freezing conditions experienced by bailed German pilots who were perishing in the North Sea during the Battle of Britain. Rascher's freezing experiment saw subjects submerged in ice water for various lengths of time; then different methods of "rewarming" were attempted. The rewarming methods included massage, heaters or a warm bath; Himmler's conjecture that the folk-tale based belief of using naked bodies for rewarming resulted in a transfer of female prisoners from Ravensbrück. The *Luftwaffe* misfortunes in the English Channel were not the only motivation for the research, as confirmed by Allied interrogation by Prosecutor McHaney of Siegfried Handloser, Chief of the medical services to the Armed forces:

McHaney:	As a result of the Eastern campaign, weren't you very much interested in 'Cold problems?'
Handloser:	Yes . . . We were always interested in cold problems . . . mainly because of the terrible winter of 1941/42.
	. . .
Q:	. . . there is no doubt that great importance was attached to the results of this experiment in Dachau by Rascher . . .
	. . .
A:	. . . we wanted to do everything and . . . wanted to concentrate our entire interest on the front where freezing took place in order to help our soldiers.[19]

With the turn of fortunes on the Eastern front in Soviet favour, it was apparent that those Soviet prisoners in Nazi hands would find themselves feeling the brunt of frustration and increasingly desperate measures to use any means to turn the tide. Science had to meet the demands of the military. With the Allies scientific advances placing their troops at a number of advantages, the pressure was on the German medical field to push ahead and secure the combative advantage. Indeed, Weindling has noted that "the sense that Germany was losing the medical war meant pressure for systematic experiments".[20] In fact, it is this inter-connectedness of circumstances that were to define the Soviet experience of Nazi medicine at the hands of Rascher in Dachau: Rascher's experiments were all motivated by military needs, as opposed to other Nazi doctors who based experimental series on racial or anthropological theories, or on personal medical interests and curiosity.[21] A basis of racial hatred and contempt meant this class of prisoners were not regarded with any ethical consideration, which was exacerbated by frustrations and fear as the Soviet campaign unravelled and military victories stalled. We learn from Neff's testimony that during this testing phase of 1942 to 1943, two Russian officers were selected from among the inmate population as experimental subjects for for freezing and placed in the ice water of Rascher's experimental basins. The account is worth relaying at some length:

> It was the worst experiment which was ever carried out. Two Russian officers were carried out from the bunker. . . . Rascher had them undressed and they had to go into the basin naked. Hour after hour passed and while usually after a short time, 60 minutes, freezing had set in, these two Russians were still conscious after two hours. All our appeals to Rascher asking him to give the injection were of no avail . . . The experiment lasted at least 5 hours until death occurred.[22]

As with so much of the evidence that has emerged from Rascher's experimental work, the degree of cruelty is stark, as is the ability of someone trained in the healing profession to deliberately propagate the suffering of his subjects without conscience. What facilitated this mind-set was of course the indoctrination of Nazism with its fervent racial chauvinism; this is what condemned Soviet prisoners to such appalling treatment. In his observations, the Italian survivor of Auschwitz, Primo Levi succinctly attests to the reality of their position: ". . .the pariahs of the Nazi universe . . . Soviet prisoners . . . demoralised, they were weakened by hunger and maltreatment; they were, and knew they were, considered worth less than beasts of burden".[23]

Within the parameters of medical experimentation in Dachau, there was no facility for mercy for this prisoner group. Rascher expanded his "wet" freezing experiments into a dry series where prisoners were exposed to the elements for extended periods of time. As was his normal procedure, Rascher appealed again to Himmler to get the support and validation for his work, especially in the face of scepticism from his rivals, and in doing so revealed that prisoners had already been subjected to extreme conditions:

> . . . I am attempting to prove through experiments on human beings that it is possible to warm up people cooled off by dry cold just as fast as people who were cooled off by rewarming in cold water. . . Up to now I have cooled off about 30 people stripped in the open air during 9–14 hours at 27°–29°.[24]

As German soldiers in the East perished at the metaphorical hands of "General Winter", in the Reich, Rascher was working on their behalf by exacting desperate and cruel scientific revenge on the prisoner population.

The final experimental series undertaken by Rascher at Dachau was testing a blood coagulant called "Polygal", designed to assist in stemming blood loss from wounds received on the battlefield. Plagiarising the work of the Jewish chemist Robert Feix who had been imprisoned in Dachau, Rascher coerced Feix into a forced collaboration, even appealing to the SS to have Feix's "half-Aryan" status restored. The most detailed insight into this experimentation comes from the testimony of Fritz Rascher, Sigmund's uncle who visited him in the camp. Fritz provided detailed testimony to the Allies after the war about the documentation he had seen connected to the Polygal experimentation. Within his statement, the murder of a Soviet prisoner is described, as the elder Rascher saw documentation that detailed:

> ... a report about the shooting (execution) for the purpose of experimenting with the homeostatic preparation "POLYGAL 10". As far as I remember they were a Russian COMMISSAR ... The Russian was shot in the right shoulder from above by an SS man who stood on a chair. The bullet emerged near the spleen. It was described how the Russian twitched (convulsively), then sat down on a chair and died after about 20 minutes.[25]

After death, the Russian victim was autopsied where it was found that there had indeed been a degree of blood-clotting, which was regarded as the cause for the long period before death; this fed into the increasingly futile belief that Polygal really could be used to turn the tide of military casualties. After discovering this report, Fritz Rascher had turned to his nephew and interrogated him on his moral and scientific conscience, only to have Sigmund reply that it was too late to pull himself out of the work. Polygal research was another avenue where Rascher could utilise the prisoner population with impunity: he had already outlined to Himmler in his first discussions about the altitude tests that there was a risk of fatality and the fact that Rascher was now willing to have prisoners shot at point blank range was indicative of the degree of obscenity that had come to characterise his research. We can never know more about the unfortunate Russian (or even if his nationality was correctly identified), but he became a part of the increasingly frantic efforts to turn the war back in the Nazis favour.

A new perspective – discovering the victim in perpetrator sources

With the altitude, freezing and Polygal experiment series, Rascher had subjected the test subjects to the most cruel procedures; and while the Soviet prisoner group was by no means the exclusive "nationality" used in testing, again and again it is the story of their fate that emerges in the source material. In the key examples of the selection of prisoners for altitude testing, in the description of two "commissars" submerged in freezing water until death, and in the reporting of the shooting of a prisoner to test the Polygal coagulant, Soviet prisoners are

Surname	Name	Date of birth	Place of birth	Nationality	Prisoner number	Date of death (if known)	Additional information
Kowaltschuk	Vassily	24.3.1918	Alinkin	Russian	34885	10.6.1945	Arrived Dachau 20.8.42 from Stapo-Karlsruhe. Cause of death listed as pulmonary tuberculosis; died in the 127th Evacuation Hospital, Dachau. First name also spelled 'Wassilij' and 'Wassil'.
Lukaschenko	Sacharko	26.2.1924	Bobrik	Ukrainian	33740		Arrived KL Dachau 8.8.42 from Stapo-Munchen
Poschitajew/Poschidaew	Alexander	6.8.1921	Krasilowka	Ukrainian	32588		Arrived KL Dachau 30.7.42
Midow	Anatolji	7.12.1918	Tachyk	Ukrainian	34785		Arrived Dachau 19.8.42 from Stapo-Munchen
Kowalenko	Ivan	19.10.1921	Orsyhe/Orsytze	Ukrainian	32221		Transferred to Neuengamme on 14.12.1942
Beletzky	Andrean	9.12.1915	Tomsk	Russian	34917	4.11.1943	Resided in Leningrad

Figure 12.1 List of KZ Dachau prisoners who "volunteered" for Rascher's altitude experiments

Source: Washington, DC, United States Holocaust Memorial Museum, inventory number 2349: International Tracing Service document: KL–Dachau GCC3/228 Ordner 277, Medical Experiments on prisoners of KL Dachau, who a) for experimental purposes were chosen by Dr Rascher (no date) b) voluntarily made themselves available for altitude experiments

specifically referred to. The historical record of Rascher's experimental undertakings at Dachau are characterised by a marked use of Soviet victims; but who were these prisoners? We have looked briefly at Wassilij Kowaltschuk: who survived experimentation in Rascher's workrooms only to die after liberation. This knowledge can be gathered from the marrying of the contemporary sources, both perpetrator and liberator created. The starting point for learning about Kowaltschuk as a Soviet victim of experimentation is on a Dachau document where his name is listed with five other prisoners as volunteers for Rascher's experimental work.

The list describes these names as "selected" for the experimental work being undertaken by Rascher. It is also possible that they volunteered, believing that volunteering would be the means to a more favourable existence in Dachau, ignorant that Rascher and Himmler had already conferred and agreed on their racial and social exemption from any kind of pardon. Indeed, Kowaltschuk would remain in Dachau, and his death would be recorded by the liberating forces. This list presents an opportunity to start learning more about the victims of these experiments; it is a starting point for investigating the biographies of names listed and making the human experimentation subjects at Dachau more than just the number assigned to them by the Nazis. Using this perpetrator-created source as a prompt for approaching accessible prisoner information in the central name index of the ITS, we can learn more about an individual life than just the coerced service that a subject was forced to give to the Reich. Access to the ITS materials means that, after decades of inaccessibility, we can start to add the "victim" to the more established and prevailing history of perpetrators. We can add the benefit of modern search techniques to draw together materials. In the case of Dachau, human experimentation programmes cannot be understood without understanding the motives, personality and chronicle of Rascher himself. But his is just one part of the account: for a more balanced approach we must look at the prisoners who were used as little more than material; that is particularly pressing in the case of Soviet victims, already so under-represented and examined in this complex history. With survivors becoming fewer, and following decades of being forced to repress their experiences for fear of reprisals, we are increasingly reliant on the surviving source materials – both left by Rascher and his associates, and yet to be discovered in collections such as the ITS holdings. In terms of the focused "micro-study" undertaken in this chapter, further examination of the list above reveals that all of these experimental subjects were Soviet prisoners.

The arrival dates for these prisoners put them in the camp for Rascher's freezing experiment series: perhaps Andrean Beletzky died as a result of the experimentation. Perhaps Wassilij Kowaltschuk – whose historical traces inform this chapter – was weakened to such an extent by testing that he was left physically vulnerable to the tuberculosis that finally claimed his life even as liberation came. But what the ITS card documentation facilitates is the ability to add the personal dimension to the original Dachau list. We cannot know the complete biography of these victims, but we can make them more than a number. As for the details of their lives, or the specifics of their interactions with Rascher, all we have is educated conjecture: that is the reality of the Nazi human experimentation programme and of a concentration camp system that destroyed individual identity. It is the consequence of a post-war Soviet culture that actively sought to crush any emergence of a victim-based solidarity and even persecuted those who returned.

Conclusion

For Sigmund Rascher, the prisoner populace of Dachau represented a resource to be exploited. Much has been written about how the Nazis regarded prisoners in terms of their utility, as slave labourers and workers, and of course most horrifyingly as organic materials. For Rascher the utility of Soviet prisoners, and others regarded with similar racial contempt, stemmed from his ability to subject them to any extremity of experimentation. Not only was there no consequence for this, but it was officially sanctioned, supported and funded.

In the end, Rascher's desperate efforts to curry favour with his superiors and secure an academic legacy would prove wasted. He assumed his favour was limitless, but intercessions on racial matters served to anger Himmler. Revelations that his three children were in fact taken from orphanages after Nini faked her pregnancies also contributed to his fall from high-approval. Rascher had wanted to present the picture of the ideal Aryan family, with multiple children, and a career spent ascending political and academic ladders through Nazi-favoured actions. Ultimately, Nini Rascher would end up in Ravensbrück while Rascher himself was shot by the SS in 1945: he had made too many enemies and his protector Himmler had been marked out as a traitor for attempting to sue for peace with the Allies. In terms of any worth that came from the unspeakable suffering meted out during his experiments, there were negligible results, and hundreds of pressurised and frozen prisoners could do nothing to stop the military tides that had already turned against the Nazis. Rascher caused approximately 150 deaths that Neff records, and possibly countless more that were not recorded or remembered. But all of it was essentially for nothing in his terms when we consider the ignominy of his fall from grace and execution, and from scientific terms considering the questionable methods of experimentation and the problematic nature of his results. As Weindling has summarised: "Most of the coerced experiments on the German side were scientifically derivative and unnecessary . . . The deaths produced meagre results in terms of lasting scientific value".[26]

Rascher had failed to deliver solutions for the military-based afflictions that continued to thwart Germany's beleaguered troops. Derided by his superiors and regarded with suspicion by his peers, his experiment series, marked by extreme cruelty and numerous fatalities, was in the end for nothing. Wassilij Kowaltschuk did not survive to tell the story of his time as a subject in Rascher's laboratory: it falls to us to try to rescue him and his fellow Soviet victims of human experimentation from obscurity; otherwise, the forces that guided and prompted Rascher to regard them as expendable and marked for eradication will have succeeded.

Notes

1 Kowaltschuk materials – card materials from the ITS collection at the United States Holocaust Memorial Museum: cross reference prisoner number, date of birth and name
2 See, for example, Hans-Joachim Lang, *Die Namen der Nummern. Wie es gelang, die 86 Opfer eines NS-Verbrechens zu identifizieren,* Hamburg: Hoffmann und Campe, 2004. There has also been extensive work by the C.A.N.D.L.E.S group in identifying twin/multiple birth victims of Mengele in Auschwitz: www.candlesholocaustmuseum.org/learn/about-survivors.htm.
3 Alexander Mitscherlich and Fred Mielke, *Doctors of Infamy – The Story of Nazi Medical Crimes,* New York: Henry Schuman, 1949. This is an English edition of the original German work, *Das Diktat der Menschenverachtung – eine Dokumentation,* Heidelberg: Lambert Schneider, 1947.
4 See, for example, Robert Jay Lifton, *The Nazi Doctors – Medical Killing and the Psychology of Genocide,* New York: Basic Books, 2000.
5 Paul Julian Weindling, *Nazi Medicine and the Nuremberg Trials – From Medical War Crimes to Informed Consent,* Houndmills, Basingstoke: Palgrave Macmillan, 2004, p. 240.
6 See, for example, Lang, *Die Namen der Nummern.*
7 Laurence Rees, *Auschwitz – The Nazis and the "Final Solution",* London: BBC Books, 2005, p. 344.
8 For more on the background on the efforts to open up the ITS to researchers see: www.ushmm.org/information/press/press-releases/united-states-holocaust-memorial-museum-to-begin-providing-holocaust-surviv and www.ushmm.org/remember/the-holocaust-survivors-and-victims-resource-center/international-tracing-service/about-the-international-tracing-service/its-frequently-asked-questions.
9 Karel C. Berkhoff, 'The "Russian" Prisoners of War in Nazi-Ruled Ukraine as Victims of Genocidal Massacre', *Holocaust and Genocide Studies,* 15.1 (2001), p. 1.
10 Ibid., p. 3.
11 Paul Weindling, *Victims and Survivors of Nazi Human Experiments – Science and Suffering in the Holocaust,* London: Bloomsbury, 2015, p. 85.
12 Letter from Rascher to Himmler, 15 May 1941, concerning High-Altitude Experiments on Human Beings, Document 1602-PS, in Trials of War Criminals before the Nuernberg Military Tribunals under Control Council Law No.10. Nuernberg October 1946–April 1949. Vol. I: The Medical Case, Washington, DC: US Government Printing Office, 1949, p. 142.
13 In reality, this only occurred on one occasion, and the reprieved prisoner was in fact sent to a harsh SS detachment. See the testimony of Walter Neff, in ibid., pp. 180–181.
14 Teletype from Rudolf Brandt to Schnitzler, 21 October 1942, concerning the pardon granted by Himmler: Document 1971-E-PS, in ibid., pp. 149–150.
15 From the Testimony of Tribunal Witness Walter Neff, in ibid., p. 178.
16 Ibid.
17 Ibid., p. 182.
18 Weindling, *Victims and Survivors,* p. 81.
19 Extract from the Testimony of Defendant Handloser, in *Trials of War Criminals,* pp. 265–269.
20 Weindling, *Victims and Survivors,* p. 79.
21 For example, sterilisation experiments to prohibit Jewish reproduction, the selection of prisoners as anatomical specimens to demonstrate alleged racial difference, or the practice of unnecessary surgery.

22 Extracts from the Testimony of Walter Neff, in *Trials of War Criminals*, p. 263.
23 Primo Levi, *The Drowned and the Saved*, London: Abacus 2000, p. 124.
24 Letter from Rascher to Himmler, 17 Feb 1943, and summary of experiments for rewarming of chilled human beings by animal warmth, 12 Feb 1943, Document 1616-PS, in *Trials of War Criminals*, p. 249.
25 Cambridge, MA, Harvard Law School Library, item no.2267, Nuremberg Document NO-1424.
26 Weindling, *Victims and Survivors*, p. 210.

Bibliography

Archival sources

USA

Cambrdige, MA, Harvard Law School Library, item no.2267, Nuremberg Document NO-1424: Affidavit concerning Sigmund Rascher's polygal experiments at Dachau, and the execution of the Raschers during the war, available at: http://nuremberg.law.harvard.edu/php/pflip.php?caseid=HLSL_NMT01&docnum=2267&numpages=3&startpage=1&title= per cent28Sworn per cent29+Affidavit.&color_setting=C
Washington, DC, United States Holocaust Memorial Museum:
Card materials from the International Tracing Service collection
Inventory number 2349, International Tracing Service document: KL-Dachau GCC3/228 Ordner 277

Literature

Berkhoff, Karel C., 'The "Russian" Prisoners of War in Nazi-Ruled Ukraine as Victims of Genocidal Massacre', *Holocaust and Genocide Studies*, 15.1 (2001), pp. 1–32
Lang, Hans-Joachim, *Die Namen der Nummern. Wie es gelang, die 86 Opfer eines NS-Verbrechens zu identifizieren*, Hamburg: Hoffmann und Campe, 2004
Levi, Primo, *The Drowned and the Saved*, London: Abacus, 2000
Lifton, Robert Jay, *The Nazi Doctors – Medical Killing and the Psychology of Genocide*, New York: Basic Books, 2000
Mitscherlich, Alexander and Fred Mielke, *Das Diktat der Menschenverachtung – eine Dokumentation*, Heidelberg: Lambert Schneider, 1947
—— *Doctors of Infamy – The Story of Nazi Medical Crimes*, New York: Henry Schuman, 1949
Rees, Laurence, *Auschwitz – The Nazis and the 'Final Solution'*, London: BBC Books, 2005
Trials of War Criminals before the Nuremberg Military Tribunals under Control Council Law No.10. Nuremberg October 1946-April 1949. Vol.1: The Medical Case, Washington, DC: US Government Printing Office, 1949
Weindling, Paul Julian, *Nazi Medicine and the Nuremberg Trials – From Medical War Crimes to Informed Consent*, Houndmills, Basingstoke: Palgrave Macmillan, 2004
—— *Victims and Survivors of Nazi Human Experiments – Science and Suffering in the Holocaust*, London: Bloomsbury, 2015

13 Heißmeyer's forgotten victims

Tuberculosis experiments on adults in Neuengamme 1944–45[1]

Anna von Villiez

In February 2000 Aleksandr Choroschun decided to send a letter to the Mayor of Hamburg. He had already written to the Red Cross in Hamburg, but had not received the answer for which he was hoping. He wrote the following: "I was deported to the KZ Neuengamme and I was used as material for medical experiments together with 28 men".[2] His letter was forwarded to the Neuengamme concentration camp Memorial where it finally found an echo. Herbert Diercks, historian at the Memorial, realised that Choroschun was in fact the first survivor of the infamous Kurt Heißmeyer's tuberculosis experiments ever to get in touch with the Neuengamme Memorial. Choroschun's letter was the first trigger for research into this victim group who until then had been neglected and much understudied.

This late interest is surprising given that they are one of the best-documented groups among the many forgotten victims of medical experiments. The trial of Kurt Heißmeyer in Magdeburg from 1963 to 1966 was one of the biggest on Nazi perpetrators in the former German Democratic Republic (GDR). The court went to a great deal of effort to clarify and obtain evidence for the case, compared with many trials carried out half-heartedly across the border in West Germany. In the preparation for the trial there was an attempt to contact various families of the victims and many witness statements were accumulated. The documentation is even more robust because of the rare survival of original material from the experiments themselves. During his trial in 1964 Heißmeyer revealed the location of a box he had buried in 1945 on the grounds of Hohenlychen sanatorium where he had been working. The box included the files and other documentation from 32 victims of the deadly experiments he conducted.[3] The prisoner doctor Tadeusz Kowalski had reported on Heißmeyer's experiments as early as November 1946 in a Polish medical journal, making their turning of a blind eye to Heißmeyer's conduct while he worked as a chest physician in the GDR all the more remarkable.[4]

Remembrance and neglecting of victims of human experiments

One can only guess why until today the adult victims of Heißmeyer have generated so little interest in the public and the academic communities despite the excellent source material. One reason is certainly the enormous emotional response created by publications on the 20 children who were among Heißmeyer's victims. The children's fate was first publicised by the Hamburg journalist Günther Schwarberg who over many years researched the families of the children who were killed – indeed many families had never known the tragic fate of their children. His books *Der SS-Arzt und die Kinder. Bericht über den Mord vom Bullenhuser Damm* published in 1979 and *Meine 20 Kinder* published in 1996 were for many years the fullest biographical accounts of any victims of Nazi medical experiments.[5] The detailed account of the experimentation on and killing of 20 children – some of them as young as five years old – became symbolic for medical atrocities conducted by German physicians in the Third Reich. The adult victims remained hidden in the shadow of Schwarberg's tragic biographies of the children, which he compiled. In reality, the so-called adult group was not that different in age from the children. The youngest of the identified test persons was Wassilij Schtscherbak, who was only 17 when experimentation started and had just turned 18 when he died of tuberculosis in January 1945. There is only a five-year gap between him and the eldest of the children, the French boy Georges-André Kohn, who was 12 when he arrived at Neuengamme. Many of the adult victims were very young men under the age of 25. Most of them had lived with their families before they were brought to Germany, mostly to work as forced labourers.

A second reason for the long silence on Heißmeyer's adult victims might be the fact most of them were Polish and Soviet prisoners. During the Cold War and until the collapse of the Soviet Union research in Russia or Poland was very complicated or impossible. Although there were full case files for the adult victims, Schwarberg chose to do his research project on the children for which he had merely names and ages.

Another factor in the lack of interest in or commemoration of the adult victims is they were not Jewish as all of the children were. The adults fell out of the better-known categories of Nazi victim groups, which might have made it hard for the public to engage in their stories. The memorialisation of human experiments in concentration camps has been focused on certain perpetrators and atrocities. The most prominent is certainly Josef Mengele who used mainly children for his anthropological and genetic research in Auschwitz. Historians have largely ignored other perpetrators, their experimental research and their victims. This is true for the non-Jewish German victims who were mostly stigmatised as "notorious criminals". They were used in typhus experiments in Buchenwald. This neglect is also true for example of the male victims used in the Ravensbrück sulphonamide experiments.[6]

A last reason for the lack of information on Heißmeyer's victims is of course the sad and simple fact that most victims were murdered or died in the experiments and never left Neuengamme alive. Post-war sources – if they exist at all – were often overlooked, again due to difficulties in academic cooperation and language difficulties when dealing with Russian, Ukrainian or Polish sources until the end of the Cold War.

Heißmeyer's network

Kurt Heißmeyer was not an isolated figure, but well connected with a group of experts in hereditary pathology who were deeply intertwined with Nazi ideologies on eugenics, racial segregation and "euthanasia".[7] Since 1928 Kurt Heißmeyer held a post as consultant at Hohenlychen under the orthopaedic surgeon Karl Gebhardt. The sanatorium in Lychen was a perfect place for Heißmeyer who had been a specialist in lung diseases – especially tuberculosis – during his earlier career. Hohenlychen had been the model sanatorium for tuberculosis since its foundation in 1902. With the decline of tuberculosis incidence due to improved living and working conditions, therapeutic innovations and vaccination (see below) the hospital later became a well-known sanatorium with a focus on sport injuries. The latter was fashionable with celebrities such as national football players, politicians and even royalty, who all came to recover and relax. Under Karl Gebhardt, a leading figure in Nazi medicine who served as the Consulting Surgeon of the *Waffen-SS*, Chief Surgeon in the Staff of the Reich Physician SS and Police, and personal physician to Heinrich Himmler, Hohenlychen had become a popular meeting point for vacationing top ranking Nazi medical functionaries. And since the outbreak of the war Hohenlychen had become a military hospital. Gebhardt then seized the hour to further his wish to expand Hohenlychen into a medical research centre. He had been appointed to find a cure for wound infections, which were killing German soldiers by the thousands. Until 1945 Hohenlychen turned into a centre for the planning and management of human experiments in concentration camps.

Tuberculosis research under National Socialism

Heißmeyer's experiments were part of the global competition for a preventive vaccine or remedy against tuberculosis. Tuberculosis was one of the most feared infectious diseases until after 1945. In France Albert Calmette and Camille Guérin found the first effective vaccine in 1906 with their vaccination formula called BCG (after the two discoverers). The introduction of BCG encountered many problems and much scepticism, not least because of the Lübeck disaster of 1930 due to a contaminated batch of vaccine. The effect was the introduction of research guidelines in 1931.[8] Heißmeyer's experiment happened in the setting of Second World War in which a feverish race for drugs and vaccines against the diseases that killed many soldiers was occurring. Heißmeyer was not the only German scientist to take advantage of the Nazi regime that persecuted and imprisoned thousands. Tuberculosis was one of the most common causes of illness and death in concentration camps and German scientists took advantage of this massive pool of involuntary test subjects. A group of scientists coalescing around the Kaiser Wilhelm Institute for Anthropology, Human Hereditary Science and Eugenics (*KWI für Anthropologie, menschliche Erblehre und Eugenik*) was very active in linking heredity pathology with tuberculosis research.[9] The protagonists were the anthropologist Otmar von Verschuer und his assistant Karl Diehl. The basis for this was that tuberculosis was seen as a disease of the poor, the lazy and the retarded, beliefs ingrained in medicine since the prospering of eugenic ideas at the turn of the century. The social hygienist Alfred Grotjahn had characterised tuberculosis as "the disease of the physically inferior people" in 1923.[10]

Tuberculosis research took place in most large concentration camps.[11] Waldemar Hoven experimented in Buchenwald with coal dust as a treatment of prisoners. At least five died. Tuberculosis experiments were also carried out in Sachsenhausen by the Dutch doctor Gualtherus Zahn, and this was known at the time as *Vergleichskur*, or comparative clinical trial. Experiments also took place in Auschwitz and Majdanek.[12]

Vaccination experiments were also carried out on disabled children within the "euthanasia" system: at the child neuropsychiatric clinic of Berlin Wittenau/Wiesengrund (by Ernst Hefter, Gertrud Reuter and Gerhardt Kujath) and at the paediatric clinic of the Charité in Berlin-Buch (by Georg Bessau), at the Kinderheilanstalt Kaufbeuren (by Georg Hensel and Valentin Falthauser), and in Vienna on children at the children's clinic of the University (by Elmar Türk). Many of the children were dissected after their murder in order to complete the research on the effect of the various vaccinations.[13]

It was in 1944, when Selman Abraham Waksman at Rutgers University in New Jersey developed the antibiotic Streptomycin, which proved to be a significant breakthrough against tuberculosis, that the scientific race for a therapeutic drug came to a halt.

Heißmeyer's tuberculosis experiments in Neuengamme

Heißmeyer had previously wished to perform experiments in Ravensbrück on work therapy for the tuberculous, but these were not approved.[14] Heißmeyer, not a leading expert in his field, had ambitions echoing those of Gebhardt to use Hohenlychen as a research hub to further his career. He had to fall back on his personal connections to the SS elite to pursue his ideas. His uncle, August Heißmeyer, was a general in the *Waffen-SS*, as was a friend of his, the powerful head of the SS economic administration Oswald Pohl.[15]

In June 1944 Kurt Heißmeyer was allowed to experiment on KZ prisoners in Neuengamme. He was looking for a cure for bacteriological tuberculosis.

He wanted to prove his hypothesis that tuberculosis was in fact not an infectious disease but a condition caused by exhaustion or "racial inferiority", and his second hypothesis that it could be cured by implementing a second, artificial centre of infection. He referred to the Austrian Hans Kutschera von Aichbergen who had argued the implementation of tuberculosis of the skin would heal tuberculosis of the lungs. Kuchera von Aichbergen had already been disproved in his ideas by the scientific community by the time that Heißmeyer started his experiments.[16]

Because of his connections with the SS leadership, Heißmeyer was well received at Neuengamme concentration camp, where its SS management was eager to meet his needs. One part of the sick bay was reserved for him and equipped with a separate entrance and visual blinds for the little courtyard next to it. Between June 1944 and April 1945 around 100 adults and 20 children were subjected to his experiments.

Heißmeyer used various techniques to infect his test subjects, many of whom had been completely healthy beforehand. He injected tuberculosis bacteria into the shoulder, rubbed it into the skin or infused the victim's lung with a tube and injected the bacteria through this.

The German photographer Josef Schmitt, born 1886 in Schwetzingen near Heidelberg, worked as the official camp photographer of Neuengamme. Heißmeyer ordered him to take pictures of the test persons in various stages of their ordeal for documentation purposes.[17] Due to his photographs, of which many have been restored from Heißmeyer's box, this evidence is powerful source material to give account not only of what Heißmeyer tried to do but also of the people he used and abused for this. The distressed faces in the pictures leave no doubt of the cruelty of Heißmeyer's experiments.[18]

Heißmeyer's Nazi beliefs led him to have no concern experimenting on "racially inferior" individuals, which included Jews as well as Eastern Europeans. The prisoner doctor Zygmunt Szafranski who worked at the sick bay next to Heißmeyer's block reported at the trial on many details of the experiments.[19] Heißmeyer had ordered that no "Aryans" should be used as test persons because of his assumption of a relation between the "racial inferiority" of "Non-Aryans" and tuberculosis infections.

According to Szafranski four groups were used as test persons:

Group 1: prisoners with tuberculosis
Group 2: prisoners who had one lung affected by tuberculosis
Group 3: patients with various types of tuberculosis in different organs
Group 4: healthy prisoners of good constitution

The first test persons were chosen and examined by Heißmeyer personally. He decided which prisoners he wanted in his experiment and sent the others back to the sick bay in Block 4 if they were too weak. In their place he chose other prisoners. This is how he operated throughout his experiment: There was a constant exchange of patients between the sick bay and his experimental block. Some of the adult victims volunteered because they were promised better and more food in Heißmeyer's block. Test persons for groups 2 and 4 were ordered and brought in especially for the experiment from other camps. Heißmeyer ordered his prisoner assistants to remove the lymph glands surgically from his test persons in order to see the extent of the tuberculosis infection. Heißmeyer closely cooperated with the pathologist Hans Klein. It was Klein who analysed the glands Heißmeyer sent from Neuengamme. Klein was a leading pathologist under neuropathologist Berthold Ostertag at Rudolf-Virchow-hospital in Berlin, but was transferred to Hohenlychen because of the bombing of Berlin.

Aleksandr Choroschun gave an account of how he experienced the experiments:

> It was eight of us in one room. We were very well fed. First various samples were taken. A little later, when we had gained weight, I got injected . . . Others were injected some liquid through a tube into their noses. After ten days the people who got me there came back. In their presence I was operated on several times. From under my arm they cut something similar to a sparrow's egg and a gland from my neck. They took everything with them. Two weeks later I was discharged to the sick bay . . . The other seven were already spitting blood. From then I had to nurse 28 patients, to hand them medication, food and fish oil. When one of them died I called for a helper from the other department of the sick bay and together we carried the deceased to the postmortem room. This is where I saw one of my former "colleagues" with cut open chest without his lungs. The same happened to the other six "rabbits". Only I survived and I waited for a similar end.[20]

Resistance against Heißmeyer and his experiments has not been reported. In various accounts it is stated that prisoners were tricked into Block 4 by promising them better food. It was never disclosed to the test persons what the experiment involved, its purpose and how it could affect them.

The test persons

The number of individuals involved has not been confirmed until today. In the report by Otto Prokop and Ehrenfried Stelzer more than 100 persons are estimated to have been victims.[21] The majority of these were Poles and Russians, but also four Ukrainians, one Croat and one Dutch research subject. All the adults were non-Jewish victims, mostly Catholic and one Russian was of Muslim faith.[22] Most victims were in their 20s. The eldest was the Russian Grigorij Goz, born 1893 who had turned 50 before he was recruited into the experiment.

Surname	First name	Date of birth	Birth place	Nationality	Date of death
Alexejew/ Aleksejews	Roman	07/07/1924*	*Latria, district of Jaduoa**	Russian	27/01/1945
Bolands/ Bolenin/ Bolensen/ Bolensch/ Batensch/ Bollands	Adolf	12/06/1916	*Solizski, district of Lida*	Polish	
Choroschun/ Choroszyn	Aleksandr	23/04/1917	Krasnojarsk	Ukrainian	29/06/1905
Danilschuk/ Daniltschuk	Iwan	23/10/1924		Russian	06/07/1944
Denisenko	Grizko Gregori Georgi	02/05/1924	Bilmatschow, Bachmac region (perhaps Bil'machivka near Bakhmach)	Ukrainian	05/03/1945
Derij	Iwan	08/12/1924	Dniepropetrowask (probably Dnipropetrovsk)	Ukranian	
Goz/Gots	Grigorij	29/09/1893	*Petrowo district of Swistunowo (Saproshe)*	Russian	
Jacubowski/ Jakubowksi	Josef	02/02/1911	Zolotniki, Kalisch (probably: Złotniki, Kalisz County)	Polish	21/04/1944
Kalyn	Wasil/ Wassyl	16/02/1916	*Bujanow, district of Stryi (Ukraine)*	Ukrainian	
Karnabal/ Karnabul	Ignacy	21/07/1906	*Sady*	Polish	03/05/1945

Figure 13.1 Confirmed adult test persons of Heißmeyer's tuberculosis experiments at KZ Neuengamme 1944–45

* The place of birth as noted in Heißmeyer's files has been matched with today's name of the place. Places that could not be verified are marked in italics.

Place of death	Cause of death	Religion	Occupation	Victim number	Sources
Neuengamme	Lung tuberculosis	Russian Orthodox	Labourer	38457	BStU: ZUV 46, file 104-107; NGA: Krankenrevier-Totenbuch Stammlager VII
		Catholic	Farm hand	26506	BStU: ZUV 46, file 72-74; NGA: Effektenliste
		Russian Orthodox	Agricultural labourer/ Locksmith	322450	BStU: ZUV 46, file 54-57 and 151
Neuengamme	Tuberculosis			14409	BStU: ZUV 46, file 28, 122
Neuengamme	Tuberculosis			10574	BStU: ZUV 46, file 20
				32238?	BStU: ZUV 46, file 90-91 and 120
		Russian Orthodox		19531	BStU ZUV 46: file 66-69, 151; NGA: Laborunter-suchungen
Neuengamme	Hanged	Catholic	Painter	17366	mentioned in Kloszinski (1962), BStU; ZUV 46, file 86; NGA: Laborunter-suchungen, Krankenrevier-Totenbuch Stammlager V
		Russian Orthodox	Locksmith	10454	BStU: ZUV 46 file 16
	died during bombard-ment of the vessels Cap Arcona or Thielbek		Farmhand	23129	BStU: ZUV 46 , file 12-15; NGA: Totenbuch

Figure 13.1 Continued

Surname	First name	Date of birth	Birth place	Nationality	Date of death
Kowalski	Alois	29/11/1916	*Toruń*	Polish	01/11/1944
Kritschalow	Aransij/ Afanassij Maximo- witsch	18/01/1907		Russian	
Lyschtwa/ Lychtra	Aleksej/ Alexi				
Molenda	Wacław	14/08/1917	Warthenau O. (Silesia)/Zawiercie	Polish	28/07/1944
Nędza	Stanisław	10/04/1913	Mirkowitz, township Mieścisko in Greater Poland Voivodeship near Posen	Polish	08/11/1944
Oldziobaj	Stoubaj	12/03/1908	*Achsaj, district of Tulubas*	Russian	
Ponomarenko	Nikolaj	21/05/1920	*Smorschki/ Nowosibirsk*	Russian	
Prokopenko	Pawlo/ Pawel/ Paul	13/01/1929	*Golgoiwko, district of Suma*	Russian	22/02/1945
Rytschalow	Andrej	16/11/1913	Mikhaylov/ Michailow near Moscow	Russian	18/10/1944
van Sabben	Pieter	19/04/1924	Den Haag	Dutch	26/02/1945
Schtscherbak/ Schtscheiback	Wassilij	24/11/1926	Novopetrivka near Saporischschja	Russian	07/01/1945
Sejdo/Sejto	Zenil	1922 or 1921	Sarajewo	Croatian	
Senko/Lenko	Alexander				

Figure 13.1 Continued

Place of death	Cause of death	Religion	Occupation	Victim number	Sources
Neuengamme					BStU: ZUV 46, file 1-5
				15308	BStU: ZUV 46, file 37; NGA-Datenbank (Liste überlebender Russen aus Haffkrug)
				19833	BStU: ZUV 46 file 37, NGA: Laborunter-suchungen
Neuengamme	Tuberculosis	Catholic	Mechanic	35757	BStU: ZUV 46, file 75-77
Neuengamme	Executed			35984	BStU: ZUV 46, file 82-85
		Muslim		32239	BStU: ZUV 46, file 58-61
				21482	BStU: ZUV 46, file 33
Neuengamme	Tuberculosis, meningitis			21372	BStU: ZUV 46, file 48
Neuengamme				22595	BStU: ZUV 46, file 27
Neuengamme	Tuberculosis	Protestant	Student at Polytech Delft until 1943	29927	BStU: ZUV 46, file 48-52; NGA: correspondence with brother Dies van Sabben (2001 to 2006), Sektionsprotokoll des Neuengammer Lagerarztes
Neuengamme	Tuberculosis		Student	15177	BStU: ZUV 46, file 42, 121
			Farm hand/ Cook	24335	BStU: ZUV 46, file 78-81; Barch: NS 3/1577, file 063534; Prokop/ Stelzer p90; Effekte at International Tracing Service
				8367	BStU ZUV 46, file 37; NGA: Laborunter-suchungen

Figure 13.1 Continued

Surname	First name	Date of birth	Birth place	Nationality	Date of death
Solow/ Zolow/ Solov/ Zolto	Mitrowan/ Mibrowan/ Metrowan/ Mitrofan	04/06/1923	*Weilandska/ Imminga*	Russian	
Szatunow/ Schatunow	Walentin	17/12/1923		Russian	15/11/1944
Terletzki / Terleckij/ Terlezkij	Joseph	07/01/1921	Dyniw, district of Drogowidsch (perhaps Dynów)	Polish	
Trotz/Troc	Jakob	10/12/1919	*Scherme, district of Belks*	Polish	
Tschamlai/ Schamlaj	Peter/ P.S./Petr	06/03/1921	*Batum, district of Batura*	Russian	1950
Tschmyr/ Tschsyr	Wassilij	02/06/1924	Zvenyhorodka	Russian	24/01/1945
Tschurkin/ Churkin	Iwan	30/10/1922	*Kalinin, distric of Koslowa*	Russian	08/11/1944
Wesołowski/ Wessolowski	Tadeusz	26/04/1910	Opatów near Ostrowiec	Polish	08/11/1944
Wójcik	Franciszek/ Franz	17/08/1914	*Krauszwo, near Łódź*	Polish	
Wolniewicz/ Wolnewitsch	Bronisław	06/02/1920	Żelechlinek near Tomaszów	Polish	08/11/1944

Figure 13.1 Continued

Place of death	Cause of death	Religion	Occupation	Victim number	Sources
			Farmer	41370	BStU: ZUV 46, file 100-103
Neuengamme	Tuberculosis			52231 or 32241	BStU: ZUV 46, file 50, 70, 71, NGA: Reviertotenbuch
		Russian Orthodox	Locksmith	17222	BStU: ZUV 46, file 63-65
			Carpenter	29204	BStU: ZUV 46, file 96-99
	Died after a traffic accident				BStU: ZUV 46, file 92-95 and 139 (expert statement Prokop/ Stelzer p31); NGA: Buchenwald Database
Neuengamme	Died of cardiac insufficiency			11571	BStU: ZUV 46, 41 (case file) and file 149 (witness report of his mother Chavitina Tschmyr)
Neuengamme	Executed in Neuengamme	Russian Orthodox	Blacksmith	35736	BStU: ZUV 46, file 108-111 (case files); Prokop/ Stelzer p81-85; NGA: Reviertoten-bücher
Neuengamme	Executed in Neuengamme	Catholic	Forester	48639	BStU: ZUV 46, case files 112-115, NGA: Reviertoten-bücher
				5292	BStU: ZUV 46, file 8-11; NGA: Laborunter-suchungsbuch III des Krankenreviers
Neuengamme	Executed	Catholic		48662	BStU: ZUV 46, files 116-119

Figure 13.1 Continued

Most of the victims had been forced labourers and came from rural or worker backgrounds. The mother of Wasilij Tschmyr gave a witness account of how her son came to Germany:

> In spring 1942 my daughter Jewgenika was deported to Germany for forced labour and approximately in June 1942 my son Wasilij Tschmyr was taken to Germany too. For the deportation my son was picked up by policemen unknown to me and taken to a collecting point which was located in the school of Swnigorodka. From there he was taken together with many others . . . by train to Germany. I never received a letter or heard from him again.[23]

She found out after the war he had been working in the satellite camp Drütte and tried to escape after which he was taken to Neuengamme. Wasilij Tschmyr died in January 1945 in Neuengamme aged only 21 years old.

Four of Heißmeyer's test persons were hanged in Neuengamme on the same day: Bronisław Wolniewicz, Tadeusz Wesołowski, Iwan Tschurkin and Stanisław Nędza.[24] Most of the test persons in Heißmeyer's project had been sentenced to death earlier. It was stated during his trial that Heißmeyer actively ordered the killing of many of his test persons because he needed the results of their autopsies. The fact that these Neuengamme prisoners were all "convicts with death sentences" was often stressed by Heißmeyer during his defence. One should bear in mind though the absurdity of these "death sentences". Most Polish or Russian prisoners in Neuengamme would have been forced labourers in Germany who had somehow broken Nazi law, most often by trying to escape. Stanisław Nędza had worked in Germany since 1940 and had been transferred to Neuengamme by the Gestapo prison Berlin-Alexanderplatz in July 1944. He was 31 years old at the time of his death. Iwan Tschurkin had been in the camp for two years until he was used for Heißmeyer's experiments. He had been completely healthy but Heißmeyer injected tuberculosis bacteria into his left lung on 11 October 1944. Three weeks later shadows on the X-ray proved the tubercular infection of his lungs. According to the Prokop report this would have put his life in danger or at least damaged his health heavily. Two weeks after this X-ray Iwan Tschurkin was hanged and autopsied. He was 22 years old at the time.

Of the corroborated 33 victims, 16 were dead when the camp was cleared in May 1945 and the surviving prisoners sent on a death march toward the shore. As the documentation in Heißmeyer's files was kept until February 1945 it is clear that 17 victims had survived until then and were sent on the death march. When they reached the bay of Lübeck, SS guards forced them onto the vessel *Cap Arcona* together with around 10,000 other Neuengamme prisoners. The *Cap Arcona* was tragically bombed by British aircraft the same night because of false information and sank. Very few survived.

In some of the Polish compensation claims from the 1970s claimants stated they were in Heißmeyer's experiments. Not every case could be corroborated due to the lack of pre-1945 material with which to match the data.[25]

The story after

Very few witness reports give an account of Heißmeyer's experiments. This is probably due to the fact that (apart from the Dutch victim) the only survivors lived behind the "iron curtain" for decades. A couple of prisoners who worked in the sick bay, but not directly with Heißmeyer in the experimental block, were interviewed during the Magdeburg trial of Heißmeyer.

The only family of a victim who contacted the concentration camp Memorial after 1945 was the Dutch family van Sabben.[26] It is probably not a coincidence that it was a family from Western Europe rather than Russia or Poland who had heard of the commemoration of the 20 children used as test persons. Communication with the families in Russia did not occur. It took until 2001 to establish contact with one of the survivors themselves and with the Memorial through Aleksandr Choroschun's letter to the Mayor of Hamburg. Choruschun survived the experiments and went on the death march on which the remaining Neuengamme prisoners were sent in the beginning of May 1945. Choroschun was one of the very few on the *Cap Arcona* who did not drown. He passed away in 2006.

Until today there has not been any official commemoration of this victim group in Hamburg or Neuengamme in the form of a ceremony or a monument. While there is the site of the "Bullenhuser Damm Memorial"[27] including an exhibition for the 20 children in Hamburg, the adult victims have remained unnamed until today.

Notes

1 I would especially like to thank Herbert Diercks (Research Centre, Neuengamme Memorial Archive) for his help in finding sources and his willingness to share his expertise in the field. I would also like to thank: Alyn Beßmann (Neuengamme Memorial Archive) for her patience, Lawrence Zeidman (University of Illinois College of Medicine at Chicago) who kindly offered to correct my English, Ronja Steffensky (Leopoldina, Halle) for proofreading and lastly Paul Weindling (Oxford Brookes University) who supported the research for this chapter and made helpful comments.
2 Hamburg, Neuengamme Camp Memorial Archive (hereafter NGA), correspondence with Aleksandr Choroschun, Letter to the Mayor of Hamburg by Aleksandr Choroschun, 21 Feb 2000.
3 The contents of the box are archived in the trial files at Berlin, Archives of the Federal Commissioner for the Records of the State Security Service of the former German Democratic Republic (hereafter BStU), ZUV 46, files 1–169. Other archival material (pre- and post-1945) is found at the NGA such as prisoner cards and documents of the former sick bay; witness reports.
4 Tadeusz Kowalski, 'Report on tuberculosis experiments in Neuengamme', *Śląska Gazeta Lekarska* (1946), cited from BStU, ZUV 46, file 139.
5 Günther Schwarberg and Daniel Haller, *Der SS-Arzt und die Kinder: Bericht über den Mord vom Bullenhuser Damm*, Hamburg: Gruner & Jahr, 1979; Günther Schwarberg, *Meine zwanzig Kinder*, Göttingen: Steidl, 1996.
6 Paul Weindling, *Victims and Survivors of Nazi Human Experiments: Science and Suffering in the Holocaust*, London: Bloomsbury, 2015, p. 89.

7   Paul Weindling unraveled Kurt Heißmeyer's network in genetic and racial research in his paper on Hans Nachtsheim: Paul Weindling, 'Genetik und Menschenversuche in Deutschland 1940–1960. Hans Nachtsheim, die Kaninchen von Dahlem und die Kinder vom Bullenhuser Damm', in Hans-Walter Schmuhl and Petra Terhoeven (eds), *Rassenforschung an Kaiser-Wilhelm-Instituten vor und nach 1933 [Workshop Rassenforschung im Nationalsozialismus: Konzepte und Wissenschaftliche Praxis unter dem Dach der Kaiser-Wilhelm-Gesellschaft, am 3./4. Dezember 1999 in Berlin]*, Göttingen: Wallstein, 2003, pp. 245–274.

8   See the chapter in this volume by Volker Roelcke.

9   Hans-Walter Schmuhl, *Grenzüberschreitungen: Das Kaiser-Wilhelm-Institut für Anthropologie, menschliche Erblehre und Eugenik 1927–1945*, Göttingen: Wallstein, 2005.

10 Cited after Christine Wolters, *Tuberkulose und Menschenversuche im Nationalsozialismus: Das Netzwerk hinter den Tbc-Experimenten im Konzentrationslager Sachsenhausen*, Stuttgart: Franz Steiner, 2011, p. 47. Christine Wolters wrote a detailed analysis on tuberculosis and human experiments under National Socialism in 2011 with a focus on Sachsenhausen. The Neuengamme experiments are completely absent in her book though for unclear reasons. Her analysis provides a very useful overview on the general topic though.

11 See ibid.

12 Weindling, *Victims and Survivors*, pp. 62 (on Hoven), 106–107 (on Auschwitz and Mauthausen) and 113–115 (on experiments on children in psychiatric clinics).

13 See Thomas Beddies and Heinz-Peter Schmiedebach, ' "Euthanasie"-Opfer und Versuchsobjekte: Kranke und behinderte Kinder in Berlin während des Zweiten Weltkriegs', *Medizinhistorisches Journal*, 39.2/3 (2004), pp. 165–196 for Georg Bessau's vaccination experiments and coercive experimentation in the *Kinderfachabteilungen* in Berlin generally. See Petra Schweizer-Martinschek, 'Tbc-Versuche an behinderten Kindern in der Heil- und Pflegeanstalt Kaufbeuren-Irsee 1942–1944', in Andreas Wirsching (ed.), *Nationalsozialismus in Bayerisch-Schwaben: Herrschaft – Verwaltung – Kultur*, Ostfildern: Thorbecke, 2004, pp. 231–259 for Kaufbeuren-Irsee and Georg Hensel's experiments there. For tuberculosis experiments at the "special children's unit" Am Spiegelgrund see Herwig Czech, 'Forschen ohne Skrupel. Die wissenschaftliche Verwertung von Opfern der NS-Psychiatriemorde in Wien', in Eberhard Gabriel, Wolfgang Neugebauer, Siegwald Ganglmair and Wolfgang Lamsa (eds), *Von der Zwangssterilisierung zur Ermordung: Zur Geschichte der NS-Euthanasie in Wien Teil II*, Vienna: Böhlau, 2002, pp. 143–164; and eadem, 'Abusive Medical Practices on "Euthanasia" Victims in Austria during and after World War II', in Sheldon Rubenfeld and Susan Benedict (eds), *Human Subjects Research after the Holocaust*, Cham: Springer, 2014, pp. 109–125.

14 Fischer affidavit, 19 Nov 1945, in Klaus Dörner, Angelika Ebbinghaus and Karsten Linne (eds), in cooperation with Karl Heinz Roth and Paul Weindling, on behalf of the Stiftung für Sozialgeschichte des 20. Jahrhunderts, *The Nuremberg Medical Trial. Transcripts, Material of the Prosecution and Defense, Related Documents. English Edition*, Microfiche ed., Munich: Saur, 1999, (MF) 3/673 and 676; Schiedlausky affidavit, 7 Aug 1945, in ibid. (MF) 3/688.

15 The story of Heißmeyer's infamous experiments has been told before: the first thorough report is by Otto Prokop and Ehrenfried Stelzer, 'Die Menschenexperimente des Dr. med. Heißmeyer', in Ehrenfried Stelzer (ed.), *Kriminalistik und forensische Wissenschaft: Beiträge zur Theorie und Praxis der sozialistischen Kriminalistik und der forensischen Wissenschaft*, Vol. 3, Berlin: Deutscher Verlag der Wissenschaften, 1970, pp. 67–104; a newer overview is by Herbert Diercks, 'Gesucht wird: Dr. Kurt Heißmeyer', in idem (ed.), *Schuldig: NS-Verbrechen vor deutschen Gerichten*, Bremen: Ed. Temmen, 2005, pp. 102–115; and Weindling, 'Genetik und Menschenversuche'.

16 Hans Kutchera-Aichbergen, 'Die Bekämpfung schwerer Lungentuberkulose mit künstlich erzeugter Hauttuberkulose', *Wiener klinische Wochenschrift*, 45 (1937) and 46

(1937). See also Prokop and Stelzer, 'Menschenexperimente des Heißmeyer', pp. 91–96.

17 Kew, The National Archives, WO 235/167, (Curiohaus-trial): Exhibit 4: Deposition of Joseph Schmitt.

18 For one of the photographs, see Weindling, *Victims and Survivors*, p. 169.

19 BStU ZUV 46, file 156, Witness reports of Zygmunt Szafranski, prisoner doctor at the sick bay, Block 4.

20 NGA, Letter by Aleksandr Choroschun to Herbert Diercks, 11 May 2000, translation by the author of this paper.

21 Prokop and Stelzer, 'Menschenexperimente des Heißmeyer', p. 78; see also Iris Groschek and Kristina Vagt, *". . . dass du weißt, was hier passiert ist": Medizinische Experimente im KZ Neuengamme und die Morde am Bullenhuser Damm*, Bremen: Ed. Temmen, 2012, p.33, who base their numbers on the witness statement of Eugène Marcel Prénant, in NGA, Häftlingsbericht (prisoner report) 857.

22 The underlying sources for my analysis of the test person's biographies are: the case files compiled by Heißmeyer 1944 to 1945, which were found during the investigation against him in 1962 (BStU, ZUV 46, file 1 to 123); trial files of the Heißmeyer trial in Magdeburg 1962/1963 (BStU, ZUV 46). The data from these sources was matched with archival material and witness reports from NGA, Krankenrevier-Totenbuch Stammlager V (death book of the sick bay); Laboruntersuchungsbücher III des Krankenreviers (lab records from Neuengamme); the archives database (including biographical details from prisoner cards and alike), witness reports/interviews: Aleksandr Choroschun (video archive reference: 2002/4273) and letter from 11 May 2000; an additional source are the compensation files for Polish victims of medical experiments from Warsaw, Central Archives of Historical Records, holdings of The Office of the Special Commissioner with the Ministry of Public Health, EPM/I-II (hereafter OSCMPH).

23 BStU, ZUV 46, file 149, affidavit Charitina Tschmyr, 18 Aug 1964.

24 NGA, Krankenrevier-Totenbuch Stammlager V, entry date 8 Nov 1944.

25 The following Neuengamme prisoners could not fully be corroborated as test persons of Heißmeyer although there is certain evidence in the sources: OSCMPH, GK 927/I/3387; OSCMPH, GK 927/I/3396: Telesfor Kowalewski; OSCMPH, GK 927/I/3403: Stanisław Małkowiak; Koblenz, Bundesarchiv Koblenz, B 126/121503: Anton Poetzl; OSCMPH, GK 927/I/3410: Piotr Starnowski; OSCMPH, GK 927/II/I/459: Tadeusz Tworzydło; OSCMPH, GK 927/I/3401–3402: the brothers Henry and Zenon Łaszek; BStU, ZUV 46, file 156 III, witness report of Witalij Semjonow; NGA, Video interview 1997/3162, prisoner reports 1599 and 1600.

26 NGA, 36–550.3–6, correspondence with Dies van Sabben, 2 Feb 2001 to 22 Mar 2006.

27 www.kz-gedenkstaette-neuengamme.de.

Bibliography

Archival sources

Germany

Berlin, Archives of the Federal Commissioner for the Records of the State Security Service of the former German Democratic Republic (BStU), ZUV 46, files 1–169
Hamburg, Neuengamme Camp Memorial Archive (NGA):

  36–550.3–6, correspondence with Dies van Sabben
  Correspondence with Alexandr Choroschun

Häftlingsberichte 857, 1599 and 1600
Krankenrevier-Totenbuch Stammlager V
Laboruntersuchungsbücher III des Krankenreviers
Video interviews 1997/3162 and 2002/4273

Koblenz, Bundesarchiv Koblenz, B 126/121503

Poland

Warsaw, Central Archives of Historical Records, holdings of The Office of the Special
Commissioner with the Ministry of Public Health, EPM/I-II (OSCMPH):

GK 927/I/3387, 3396, 3401–3403, 3410
GK 927/II/I/459

United Kingdom

Kew, The National Archives, WO 235/167

USA

College Park, MD, National Archives and Records Administration, M 1019/17

Literature

Beddies, Thomas and Heinz-Peter Schmiedebach, ' "Euthanasie"-Opfer und
    Versuchsobjekte: Kranke und behinderte Kinder in Berlin während des Zweiten
    Weltkriegs', *Medizinhistorisches Journal*, 39.2/3 (2004), pp. 165–196
Czech, Herwig, 'Forschen ohne Skrupel. Die wissenschaftliche Verwertung von Opfern
    der NS-Psychiatriemorde in Wien', in Eberhard Gabriel, Wolfgang Neugebauer,
    Siegwald Ganglmair and Wolfgang Lamsa (eds), *Von der Zwangssterilisierung zur
    Ermordung: Zur Geschichte der NS-Euthanasie in Wien Teil II*, Vienna: Böhlau, 2002,
    pp. 143–164
—— 'Abusive Medical Practices on "Euthanasia" Victims in Austria during and after
    World War II', in Sheldon Rubenfeld and Susan Benedict (eds), *Human Subjects
    Research after the Holocaust*, Cham: Springer, 2014, pp. 109–125
Diercks, Herbert (eds), *Schuldig: NS-Verbrechen vor deutschen Gerichten*, Bremen: Ed.
    Temmen, 2005
Dörner, Klaus, Angelika Ebbinghaus and Karsten Linne (eds), in cooperation with
    Karlheinz Roth and Paul Weindling, on behalf of the Stiftung für Sozialgeschichte
    des 20. Jahrhunderts, *The Nuremberg Medical Trial. Transcripts, Material of the Prosecution
    and Defense, Related Documents. English Edition*, Micorfiche ed., Munich: Saur, 1999
Groschek, Iris and Kristina Vagt, ". . . *dass du weißt, was hier passiert ist": Medizinische
    Experimente im KZ Neuengamme und die Morde am Bullenhuser Damm*, Bremen: Ed.
    Temmen, 2012
Prokop, Otto and Ehrenfried Stelzer, 'Die Menschenexperimente des Dr. med.
    Heißmeyer', in Ehrenfried Stelzer (ed.), *Kriminalistik und forensische Wissenschaft:
    Beiträge zur Theorie und Praxis der sozialistischen Kriminalistik und der forensischen
    Wissenschaft*, Vol. 3, Berlin: Deutscher Verlag der Wissenschaften, 1970, pp. 67–104

Rubenfeld, Sheldon and Susan Benedict (eds), *Human Subjects Research after the Holocaust*, Cham: Springer, 2014

Schmuhl, Hans-Walter, *Grenzüberschreitungen: Das Kaiser-Wilhelm-Institut für Anthropologie, menschliche Erblehre und Eugenik 1927–1945*, Göttingen: Wallstein, 2005

Schwarberg, Günther, *Meine zwanzig Kinder*, Göttingen: Steidl, 1996

—— and Daniel Haller, *Der SS-Arzt und die Kinder: Bericht über den Mord vom Bullenhuser Damm*, Hamburg: Gruner & Jahr, 1979.

Schweizer-Martinschek, Petra, 'Tbc-Versuche an behinderten Kindern in der Heil- und Pflegeanstalt Kaufbeuren-Irsee 1942–1944', in Andreas Wirsching (ed.), *Nationalsozialismus in Bayerisch-Schwaben: Herrschaft – Verwaltung – Kultur*, Ostfildern: Thorbecke, 2004, pp. 231–259

Weindling, Paul, 'Genetik und Menschenversuche in Deutschland 1940–1960. Hans Nachtsheim, die Kaninchen von Dahlem und die Kinder vom Bullenhuser Damm', in Hans-Walter Schmuhl and Petra Terhoeven (eds), *Rassenforschung an Kaiser-Wilhelm-Instituten vor und nach 1933 [Workshop Rassenforschung im Nationalsozialismus: Konzepte und Wissenschaftliche Praxis unter dem Dach der Kaiser-Wilhelm-Gesellschaft, am 3./4. Dezember 1999 in Berlin]*, Göttingen: Wallstein, 2003, pp. 245–274

—— *Victims and Survivors of Nazi Human Experiments: Science and Suffering in the Holocaust*, London: Bloomsbury, 2015

Wolters, Christine, *Tuberkulose und Menschenversuche im Nationalsozialismus: Das Netzwerk hinter den Tbc-Experimenten im Konzentrationslager Sachsenhausen*, Stuttgart: Franz Steiner, 2011

Part Four

Legacies

14 From witness to indictee

Eugen Haagen and his court hearings from the Nuremberg Medical Trial (1946–47) to the Struthof Medical Trials (1952–54)

Christian Bonah and Florian Schmaltz

The question of the prosecution of Nazi medical war crimes and their relationship to the reconstruction of biomedical research and development in the western world after 1945 is a complex issue. Intelligence services and prosecutors had to identify potentially compromised persons; they had to localise and arrest them, interrogate and decide about further custody; they had to reconstruct piece by piece the dimensions of a criminal system of medical research and responsible individuals within it. Finally, they had to gather and secure sufficient evidence for courtroom procedures staging war crime trials concerning medicine and experiments, involving coerced human subjects. Investigations and prosecution in this immediate post-war period were complicated by the fact that they were undertaken by individual nations and their respective intelligence agencies and war crimes services. The four allied powers accordingly investigated and tracked potential perpetrators rolling forward as they liberated Germany and then in the four zones of occupied Germany (and again in the four zones of occupied Austria). Allied powers cooperated on these issues, but at the same time investigations and procedures were tainted by national priorities and interests that at times could be competing or conflicting as well.

Evidence gathered during the prosecution and the trials was relayed in the public sphere in press reports and through publications. Early accounts of the Nuremberg Medical Trial (NMT) observers include a shorter and then a fuller overview from the German side Mitscherlich and Mielke (1947) and in their revised and extended edition (1949)[1] and from the French point of view Bayle (1950)[2] in order to inform, document and reeducate the German population.[3] If these were early documents about the perception and the reception of the 1946–47 Nuremberg War Crimes Trial against (Nazi) doctors, these accounts at the same time overlapped and thus interfered with further still ongoing legal procedures including US and British trials[4] concerning medical war crimes committed for example at Ravensbrück[5] and French military trials in the French zone of occupied Germany, as well as the Struthof[6] medical war crimes trials

(SMT), held in Metz and Lyon in 1952 and 1954, and named after the location of the Nazi concentration camp on French territory in Alsace.[7]

So far later historical accounts of the prosecution of medical war crimes have been predominantly written from the perspective focusing on the NMT.[8] This contribution intends to draw attention to the need to better understand the interaction and connections between the American and the French prosecution and the contemporary press and observer accounts. To exemplify these, we will use a single significant case: Eugen Haagen's testimonies and trial examinations first at the NMT (1946–47) and then at the Struthof Medical Trial of the French Military Tribunals in Metz and Lyon against perpetrators involved in medical war crimes in the Natzweiler concentration camp. To include the SMT opens a perspective for a wider timeframe between 1945–1954 that implies that trials from NMT to SMT and early accounts of the NMT and press reports were highly related and influenced each other. Furthermore we intend to take a practical turn analysing prosecution at work, meaning here to ask questions not only about the historical facts of the medical war crimes but also about how the prosecution pursued and documented in practice medical research in concentration camps. This means that our contention is that present historical analysis would benefit from taking more into account a perspective from legal history, in particular beyond the 1946–47 Nuremberg War Crimes Trial against (Nazi) doctors, thus acknowledging more strongly the complexities of prosecution over a longer timespan as well as the not always evident encounter of professional cultures of law and medicine following approaches such as those proposed by Sheila Jasanoff[9] translated here as: medicine at the bar.

Eugen Haagen – a biographical sketch

Born in 1898 in Berlin, Eugen Haagen started medical school at the University of Berlin where he obtained his medical license (*Approbation*) in 1924. After two years as a medical assistant at the First Clinic for Internal Medicine at the Charité (the main university hospital in Berlin), he joined the Reich Health Office (*Reichsgesundheitsamt*) in 1926 where he conducted research on viruses and cancer. In 1928 after several attempts he was awarded a research fellowship at the Rockefeller Institute for Medical Research in New York where he perfected his technique with tissue cultures. After a short second stint at the Imperial Health Office in 1929–30, Haagen was again recruited for two years at the Yellow Fever Laboratories of the International Health Division of the Rockefeller Foundation, working with Max Theiler. After returning to the Imperial Health Office between 1934 and 1936, he eventually joined the Robert Koch Institute in 1936 where he stayed until 1941. In October 1941 Haagen received a position as professor for hygiene and bacteriology at the newly created National Socialist Reich University of Strasbourg where he collaborated with Hellmut Erich Gräfe and his technical assistant Brigitte Crodel on an ambitious research programme on yellow fever (1941–43), typhus (i.e. *Fleckfieber*) (1943–44), influenza (1943–44), epidemic hepatitis (1944), sulfonamides (1944) and penicillin (1944).[10]

This research programme led Haagen in 1942 to the concentration camp of Natzweiler/Struthof and its nearby sub-camp at Schirmeck. According to Raphael Toledano's thesis, experiments on camp inmates started in June 1942 in the Schirmeck camp testing yellow fever vaccines. The year 1943 witnessed Haagen expanding his use of Schirmeck camp inmates for typhus, influenza and hepatitis research alongside the continued yellow fever investigations. Originally his scientific aims consisted of human vaccine trials testing new or "improved" versions of vaccines developed at Haagen's bacteriological institute at the *Reichsuniversität Straßburg*. In January 1944 Haagen started using camp inmates in the main camp Struthof/Natzweiler, according to Toledano, for experimental series on larger groups of subjects on typhus, hepatitis and pneumonia research. Best documented is the human experiment with 80 Roma who had been "ordered" from Auschwitz especially for the purpose of Haagen's typhus vaccine testing.

As Allied forces approached Strasbourg in September 1944, Haagen evacuated part of his institute and left the city in November. He was arrested for the first time on 3 May 1945 by members of the Alsos Mission, a military intelligence unit of Allied scientific experts evaluating German war-time research on chemical, biological and nuclear weapons.[11] As Paul Weindling has described, Haagen was interrogated, released and after he moved to work in the Soviet zone he was arrested again by the British.[12] The French Military Tribunal at Metz issued an arrest warrant for Haagen and took him into custody after the British arrest. While awaiting his trial, Haagen was transferred to Nuremberg in May 1947 where he served between 17 and 20 June 1947 as a defence witness in the Nuremberg doctors' trial. He remained imprisoned for further eight years until his final conviction in Lyon in 1954. He was then granted amnesty and released in September 1955. After having returned to West Germany, Haagen was able to complete his professional rehabilitation by being re-employed by the Federal Research Center for Viral Animal Diseases, where he worked until his retirement in 1965. Haagen died in 1972 and has been recognised as one of Germany's founders of virology.[13]

Haagen at the Nuremberg Medical Tribunal

In the NMT 13 of the 23 defendants were tried for their knowledge, responsibility and support of human experiments with typhus vaccines that had been conducted in the concentration camps of Buchenwald and Natzweiler.[14] Eugen Haagen was called upon as a key witness for the Natzweiler experiments. The case of Haagen provides interesting insights into prosecution practices and allows one to juxtapose the American-conducted Nuremberg Trial and the French-conducted Struthof medical case. Three elements encourage such a comparison. First, in contrast to most other witnesses Haagen did not come to the NMT as a free man but was summoned from a prison cell at Nuremberg, where he had been transferred by French authorities on 16 May 1947.[15] As a war crime suspect accused of poisoning concentration camp inmates, he was awaiting his own trial before the French Military Court and had to be extremely careful in his testimonies not to incriminate himself. Second, no other witness was interrogated for as long a period during the NMT as Haagen was. As a witness for the defence he was expected by the lawyers to exonerate several defendants, especially the Luftwaffe officers Oskar Schröder, Gerhard Rose and Hermann Becker-Freyseng. The examination of Haagen in the Nuremberg Medical Trial lasted from 17 to 20 June 1947, resulting in a transcript exceeding 300 pages, underlining the great importance his testimony had for the defence. Third, Haagen's examination had obviously been scripted with the lawyers. This became clear when the prosecutor Alexander G. Hardy interrupted the examination of Haagen on the second day under the impression that the witness used written notes with precise formulations answering the questions asked by the defence. Hardy requested to see the notes and suggested stopping further questioning by handing over the notes in the form of a written affidavit to shorten the expectedly long examination. After consultation, the judges asked Haagen if a third party prepared the notes. When Haagen assured them that he had written the notes to enable him to answer precisely questions of a complex scientific nature, the judges dismissed the prosecutor's request to see the notes and abandoned the examination of the witness.[16]

Concerning the typhus experiments the court finally found eight defendants guilty and acquitted five.[17] With regards to their organisational affiliation the defendants can be divided into two groups: officers and physicians of the *Luftwaffe*, who brought in their scientific expertise in virology, and SS-Officers, who sought influence in the sciences, and were in a powerful position to allow access to concentration camp inmates as subjects for human experimentation. Collaboration of both groups, although never free from competition, led to a division of responsibilities concerning the medical war crimes committed at Natzweiler. Although medical war crimes were crimes committed by a collective, the juridical aim of the prosecution in Nuremberg was to show the individual responsibility of the defendants, who fostered, ordered, approved or supported the typhus experiments. The case of the defendant Gerhard Rose, former *Generalarzt* and Adviser for Tropical Medicine to the Chief of the Medical Service of the Luftwaffe; Vice President and Chief of the Department for Tropical Medicine at the renowned Robert Koch Institute gives us a better insight and provides a precise example of the collaboration between American and French authorities during the NMT. One of the main charges against Rose concerned his participation in Haagen's typhus experiments in Natzweiler. The examination of Rose took place in April 1947 a few weeks before Haagen was called as a witness. By the end of the month, after examination of Rose had been completed, prosecutor James M. McHaney wrote to the French trial observer François Bayle asking him for urgent support:

The prosecution contends that these experiments by Haagen were for the purpose of testing the effectiveness of typhus vaccines and that after the experimental subject had been vaccinated, he was then infected with virulent typhus to test the vaccine. Rose on the other hand, contends that so far as he knows, Haagen never artificially infected his experimental subjects in the way urged by the prosecution. Several documents introduced by the prosecution concerning the Haagen experiments, and in which the word "infection" is used, are explained by Rose as meaning nothing more than vaccination, attenuated avirulent typhus vaccine, that is to say, a living vaccine necessarily involved in the infection. While this, of course, is quite true and conceded by the prosecution, we still maintain that the word "infection" would not be used by anyone as synonymous with vaccination, even with an avirulent vaccine.[18]

Earlier, in January 1947, Haagen's former assistant Edith Schmidt had testified before the court that about 50 concentration camp inmates had died as a result of Haagen's typhus experiments.[19] However, the prosecution did not want to rely on this oral account alone and found it "highly desirable" to receive "further documentary and testimonial evidence on the Haagen experiments" from the French to show "beyond any doubt that Haagen actually carried out infections with virulent typhus".[20] At this point the prosecution expecting that Haagen would follow the same line of argumentation as Rose and therefore facing stalled accusations, the court was weary to find new (French) documentary evidence calling for legal allied cooperation.

The French authorities were able to provide three important documents before the examination of Haagen began. The first one was a list (Exhibit 519)[21] and the second a pocket book of Haagen's expenditures for his typhus research (Exhibit 542),[22] indicating the dates of his trips to and phone calls with the concentration camps of Schirmeck and Natzweiler. The third, and even more incriminating, document was a laboratory diary of Haagen's assistant Brigitte Crodel (Exhibit 521)[23] with notes on the inoculations of humans at Schirmeck and Natzweiler. These documents, introduced by the prosecutor James M. McHaney during his cross-examination of Haagen on 19 and 20 June 1947, came as a complete surprise for Haagen.

Previously Haagen had insisted on several occasions under oath before the court that his vaccinations in Schirmeck had ended in May 1943[24] and in Natzweiler in January 1944.[25] With the notebook written by Brigitte Crodel,[26] the prosecution was able to show that further vaccinations had taken place in 1944, proving that Haagen had lied under oath. In addition to that Haagen now was confronted with the notes of Crodel that two of the persons he had inoculated were "not available", interpreted by the prosecution as a camouflaged note that two concentration camp inmates had died as a result of the experiments, while Haagen was defending himself with the explanation that the notation only referred to blood samples for in vitro-tests and not persons.[27]

Even though the aim of the NMT was not to convict Haagen for his typhus experiments, the US Military Tribunal was able to establish some important findings related to and anticipating Haagen's own trial. For the time being they were essential for the Nuremberg verdict. First, the experiments at Schirmeck and Natzweiler were of comparative nature, examining vaccines that had already been in use for some time with a new typhus vaccine developed by Haagen and his assistant Brigitte Crodel from a virulent virus. Second, as contemporary documents introduced by the prosecution had shown, the exploitation of concentration camp inmates as experimental subjects resulted from an initiative of Haagen, and had not been imposed on him by superior Luftwaffe authorities. His rank as Stabsarzt and Consulting Hygienist of the Luftwaffe enabled him to conduct the experiments on his own initiative. Third, Haagen admitted that the concentration camp inmates had not taken part voluntarily in the experiments. He tried to justify his actions by arguing that inoculations were a measure for active immunisation ordered by German authorities to prevent the outbreak of a typhus epidemic in the concentration camp.[28] Fourth, even though Haagen had prepared plans for a vaccine production at the Hygiene Institute of the *Reichsuniversität Straßburg*, as intended by the Medical Service of the Luftwaffe, this plan was not implemented before the liberation of Strasbourg by American Forces.

At the same time several crucial questions remained controversial or were not explicitly addressed in the judgement of the Nuremberg Medical Trial. For one thing, the acknowledged nature of the experiments remained without clear status. Haagen and the defence insisted that the inoculation had the character of an active immunisation. The prosecution, in contrast, was convinced that Haagen had vaccinated the inmates and then deliberately infected them with typhus *rickettsiae* to confirm an effective immunisation. This view was supported by the judges.[29] Second, prosecution and defence views differed with regard to the question whether or not the vaccine had been sufficiently tested in animal- and self-experiments by Haagen and his collaborators. While Haagen insisted that the experiments were without risk and conducted to study the tolerability and side reactions of his vaccine on a higher number of subjects, the prosecution was convinced that the experiments were not only harmful but bore an extremely high risk. Furthermore, the question how long the experiments had continued remained a controversial point. Haagen claimed that he stopped his typhus experiments in Schirmeck in May 1943[30] and in Natzweiler in January 1944.[31] On the contrary, the notebook of Crodel, presented by the French prosecution, showed that Haagen had inoculated prisoners at Natzweiler in July 1944 with typhus vaccine.[32] A final crucial point, especially in consideration of the coming French Military Tribunal, was the question of whether Haagen's experiments had caused any fatalities. Haagen adamantly denied that any of the concentration camp inmates had died as a result of the inoculation with his vaccine.[33] Based on a testimony from Georges Hirtz[34] and the notebook of Brigitte Crodel, the prosecution on the other side was convinced that at least two persons died between the end of May and June 1943 in the Schirmeck camp. Based on the oral examination of the Dutch survivor Gerrit Hendrik Nales, who witnessed the typhus experiments of Haagen when he had to work as male nurse in the prison clinic of Natzweiler, the prosecution also believed that approximately another 30 inmates had deceased in Natzweiler.[35] Haagen's former assistant Edith Schmidt had even claimed that approximately 50 camp prisoners, belonging to the unprotected control group, had died as a result of the experiments.[36] It is noteworthy that in the documenation of the NMT by Mitscherlich and Mielke the involvement of Haagen in the typus experiments at Struthof and Schirmeck differed remarkably between the first and the second extended edition, e.g. between 1947 and 1949.[37] Intensified interrogations of Haagen between 1947 and 1949 by the French prosecution detailed below condensed incriminations against him well before the final act of accusation was filed in December 1952. In 1949 the Colmar Court of Appeals was seized to decide whether Haagen and Bickenbach were to be indicted at the Permanent Military Tribunal in Metz. Concerning Haagen's defence strategy Mitscherlich and Mielke added new exhibits and transcripts of the Nuremberg trial to their second edition. They also added several longer comments in which they refuted Haagen's claim that his typhus experiments in Schirmeck in May 1943 and in Natzweiler in January 1944 were only protective vaccinations of therapeutic nature not putting at risk the health of the camp inmates.[38] They cited the prosecution's argument that it was unlikely that the small number of 20 vaccinated inmates at Schirmeck and 80 at Natzweiler could prevent a typhus epidemic in a camp of approximately 12,000 inmates such as Natzweiler.[39] Passages from the testimony of the former camp inmate and pharmacists Dr Hirtz, who had charged Haagen with responsibility for the death of two Polish prisoners who had died of typhus, were added. Mitscherlich and Mielke commented on the experimental notebook of Haagen's technical assistant and documented several requests by Haagen for new healthy camp inmates as research subjects.[40] They also inserted a reference to the French prosecution yet little detailed and vaguely attributed to a procedure in Strasbourg against Haagen.[41] The changes between the first and the second edition of the book by Mitscherlich and Mielke reflect the shifting role of Haagen from witness of the defence at the NMT to defendant in the French prosecution. Haagen's status as witness in the NMT did not require proof of his individual guilt, and the American judges were careful not to anticipate the French Military Tribunal, which Haagen was awaiting. However, the American judges had to take a position concerning Haagen's typhus experiments, insofar as this was necessary for the judgement of the defendants connected with the Natzweiler experiments: the Air Force officers Hermann Becker-Freyseng, Oskar Schröder and Gerhard Rose as well as the SS-Officers Wolfram Sievers and Rudolf Brandt. In the case of Hermann Becker-Freyseng, the former head of the Aeromedical Department in the Reich Air Ministry, the NMT found the evidence was "insufficient to disclose any criminal responsibility of the defendant" in regard to the typhus experiments.[42] As a medical officer of the

Air Force, Haagen was subordinate to Oskar Schröder as Chief of the Medical Service. Schröder had approved research assignments concerning the typhus experiments and had been informed about the exploitation of concentration camp inmates for typhus vaccine experiments by reports he had received.[43] The judges emphasised that it would have been his "affirmative duty", as commanding officer, "to take such steps as are within his power and appropriate to the circumstances to control those under his command for the prevention of acts which are violations of the law of war".[44] Instead

> he blindly approved a continuation of typhus research by Haagen, supported the program, and was furnished with reports of its progress, without so much as taking one step to determine the circumstances under which the research had been or was being carried on, to lay down rules for the conduct of present or future research by his subordinates, or to prescribe the conditions under which the concentration camp inmates could be used as experimental subjects.[45]

Written documents had given evidence that Gerhard Rose had worked out a plan with Haagen for the production of his typhus vaccine at his Hygiene Institute, and, even more incriminating, about the delivery of humans "for infecting the vaccinated subjects with a virulent pathogenic virus".[46] The judges therefore saw him as "directly connected with the criminal experiments conducted by Haagen".[47] According to their judgement, it had been "proven that not less than 50 experimental subjects died as a direct result of their participation in these typhus experiments".[48] The defendant Rudolf Brandt was held responsible for the "smooth operation of these experiments" as on the Personal Staff of Reichsführer SS Heinrich Himmler. The judges held Rudolf Brandt responsible for having informed Himmler about the typhus experiments "before and after their performance" to arrange "the supply of quotas of suitable human experimental material to the physicians at the scene of the experiment". Therefore he was "considered as one of the defendants responsible for performance of illegal medical experiments where deaths resulted to the nonconsenting human subjects".[49] Another SS officer, who was convicted for the typhus experiments at Natzweiler, was Wolfram Sievers, former Reich Business Manager of the *SS-Ahnenerbe*. In his case the judges explicitly referred to the monthly reports from the camp doctor at Natzweiler furnished by French authorities.[50] Concerning the controversial question of fatalities as a direct result of Haagen's typhus experiments, the judges followed the opinion of the prosecution and stated in their judgement against Sievers: "That the experiments were carried out in the *Ahnenerbe* experimental station in Natzweiler is proved by excerpts from monthly reports of the camp doctor in Natzweiler. A number of deaths occurred among non-German experimental subjects as a direct result of the treatment to which they were subjected".[51] Concerning precise numbers of Haagen's typhus experiment victims, the judgement of the NMT remained relatively vague and neither gave their concrete number nor did the NMT elucidate who the victims were. This remained an open question for the French Military Tribunal.

Haagen at the SMT, 1952–54

Official investigations for the SMT started on 19 April 1945 and lasted until 1 April 1949. Three judges were successively assigned to the case: Raymond Jadin (1945–47), Captain Margraff in 1947 and finally Captain Joseph Lorich (1947–49). The *Chambre de Mises en Accusation* of the Colmar Court of Appeals (detached to Metz) ruled on 20 December 1949 that Haagen and Bickenbach were to be sent to the TMP at Metz to face charges of poisoning.[52] An appeal against this decision by Haagen and Bickenbach was rejected on 18 July 1952, giving way to the preparation of the trial, which took place from 16 to 24 December 1952 in Metz. The SMT lasted, including an appeal, from 1952 to 1954 taking thus place respectively five to seven years after the US Nuremberg Military Trial. Four of the six indictees, professor of anatomy August Hirt (1898–1945) and his assistant Otto Bong (1901-?), Haagen's assistant Hellmut Erich Gräfe (1911–52) and Bickenbach's assistant Helmut Rühl (1918-?) were absent or not alive anymore. The two defendants the French prosecution had been able to arrest were professor of hygiene, bacteriology and virology Eugen Haagen (1898–1972) and professor of biochemistry and director of the Strasbourg polyclinic Otto Bickenbach (1901–71). Bickenbach was accused of human experimentation with the chemical warfare agent phosgene in the gas chamber of Natzweiler thereby killing four persons and injuring many more. Charges against Haagen concerned in particular his typhus experiments, whereas much of his other research activities including experiments with human subjects were less well documented and played a marginal role in the trial proceedings.

By the time the SMT was actually held in December 1952, early studies of the NMT including Mitscherlich and Mielke's 1947 account and the much more extensive book *Croix Gammée Contre Caducée* published in 1950 by the French trial observer François Bayle were available.[53] Prosecution and early reception collided when the French defence lawyer De la Pradelle on the opening day of the SMT in Metz on 16 December 1952 immediately after the accusation statement was read argued that the publication *in extenso* of secret trial documents by Bayle that had not been notified to Haagen interfered with the right of the defence and accordingly required an annulation of the whole legal procedure.[54] After secret deliberation the judges finally declared that Bayle purveyed only testimonies and documents of official character and that Bayle had wisely acknowledged in his conclusion himself: "I will stop here the reflections suggested by Haagen's work that has not yet been judged, and I will leave to his judges, possibly enlightened by further testimonies I have not known, the task to make up their own opinion".[55] The judges concluded thus that rights of the defence were not infringed. The episode raises the question to what extent the French prosecution and judges mobilised evidence and sentences from the Nuremberg Medical Trial and Haagen's testimonies there? This prompts us to turn to the initial French interrogations and testimonies gathered between 1947 and 1949.

After Haagen's second arrest on 16 November 1946 by the British and his transfer to the French authorities in Baden-Baden on 1 February 1947 and later in Strasbourg he faced an initial interrogation by Captain Margraff on 26 February 1947 without any legal assistance.[56] During the interrogation Haagen employed repeatedly the term "experimentation" for his research activities. He admitted having visited the Natzweiler concentration camp approximately ten times working on "an attenuated typhus virus administration". He underlined that no deaths had occurred during the experiments and therefore concluded that the strains he worked with could only have been non-virulent *rickettsiae* since otherwise 50 of the 80 subjects would probably have died. Haagen conceded that he knew that inmates came from Auschwitz and stated that he had been interrogated in November 1945 during his first arrest in view of the preparation for the NMT. For any further declarations he directed the judge to the scientific publication of his research results in the *Zentralblatt für Bakteriologie* of 1944.[57] For the rest, Haagen reassured the prosecutor that in Schirmeck he only vaccinated two persons with typhus desiccated Koch vaccine, that he was not aware of any deaths and had never been engaged in typhus experiments in the Schirmeck camp, claiming these had only been "preventive influenza vaccinations".[58] He insisted that he had allegedly no connections to research with Hirt or Bickenbach. The final line of his declaration was that he considered not having performed experiments with a scientific objective but that he was on the way to establish a new means to combat typhus and that there was great epidemic danger for a typhus epidemic in the Natzweiler camp. At this early stage of French interrogations the only reference to Nuremberg was Haagen's vague mentioning of his interrogation of November 1945.

It is interesting to note here that the 1947 account of the NMT by Mitscherlich and Mielke, perfectly contemporary to Haagen's first interrogation by the French prosecutor, described Haagen's "human experiments with typhus in the KL Natzweiler" on barely two pages[59] establishing that they were conducted from autumn 1943 until the liberation of the camp in autumn 1944 and insisting strongly on their organisational structures and hierarchies, stating that their initiator was Professor Eugen Haagen but that the investigations were supported by the chiefs of the *Sanitätswesens der Luftwaffe*, the *Reichsforschungsrats* and the *Reichsführer SS* personally, as well as by the *SS-Wirtschafts-Verwaltungshauptamt* and the *Institut für Wehrwissenschaftliche Zweckforschung der Waffen-SS*. Mitscherlich and Mielke concluded their two pages devoted to Haagen and typhus saying:

> A lab log book comparable to the Ding diary [for typhus experiments in Buchenwald] is not known for Natzweiler. Form and scale of experiments remain therefore in the dark. We dispose only of three concordant oral testimonies that in May 1943 twenty-five Polish persons were subjected to human experiments.[60]

Two months later the second interrogation by Captain Margraff on 25 April 1947, this time with legal assistance from his lawyer Frederic Hoffet, suggested a reinterpretation of the term "experimentation" employed by Haagen in his first testimony.[61] Haagen insisted now that whenever he had used the term "experimentation" this needed to be understood in relation to a set of self-declared restrictions considering that he had never "inoculated typhus directly" – in fact he claimed that he did not detain the virulent viral strain required for that; that he had tested the vaccine first on himself, his collaborator Mrs Crodel and seven volunteers of his institute, and that he was totally convinced by that time that the vaccine was harmless because it had been developed to a point where it was not at the stage of trial and error anymore.

Haagen claimed that his vaccine had moved beyond the point that could be properly designated as experimental. His intervention in the camp, he claimed, therefore did not have the character of an experimental "trial" anymore, but represented the application of a product and a procedure that he considered as proven. Beyond this semantical reinterpretation of the medical meaning of "experimentation" Haagen suggested that no virulent viral virus strains had been at his disposal. He declared to have contacted the camp physician to take "prophylactic measures" and they came to an agreement to start vaccination of 100 subjects with a group of Roma from Auschwitz. According to Haagen approximately 80 were declared as "vaccinated": a first group by injection, a second one by scarification.[62] A completely different atmosphere emerges from the four successive interrogations conducted with Haagen by the newly appointed French prosecutor Captain J.M. Lorich in December 1947 after Haagen's return from the NMT. Starting with the Schirmeck interventions and Haagen's former depositions, Lorich first repeated questions addressed eight months earlier by Margraff concerning influenza, typhus and yellow fever "vaccinations" to then abruptly questioning Haagen why he had denied in April having experimented in Schirmeck?[63]

For a second time Lorich turned to the question of "inoculations" in the Natzweiler camp that were, according to Haagen, requested by the camp commandant Josef Kramer. The acknowledged series of 80 "vaccinated" Roma was explained by Haagen as "the first step to vaccinate all camp inmates".[64] Lorich again challenged Haagen's account questioning why then Haagen would have requested subjects according to a letter to the SS *Wirtschafts-Verwaltungshauptamt* in August 1943, and why he would not have employed the proven vaccine of Georges Blanc from the Institut Pasteur, or why he would have subjected individuals to scarifications with "virulent germs". In his interrogations Lorich used Nuremberg documents including letters to SS authorities[65] as well as oral testimonies by former collaborators of Haagen (Edith Schmidt,[66] Alex-Nikolas Probst,[67] Alphonse Bauer,[68] and Eugen Hönig[69]).

Twelve days later Lorich intensified pressure when opening the third interrogation, bluntly confronting Haagen with his depositions made in Nuremberg that no "vaccinations" at all were conducted in Schirmeck.[70] Lorich now followed the proactive line of interrogation initiated by McHaney at the end of the four-day Nuremberg examination of June 1947. Haagen's theory of immunity, practicalities of vaccine production and anti-body evaluation were scrutinised in detail before Lorich moved to what had become a central document of accusation: the Crodel laboratory notebook. The interrogation was concluded as follows: "We allow ourselves to indicate to the accused that based on this notebook his declarations are false".[71]

Lorich's interrogations from 1947 to 1949 consisted in distancing himself from oral testimonies considered as too easily refuted or questionable in order to privilege written documentary evidence. The final interrogation in January 1949 opposed again written evidence to Haagen's oral testimonies referring this time to infection reports by the SS camp physician establishing that no typhus epidemic had occurred in the KL Natzweiler before Haagen's experimental procedure.

The act of accusation filed by the Permanent Military Tribunal in Metz on 28 October 1952 retained in its exposition of facts that Haagen, his collaborator Graefe and their laboratory assistants initiated a series of human experiments for a new vaccine against typhus in May or June 1943 in the Schirmeck camp. Observations were based on the oral testimonies of former camp inmate Dr Georg Hirtz.[72] From there, the accusation moved quickly to events at the Natzweiler camp based on oral testimonies by Georg Rosef[73] and doctors Henri Chretien[74] and Leif Poulsson[75] about prisoner transports from Auschwitz to Natzweiler of two groups of Roma of which the second one was used for experiments in "February and March 1944 including 40 unvaccinated subjects used as control group and exposed to 'control infections'". The accusation concluded that: "The non-military Eugen Haagen . . ., voluntarily made an attempt on the lives of 40 non identified persons, by the effect of substances that could kill more or less rapidly".[76]

On 24 December 1952 the jury of the Permanent Military Tribunal of the 6th regiment answered the question "The non military Eugen Haagen . . . is he guilty of having at Natzweiler, in 1944, in any case in France, during war hostilities and since less than 10 years, voluntarily made an attempt on the lives of 40 non identified persons, by the effect of substances that could kill more or less rapidly"[77] with YES.

The judgement retained one single question concerning the accused Haagen. Fifty other questions addressed to the judges for the final judgement concerned the other defendants of the SMT group trial. Charges against Haagen had been restricted to the one and single issue of the group of 40 Roma inoculated in early 1944 in the Natzweiler camp. The audience notes of the trial make no mention neither of the trial nor of the judgement of the NMT five years earlier.[78] This is not to state that the American trial exerted no direct influence on the French judges, but if it did this remains for the moment untraceable since deliberations were secret and only the final votes were transcribed in the judgement.

Conclusion

In concluding we would like to argue that our contextual cross-trial and trial-early reception approach viewed through the Haagen case at the NMT and the SMT highlights that American and French procedures were intimately linked. What our analysis suggests is that a comparative perspective beyond the Nuremberg Medical Trial provides new understanding of how the American and French Trials were in many ways linked, namely through the pre-trial investigations on war crimes, and the exchange of evidence, expert surveys and witnesses.

The prosecution included from early on the exchange of written evidence as the described cross examination of Haagen's testimonies, his written articles of 1944 and the reconstruction of typhus cases in the Natzweiler camp from the SS physician *Infektionsmeldungen* indicate. Such information was shared by French and American investigators immediately before the NMT hearings of Haagen. Bayle's 1950 publication on the NMT was cited at the opening of the SMT, German reports by Mitscherlich and Mielke were not so. And, consequences of the Bayle reference could be squarely contradictory in outcome. If the French evidence for the NMT enabled prosecution to put into question Haagen's earlier accounts, the Bayle account at the SMT was used by the defence to attempt to delay the trial for reasons of procedure.

We have not pursued in depth the question of witnesses and experts in the framework of this contribution. Nevertheless it seems that a closer reading of the role of French scientific experts like the Casablanca Pasteur Institute director Georges Blanc would be needed to better understand what provocatively and superficially summarised could be qualified here as a line of an international professional defence of bacteriologists exchanging cultures and physicians doing human subject research. International scientific cooperation and cohesion often overruled considerations about wartime enemies especially when questions of war crimes were cast as "medical" war crimes. Part of this defence addressed charges levied by Haagen at the NMT that French typhus experiments of the 1930s were "comparable" in design and practice with his activities in the Natzweiler camp. Part of it was scientist's apprehending of public opinion as in the case when a 1952 statement of the French Academy of Medicine addressed the question of guidelines for human experimentation shortly before the SMT started and was publicised by the press. Judgements and their early reception clearly need to be interpreted and reanalysed in this historical context.

Early reception of the NMT in the first edition of Mitscherlich and Mielke volume from 1947 kept much in the dark on the Natzweiler experiments. Charges against Eugen Haagen were described there as focused on 25 subjects vaccinated at the Schirmeck camp. These charges were dropped during the court proceedings, and only the vaccine experiments in Natzweiler in spring 1944 were retained as charge in the final judgement (involving the 40 Roma). The early reception history of the NMT and subsequent medical war crime trials became entangled very quickly as part of the ongoing prosecution itself. National perspectives from Mitscherlich and Mielke to Bayle indicate an interpretative spectrum ranging from a system analysis of the Nazi regime to perpetrator psychology in prosecution and trial public accounts. French and German accounts differ significantly for the Natzweiler Haagen typhus experiments – two pages in Mitscherlich and Mielke's *Diktat* book (1947), and eight in their *Wissenschaft* book (1949), versus 45 pages in the Bayle's voluminous account (1950), establishing different lines of interpretation for the crimes committed. The differences in the two editions of Mitscherlich and Mielke and later of Bayle in length and detail clearly reflect the process of Haagen having been a witness in the NMT turning into a defendant in France. It is evident at this point that a single case analysis raises the question of its representativeness. SMT was group trial and it is tempting to juxtapose the Haagen and Bickenbach case since both were present at the trial. Both were described in 1946 by the witness Camille Simonin (himself an expert in forensic medicine) as equally responsible for the *Versuchsstation* for human experiments established at the Natzweiler camp. Prosecution evidence during the investigation meant that Otto Bickenbach could not be regarded as having a similar position as that taken by Eugen Haagen. These were not merely questions of personality, but complex outcomes of trial evidence, defence strategies and perpetrator personalities. What both cases have in common as historical analysis shows is that neither of the two cases could be described as "pseudo-medical experiments". Continuing interrogation about how these non SS physicians could understand themselves and justify their crimes until the end of the SMT in Lyon pleading "not guilty" is as much a question of coming to terms with physician practices under the Nazi regime as an open question for biomedical research with human subjects ever since 1945.

Type of tested vaccine	Date	Number of experimental subjects
Yellow Fever	09/06/1943	20-30 according to Haagen
Yellow Fever	March 1943	Unknown
Epidemic Typhus	26/05/1943	10 men (2 deceased)
Epidemic Typhus	13/07/1943	20 men
Epidemic Typhus	04/10/1943	10-20 men
Influenza	November 1943	30 women according to Haagen
Hepatitis	1944	?

Figure 14.1 Experiments by Eugen Haagen at the Schirmeck Camp in 1943

Type of tested vaccine	Date	Number of experimental subjects
Epidemic Typhus	27/01/1944	80–88 men
Epidemic Typhus	25/05/1944	20 men
Epidemic Typhus	Summer 1944	Projected experiments on 200 men
Hepatitis	1944	1-5 men
Pneumonia	1944	Projected experiments were sabotaged

Figure 14.2 Experiments by Eugen Haagen at the Natzweiler Concentration Camp in 1944

Defendant	Former position	Sentence	Concentration camp
Hermann Becker-Freyseng	Chief of the Department for Aviation Medicine of the Chief of the Medical Service of the Luftwaffe	Not guilty	Natzweiler
Rudolf Brandt	Personal Administrative Officer to Reichsführer-SS Heinrich Himmler	Guilty	Natzweiler
Oskar Schröder	Chief of Staff of the Inspectorate of the Medical Service of the Luftwaffe and Chief of the Medical Service of the Luftwaffe	Guilty	Natzweiler
Wolfram Sievers	Reich Manager of the Amt Ahnenerbe and Deputy Chairman of the Managing Board of Directors of Reich Research Counsel	Guilty	Natzweiler
Gerhard Rose	Chief of the Medical Service of the Luftwaffe; Vice President of the Robert Koch Institute	Guilty	Natzweiler & Buchenwald
Karl Genzken	Chief of the Medical Department of the Waffen SS	Guilty	Buchenwald
Waldemar Hoven	Waffen-SS and Chief Doctor of the Buchenwald concentration camp	Guilty	Buchenwald
Joachim Mrugowsky	Chief of Hygiene of the Reich Physician SS and Police; Chief of the Hygiene Institute of the Waffen SS	Guilty	Buchenwald
Siegfried Handloser	Medical Inspector of the Army; Chief of the Medical Services of the Armed Forces	Guilty	Buchenwald
Helmut Poppendick/ Poppendieck	Chief of the Personal Staff of the Reich Physician SS and Police	Not guilty	Buchenwald
Karl Brandt	Reich Commissioner for Health and Sanitation	Not guilty	
Karl Gebhardt	Chief Surgeon of the Staff of the Reich Physician SS and Police; President of the German Red Cross	Not guilty	
Paul Rostock	Surgical Adviser to the Army; and Chief of the Office for Medical Science and Research under the Reich Commissioner for Health and Sanitation Karl Brandt	Not guilty	

Figure 14.3 Defendants and judgement of the NMT on the Typhus Experiments, 1947

Defendant	Sentence	Reasons
Hermann Becker-Freyseng	Not guilty	Insufficient evidence for criminal responsibility
Oskar Schröder	Guilty	As a medical officer of the Air Force Haagen was subordinate of Schröder as Chief of the Medical Service who approved research assignments pursuant to the typhus experiments
Wolfram Sievers	Guilty	Deaths at the experimental station of the SS-Ahnenerbe in Natzweiler.
Gerhard Rose	Guilty	Planning of delivery of concentration camp prisoners. Death of 50 experimental subjects.
Rudolf Brandt	Guilty	Supply of concentration camp inmates

Figure 14.4 Defendants, judgement and arguments for the legal decision of the NMT on the Typhus Experiments, 1947

Notes

1 Alexander Mitscherlich and Fred Mielke, Das Diktat der Menschenverachtung. Eine Dokumentation, Heidelberg: Verlag Lambert Schneider, 1947; idem, Wissenschaft ohne Menschlichkeit. Medizinische une eugenische Irrwege unter Dikatatur, Bürokratie und Krieg, Heidelberg: Verlag Lambert Schneider, 1949.
2 François Bayle, *Croix gammée contre caducée. Les expériences humaines en Allemagne pendant la deuxième guerre mondiale*, Neustadt: Centre de L'Imprimerie Nationale, 1950.
3 Clemens Gabriele, '"Man aus den Deutschen Demokraten machen wollte". Umerziehung durch Film. Britische und amerikanische Filmpolitik in Deutschland 1945–1949', in Harro Segeberg (ed.), *Mediale Mobilmachung II. Hollywood, Exil und Nachkrieg*, Munich: Fink, 2006, pp. 243–271; Sabine Hake, 'Erziehung zur Demokratie. Trümmerfilme made in Holywood', in Johannes Roschlau (ed.), *Im Bann der Katastrophe Innovation und Tradition im europäischen Film 1940 – 1950*, Munich: Ed. Text + Kritik, 2010, p. 85–87.
4 Paul Weindling, 'From International to Zonal Trials: The Origins of the Nuremberg Medical Trial', *Holocaust and Genocide Studies*, 14.3 (2000), pp. 367–389.
5 Nina Staehle, 'La politique des crimes de guerre médicaux: les tribulations qui conduisirent au procès de Ravensbrück, 1946–1947', in Christian Bonah, Etienne Lepicard and Volker Roelcke (eds), *La médecine expérimentale au tribunal: Implications éthiques de quelques procès médicaux du XXe siècle européen*, Paris: Editions des Archives contemporaines, 2003, pp. 215–231; Angelika Ebbinghaus and Karl Heinz Roth, 'Medizinverbrechen vor Gericht. Die Menschenversuche im Konzentrationslager Dachau', in Ludwig Eiber and Robert Sigel (eds), *Dachauer Prozesse. NS-Verbrechen vor amerikanischen Militärgerichten in Dachau 1945–48. Verfahren, Ergebnisse, Nachwirkungen*, Göttingen: Wallstein Verlag, 2007, pp. 126–159; Ulf Schmidt, '"The Scars of Ravensbrück". Medical Experiments and British War Crimes Policy, 1945–1950', *German History*, 23.1 (2005), pp. 20–49; Paul Weindling, 'Auf der Spur von Medizinverbrechen: Keith Mant (1919–2000) und sein Debut als forensischer Pathologe', *1999. Zeitschrift für Sozialgeschichte des 20. und 21. Jahrhunderts*, 16 (2001), pp. 129–139.

6 The camp is also identified by the occupiers as the Natzweiler camp named after the village closest to the location.

7 A first mention of the SMT appears in Ernst Klee, *Auschwitz, die NS-Medizin und ihre Opfer*, Frankfurt am Main: S. Fischer Verlag, 1997, pp. 385–387; Raphael Toledano, 'Les Expériences Médicales du Professeur Eugen Haagen de la Reichsuniversität Strassburg. Faits, Contexte et Procès d'un Médecin National-Socialiste', MD thesis, Strasbourg: University of Strasbourg, 2010; Christian Bonah and Florian Schmaltz, 'The Struthof Medical Trials 1952–1954. Prosecution and Judgement of Nazi Physicians Otto Bickenbach and Eugen Haagen at Military Tribunals in France', in Ulf Schmidt, Andreas Frewer and Dominique Sprumont (eds), *Human Research and the Declaration of Helsinki*, Oxford: Oxford University Press, forthcoming in 2017.

8 The literature on the NMT is extensive, for an overview see: Klaus Dörner *et al.* (eds), Der Nürnberger Ärzteprozeß 1946/47. Wortprotokolle, Anklage- und Verteidigungs-material, Quellen zum Umfeld. Erschließungsband zur Mikrofiche-Edition: Bearbeitet von Karsten Linne, Munich: K.G. Saur, 2000. For the English edition see: idem (eds), The Nuremberg Medical Trial 1946/47. Transcripts, Material of the Prosecution and Defense, Related Documents. Guide to the Mikrofiche-Edition, Munich: Saur, 2001; George J. Annas and Michael A. Grodin (eds), *The Nazi Doctors and the Nuremberg Code: Human Rights in Human Experimentation*, New York and Oxford: Oxford University Press, 1992; Klaus Dörner and Angelika Ebbinghaus (eds), *Vernichten und Heilen. Der Nürnberger Ärzteprozeß und seine Folgen*, Berlin: Aufbau Verlag, 2001; Paul Julian Weindling, *Nazi Medicine and the Nuremberg Trials: From Medical War Crimes to Informed Consent*, Houndmills, Basingstoke: Palgrave Macmillan, 2004; idem, John W. Thompson, *Psychiatrist in the Shadow of the Holocaust*, Rochester, NY: Rochester University Press, 2010; Ulf Schmidt, *Justice at Nuremberg. Leo Alexander and the Nazi Doctors' Trial*, Houndmills, Basingstoke: Palgrave Macmillan, 2004; Volker Roelcke and Giovanni Maio (eds), *Twentieth Century Ethics of Human Subjects Research. Historical Perspectives on Values, Practices, and Regulations*, Stuttgart: Steiner, 2004; Michael R. Marrus, 'The Nuermberg Doctor's Trial in Historical Context', *Bulletin for the History of Medicine*, 73.1 (1999), pp. 106–123. Volker Roelcke, Etienne Lepicard and Sascha Topp (eds.), Silence, Scapegoats, Self-Reflection. The Shadow of Nazi Medical Crimes on Medicine and Bioethics, Göttingen: V&R unipress, 2014.

9 Sheila Jasanoff, *Science at the Bar Law, Science, and Technology in America*, Cambridge, MA: Harvard University Press, 1997; eadem, 'Just Evidence. The Limits of Science in the Legal Process', *Journal of Law, Medicine and Ethics*, 34 (2006), pp. 328–339.

10 For an extensive account on Haagen, see Toledano, 'Expériences Médicales'.

11 Leo James Mahoney, 'A History of the War Department Scientific Intelligence Mission (ALSOS), 1943–1945', PhD thesis, Kent, OH: Kent State University, 1981, pp. 221–249. For the Alsos Mission see also: Samuel Abraham Goudsmit, *Alsos (History of Modern Physics and Astronomy)*, Woodbury, NY: 1996.

12 Paul Weindling, 'Virologist and National Socialist. The Extraordinary Career of Eugen Haagen', in Marion Hulverscheidt and Anja Laukötter (eds), *Infektion und Institution. Zur Wissenschaftsgeschichte des Robert-Koch-Instituts im Nationalsozialismus*, Göttingen: Wallstein-Verlag, 2009, pp. 232–249.

13 Ibid.

14 In the NMT the defendants Becker-Freyseng, Karl Brandt, Rudolf Brandt, Gebhardt, Genzken, Handloser, Hoven, Mrugowsky, Poppendick, Rose, Rostock, Schröder and Sievers were charged with special responsibility for and participation in criminal conduct involving typhus experiments. See part 6 J of the indictment: *Trials of War Criminals before the Nuernberg Military Tribunals under Control Council Law No.10. Nuernberg October 1946-April 1949. Vol. I: The Medical Case,* Washington, DC: US Government Printing Office, 1949, pp. 13–14.

15 Dörner *et al.*, *Der Nürnberger Ärzteprozeß*, (Microfiche = MF) 02/9524.

16 Vernehmung von Eugen Haagen, 18 June 1947, Wortprotokoll. 9544–9556, in ibid., (MF) 02/09554–09556.

17 Handloser, Schröder, Genzken, Rudolf Brandt, Mrugowsky, Sievers, Rose, and Hoven were convicted, while the defendants Becker-Freyseng, Karl Brandt, Gebhardt, Poppendick, Rostock, were acquitted on these counts. See: *Trials of War Criminals before the Nuernberg Military Tribunals under Control Council Law No. 10. Nuernberg October 1946-April 1949. Vol. 2. The Medical Case/The Milch Case*, Washington, DC: US Government Printing Office, 1949, pp. 177–178.

18 Paris, Centre de recherches des Archives nationales (hereafter CARAN), BB/35/276, McHaney to Bayle: Subject: Typhus Experiments by Dr Haagen in Strasbourg and Natzweiler Concentration Camp, 28 Apr 1947. See also: Toledano, 'Expériences Médicales', p. 494.

19 Vernehmung von Edith Schmidt, 9 Jan 1947, in Dörner *et al.*, *Nürnberger Ärzteprozeß*, (MF) 2/01381.

20 CARAN, BB/35/276, McHaney to Bayle: Subject: Typhus Experiments by Dr Haagen in Strasbourg and Natzweiler Concentration Camp, 28 Apr 1947. See also: Toledano, 'Expériences Médicales', p. 494.

21 Eugen Haagen: Aufstellung der Ausgaben betr. Influenza-Forschungsauftrag RdL u. ObdL, 14 Feb 1944, Exhibit 519b – NO-3450, Anklagedokumentenband = ADB 19. Addendum B, in Dörner *et al.*, *Nürnberger Ärzteprozeß*, (MF) 3/2953–2954.

22 Auszug aus dem Tagebuch von Eugen Haagen, 1942, Exhibit 542 NO-3837, ADB 18, in ibid., (MF) 3/2564–2570.

23 Auszug aus dem Tagebuch von Eugen Haagen, Apr 1943 – July 1943, Exhibit 521, NO-3852, ADB 19. Addendum B, in ibid., (MF) 3/2958–2964.

24 See for example: Vernehmung Haagen, 20 June 1947, Wortprotokoll. Bl. 9775, in ibid., (MF) 02/9775; National Archives Microfilm Publication M 887. Records of the United States Nuernberg War Crimes Trials: United States of America v. Karl Brandt *et al.* (Case I), November 21, 1946–August 20, 1947, Washington, DC: National Archives and Records Service, 1974, roll 10, Transcript, 9636.

25 Direktes Verhör des Zeugen Eugen Haagen, 20 June 1947 (124. Verhandlungstag), Wortprotokoll, in Dörner *et al.*, *Nürnberger Ärzteprozeß*, (MF) 2/09764.

26 Auszug aus dem Tagebuch von Eugen Haagen, Apr – July 1944, Prosecution Exhibit 521, NO-3852, ADB 19. Addendum B, in ibid., (MF) 3/2958–2964; Le Blanc, Dépot centrale d'archives de la justice militaire (hereafter DCAJM), TPFA Lyon, Jugement 202/2, Info 266, Cahier du Dr. Haagen. Traduction certifiée conforme de neuf feuillets, 13 Feb 1948.

27 Vernehmung Haagen, 20 June 1947, in Dörner *et al. Nürnberger Ärzteprozeß*, (MF) 2/09835–09836.

28 Vernehmung von Eugen Haagen, 18 June 1947, Wortprotokoll, Bl. 9600–9601, in ibid., (MF) 3/09600–9601.

29 "Haagen stated that he had already reported to Rose on the results of [p. 269] experiments with human beings and expressed his regret that, up to the date of the letter, he had been unable to 'perform infection experiments on the vaccinated persons'. He also stated that he had requested the *Ahnenerbe* to provide suitable persons for vaccination but had received no answer; that he was then vaccinating other human beings and would report results later. He concluded by expressing the wish and need for experimental subjects upon whom to test vaccinations, and suggested that when subjects were procured, parallel tests should be made between the vaccine referred to in the letter and the Ipsen tests. We think the only reasonable inference which can be drawn from this letter is that Haagen was proposing to test the efficacy of the vaccinations which he had completed, which could only be accomplished by infecting the vaccinated subjects with a virulent pathogenic virus", see: *Trials of War Criminals. Vol. 2*, pp. 269–270.

30 Direktes Verhör des Zeugen Eugen Haagen, 20 June 1947 (124. Verhandlungstag), Wortprotokoll, in Dörner *et al. Nürnberger Ärzteprozeß*, (MF) 2/09775.

31 Direktes Verhör des Zeugen Eugen Haagen, 20 June 1947 (124. Verhandlungstag), Wortprotokoll, in ibid., (MF) 2/09764.

32 Leo Alexander, James M. Haney, Alexander G. Hardy, Arnost Horlik-Hochwald and Esther Jane Johnson: Militärgerichtshof Nr. 1. Fall Nr. 1. Zusammenfassender Schriftsatz der Anklage gegen Hermann Becker-Freyseng, 16 June 1947, in ibid., (MF) 3/07465–07468; Auszug aus dem Tagebuch von Eugen Haagen, April–July 1944, Exhibit 521, NO-3852, ADB 19, in ibid., (MF) 3/2958–2964.

33 Vernehmung von Eugen Haagen, 18 June 1947, Wortprotokoll, Bl. 9593, in ibid., (MF) 3/09593.

34 Vernehmung Georges Hirtz, 8. Jan 1947, Wortprotokoll, Bl. 1314, in ibid., (MF) 2/1314.

35 Direktes Verhör des Zeugen Gerrit Hendrik Nales durch den Anklagevertreter Alexander Hardy, 30 June 1947 (132. Verhandlungstag), in ibid., (MF) 2/10588–10589.

36 Vernehmung von Edith Schmidt, 9 Jan 1947, in ibid., (MF) 2/01381.

37 Mitscherlich and Mielke, *Diktat*, pp. 66–69.

38 Idem, *Wissenschaft*, pp. 111–112; 115.

39 Ibid., p. 113.

40 Ibid., pp. 115–119.

41 Ibid., p. 111n1.

42 *Trials of War Criminals*. Vol. 2, p. 283.

43 Ibid., p. 211.

44 Ibid., p. 212.

45 Ibid., p. 213.

46 Ibid., p. 270.

47 Ibid.

48 Ibid., p. 239

49 Ibid.

50 Ibid., p. 261.

51 A similar vague formulation can be found in the part of the judgement that refers to Wolfram Sievers: "A number of deaths occurred among non-German experimental subjects as a direct result of the treatment to which they were subjected", see: ibid.

52 The following summary of the SMT at Metz is based on: DCAJM, TPFA Lyon, Jugement 202/2, Information 457, TMP de Metz, Notes d'audience. Affaire: Bickenbach, Haagen, Hirt, Gräfe, Rühl, Bong. Inculpés de: Empoisonnement – administration de substances nuisibles à la santé – Complicité d'empoisonnement et d'administration de substances nuisibles à la santé – recel de cadavres homocides, 16 décembre 1952, pp. 95–159.

53 Mitscherlich and Mielke, *Diktat*, pp. 67–69; Bayle, *Croix Gammée*, pp. 1148–1154. Another publication linking Haagen to human experiments in concentration camps was the book published by Goudsmit in 1947, the scientific head of the Alsos mission: Goudsmit, *Alsos*, pp. 66, 67; 73–75.

54 Bayle, *Croix Gammée*, pp. 1148–1154; 1166–1169; 1179–1181; 1182–1197; Raymond de Geouffre De La Pradelle, *Aux frontières de l'injustice*, Paris: Albin Michel, 1979, pp. 103–151.

55 DCAJM, TPFA Lyon, Jugement 202/2, Info 457, TMP Metz, Notes d'audiences du 16.12.-23.12.1952.

56 Ibid., Jugement 202/1, Info 114, Haagen, procès-verbal de première comparution, signé par Margraff et Richert, 26 Feb 1947.

57 Eugen Haagen and Brigitte Cordel, 'Versuche mit einem neuen getrockneten Feckfieberimpfstoff. I. Mitteilung', *Zentralblatt für Bakteriologie, Parasitenkunde und Infektionskrankheiten*, I Abt., 151 (1944), pp. 307–311; idem, 'Versuche mit einem neuen

getrockneten Feckfieberimpfstoff. II. Mitteilung', *Zentralblatt für Bakteriologie, Parasitenkunde und Infektionskrankheiten*, I Abt., 151.7 (1944), pp. 369–377.

58   DCAJM, TPFA Lyon, Jugement 202/1, Info 114, Haagen, procès-verbal de première comparution, signé par Margraff et Richert, 26 Feb 1947.

59   Mitscherlich and Mielke, *Diktat*, pp. 67–69, referring to a letter from Hirt to Haagen, 10 July 1944, PE 308, NO-129, ADB 12, Bl. 98, in Dörner *et al.*, *Nürnberger Ärzteprozeß* (MF) 3/01586 and Haagen to Hirt, 15 Nov 1943, PE 293, NO-121, ADB 12, Bl. 81, in ibid., (MF) 3/01569.

60   Mitscherlich and Mielke, *Diktat*, p. 69.

61   DCAJM, TPFA Lyon, Jugement 202/1, Info 129, Eugène [Eugen] Haagen, procès verbal, 25 Apr 1947.

62   Ibid., Jugement 202/2, Info 255, Eugen Haagen, procès verbal, 2 Dec 1947, signé par J.M. Lorich et Derytere.

63   Ibid.

64   Ibid.

65   Ibid., Jugement 202/2, Info 186, Professeur Haagen, Lettre au Recteur de l'Université de Strasbourg avec traduction, 7.10.1945, NO-137; Jugement 202/2, Info 188, Haagen an Sanitätsinspektion, NO-304; Jugement 202/2, Info 189, Lagerarzt KL Dachau an Haagen, 30.10.1944, NO-135; Jugement 202/2, Info 190, Haagen an Rose, 5.6.1943; Jugement 202/2, Info 191, Rascher, lettre au Prof. Haagen et traduction, 9.6.1943, NO-306; Jugement 202/2 Info 192, Scholler an Haagen, 14.7.1943; Jugement 202/2, Info 193, Prof. Rose, lettre au Prof. Haagen et traduction NO-122, 13.12.1943; Jugement 202/2, Info 194, Präsident des Reichsforschungsrates, lettre au Prof. Haagen et traduction NO-311, 12.1.1944; Jugement 202/2, Info 195, Haagen, réponse à la lettre du 12.1.1944 et traduction NO-138, 21.1.1944; Jugement 202/2, Info 196, Lettre au Dr. Krieger, 3.2.1944, non-signée; Jugement 202/2, Info 197, Dr. Grunsko Flottenarzt au Professeur Haagen, 7.3.1944 NO-139; Jugement 202/2, Info 198, Luftflottenarzt au Prof. Haagen, Fleckfieberimpfstoff et traduction NO-310, 19.4.1944; Jugement 202/2, Info 199, Haagen an Reichsminister der Luftfahrt, Fleckfieberimpfstoff et traduction NO-302, 27.4.1944; Jugement 202/2, Info 200, Haagen à Hirt, Versuche Fleckfieberimpfstoff et traduction, 9.5.1944 NO-123; Jugement 202/2, Info 201, Haagen à Hirt, Prüfung von getrocknetem Fleckfieberimpfstoff et traduction NO-127, 27.6.1944; Jugement 202/2, Info 202, Académie de Médecine de l'Armée de l'Air au Médecin de Flotte de l'Air Reich, 7.7.1944 et traduction NO-128; Jugement 202/2, Info 203, Hirt à Haagen, 10.7.1944 et traduction NO-129; Jugement 202/2, Info 204, Haagen, Bericht über die Erfolge mit den TAB-Chol-Impfstoffen NO-130, 4.8.1944; Jugement 202/2, Info 205, Oberkommando der Luftwaffe an Haagen und Lehrgruppe Akademie Saalow und Chef San. W.d.Lw. et traduction NO-131, 29.8.1944; Jugement 202/2, Info 206, Haagen an Oberkommando der Luftwaffe, Fleckfieber-Forschungsauftrag et traduction NO-132, 19.9.1944; Jugement 202/2, Info 207, Der Reichsführer SS an den Direktor des Hygienischen Institutes Reichsuniversität Straßburg, 30.9.1943 et traduction NO-120; Jugement 202/2, Info 208, Haagen an Hirt et traduction, 15.2.1943 NO-6121; Jugement 202/2, Info 209, Haagen an Lagerarzt des Konzentrationslagers, 16.11.1944, NO-136. All documents were taken from the NMT prosecution document file no. 12, see: Dörner *et al.*, *Nürnberger Ärzteprozeß*, (MF) 3/1564–1591.

66   DCAJM, TPFA Lyon, Jugement 202/2, Info 261, Edith Schmidt, procès verbal, 15 Dec 1947, signé par Lorich et Derytere.

67   Ibid., Jugement 202/1, Info 116, Alex-Nicolas Probst, procès verbal, 20 Mar 1947, signé par Grand et Huber.

68   Ibid., Jugement 202/1, Info 158, Alphonse Bauer, procès verbal, 16 Apr 1947, signé par Chary.

69 Ibid., Jugement 202/2, Info 169, Eugen Hönig, déclaration, 31 July 1947.
70 Ibid., Jugement 202/2, Info 260, Eugene [Eugen] Haagen, procès verbal, 15 Dec 1947, signé par Lorich et Derytere.
71 Ibid., p. 5. Furthermore: ibid., Jugement 202/2, Info 457, TMP Metz, Notes des audiences du 16.12.–23.12.1952.
72 Ibid., Jugement 202/1, Info 31, Georges Hirtz, procès verbal, 28 June 1945, signé par Jadin et Hertzog.
73 Ibid., Jugement 202/2, Info 290, Georg Selmer Rosef, déclaration affaire Haagen (traduction), 24 May 1948.
74 Ibid., Jugement 202/2, Info 280, Henri Chretien, procès verbal, 11 Oct 1948, signé par Boussard.
75 Ibid., Jugement 202/2, Info 290, Poulsson, Rapport affaire Haagen traduction, 9 May 1948.
76 "Le non militaire HAAGEN Eugen, . . .volontairement attende à la vie de quarante personnes non identifées, par l'effet des substances qui pouvaient donner la mort plus ou moins promptement, la dite infraction même accom lie à l'occasion ou sous pretexte de guerre n'etant pas justifiée par les lois et costumbres de guerre?", see ibid., Jugement 202/2, Info 498, Jugement rendu par le Tribunal Militaire Permanent à Metz, 27 December 1952, 8e feuillet.
77 Ibid., 10e feuillet.
78 Ibid., Jugement 202/2, Info 457, TMP Metz, Notes d'audiences du 16.12.–23.12.1952.

Bibliography

Archival sources

France

Le Blanc, Dépot centrale d'archives de la justice militaire (DCAJM), TPFA Lyon, Jugement 202/1–2
Paris, Centre de recherches des Archives nationales (CARAN), BB/35/276

Literature

Bayle, François, *Croix Gammée contre caducée. Les expérimences humaines en Allemagne pendant la deuxième guerre mondiale*, Neustadt: Centre de L'Imprimerie Nationale, 1950
Bonah, Christian and Florian Schmaltz, 'The Struthof Medical Trials 1952–1954. Prosecution and Judgement of Nazi Physicians Otto Bickenbach and Eugen Haagen at Military Tribunals in France', in Ulf Schmidt, Andreas Frewer and Dominique Sprumont (eds), *Human Research and the Declaration of Helsinki*, Oxford: Oxford University Press, forthcoming in 2017
De La Pradelle, Raymond de Geouffre, *Aux frontières de l'injustice*, Paris: Albin Michel, 1979
Dörner, Klaus, and Angelika Ebbinghaus (eds), *Vernichten und Heilen. Der Nürnberger Ärzteprozeß und seine Folgen*, Berlin: Aufbau Verlag, 2001
Dörner, Klaus, Angelika Ebbinghaus and Karsten Linne (eds), in cooperation with Karl Heinz Roth and Paul Weindling, on behalf of the Stiftung für Sozialgeschichte des 20. Jahrhunderts, *Der Nürnberger Ärzteprozeß 1946/47. Wortprotokolle, Anklage- und Verteidigungsmaterial, Quellen zum Umfeld*, Micorfiche ed., Munich: K.G. Saur, 1999

—— *Der Nürnberger Ärzteprozeß 1946/47. Wortprotokolle, Anklage- und Verteidigungsmaterial, Quellen zum Umfeld. Erschließungsband zur Mikrofiche-Edition: Bearbeitet von Karsten Linne*, Munich: K.G. Saur, 2000

—— *The Nuremberg Medical Trial 1946/47. Transcripts, Material of the Prosecution and Defense, Related Documents. Guide to the Mikrofiche-Edition*, Munich: Saur, 2001

Ebbinghaus, Angelika and Karl Heinz Roth, 'Medizinverbrechen vor Gericht. Die Menschenversuche im Konzentrationslager Dachau', in Ludwig Eiber and Robert Sigel (eds), *Dachauer Prozesse. NS-Verbrechen vor amerikanischen Militärgerichten in Dachau 1945–48. Verfahren, Ergebnisse, Nachwirkungen*, Göttingen: Wallstein Verlag, 2007, pp. 126–159

Gabriele, Clemens, ' "Man aus den Deutschen Demokraten machen wollte". Umerziehung durch Film. Britische und amerikanische Filmpolitik in Deutschland 1945–1949', in Harro Segeberg (ed.), *Mediale Mobilmachung II. Hollywood, Exil und Nachkrieg*, Munich: Fink, 2006, pp. 243–271

Goudsmit, Samuel Abraham, *Alsos (History of modern physics and astronomy)*, Woodbury, NY: 1996

Haagen, Eugen and Brigitte Cordel, 'Versuche mit einem neuen getrockneten Feckfieberimpfstoff. I. Mitteilung', *Zentralblatt für Bakteriologie, Parasitenkunde und Infektionskrankheiten*, I Abt., 151 (1944), pp. 307–311

—— 'Versuche mit einem neuen getrockneten Feckfieberimpfstoff. II. Mitteilung', *Zentralblatt für Bakteriologie, Parasitenkunde und Infektionskrankheiten*, I Abt., 151.7 (1944), pp. 369–377

Hake, Sabine, 'Erziehung zur Demokratie. Trümmerfilme made in Holywood', in Johannes Roschlau (ed.), *Im Bann der Katastrophe Innovation und Tradition im europäischen Film 1940 – 1950*, Munich: Ed. Text + Kritik, 2010, pp. 85–87

Jasanoff, Sheila, 'Just Evidence. The Limits of Science in the Legal Process', *Journal of Law, Medicine and Ethics*, 34 (2006), pp. 328–339

—— *Science at the Bar. Law, Science, and Technology in America*, Cambridge, MA: Harvard University Press, 1997

Klee, Ernst, *Auschwitz, die NS-Medizin und ihre Opfer*, Frankfurt am Main: S. Fischer Verlag, 1997

Mahoney, Leo James, 'A History of the War Department Scientific Intelligence Mission (ALSOS), 1943–1945', PhD thesis, Kent, OH: Kent State University, 1981

Marrus, Michael R., 'The Nuermberg Doctor's Trial in Historical Context', *Bulletin for the History of Medicine*, 73.1 (1999), pp. 106–123

Mitscherlich, Alexander and Fred Mielke, *Das Diktat der Menschenverachtung. Eine Dokumentation*, Heidelberg: Verlag Lambert Schneider, 1947

—— *Wissenschaft ohne Menschlichkeit. Medizinische und Eugenische Irrwege unter Diktatur, Bürokratie und Krieg. Mit einem Vorwort der Arbeitsgemeinschaft der Westdeutschen Ärztekammern*, Heidelberg: Lambert Schneider, 1949

National Archives Microfilm Publication M 887. Records of the United States Nuernberg War Crimes Trials: United States of America v. Karl Brandt et al (Case I), November 21, 1946–August 20, 1947, Washington, DC: National Archives and Records Service, 1974

Roelcke, Volker, Etienne Lepicard and Sascha Topp, *Silence, Scapegoats, Self-Reflection the Shadow of Nazi Medical Crimes on Medicine and Bioethics*, Göttingen: V&R unipress, 2014

Roelcke, Volker and Giovanni Maio (eds), *Twentieth Century Ethics of Human Subjects Research. Historical Perspectives on Values, Practices, and Regulations*, Stuttgart: Franz Steiner, 2004

Schmidt, Ulf, *Justice at Nuremberg. Leo Alexander and the Nazi Doctors' Trial*, Houndmills, Basingstoke, Hampshire: Palgrave Macmillan, 2004
—— ' "The Scars of Ravensbrück". Medical Experiments and British War Crimes Policy, 1945–1950', *German History*, 23.1 (2005), pp. 20–49
Staehle, Nina, 'La politique des crimes de guerre médicaux: les tribulations qui conduisirent au procès de Ravensbrück, 1946–1947', in Christian Bonah, Etienne Lepicard and Volker Roelcke (eds), *La médecine expérimentale au tribunal: Implications éthiques de quelques procès médicaux du XXe siècle européen*, Paris: Editions des Archives contemporaines, 2003, pp. 215–231
Toledano, Raphael, 'Les Expériences Médicales du Professeur Eugen Haagen de la Reichsuniversität Strassburg. Faits, Contexte et Procès d'un Médecin National-Socialiste', MD thesis, Strasbourg: University of Strasbourg, 2010
Trials of War Criminals before the Nuernberg Military Tribunals under Control Council Law No.10. Nuernberg October 1946–April 1949. Vol. I: The Medical Case, Washington, DC: US Government Printing Office, 1949
Trials of War Criminals before the Nuernberg Military Tribunals under Control Council Law No.10. Nuernberg October 1946–April 1949. Vol. 2. The Medical Case/The Milch Case, Washington, DC: US Government Printing Office, 1949
Weindling, Paul, 'From International to Zonal Trials: The Origins of the Nuremberg Medical Trial', *Holocaust and Genocide Studies*, 14.3 (2000), pp. 367–389
—— 'Auf der Spur von Medizinverbrechen: Keith Mant (1919–2000) und sein Debut als forensischer Pathologe', *1999. Zeitschrift für Sozialgeschichte des 20. und 21. Jahrhunderts*, 16 (2001), pp. 129–139
——*John W. Thompson, Psychiatrist in the Shadow of the Holocaust*, Rochester, NY: Rochester University Press, 2010
—— 'Virologist and National Socialist. The Extraordinary Career of Eugen Haagen', in Marion Hulverscheidt and Anja Laukötter (eds), *Infektion und Institution. Zur Wissenschaftsgeschichte des Robert-Koch-Instituts im Nationalsozialismus*, Göttingen: Wallstein-Verlag, 2009, pp. 232–249
—— *Nazi Medicine and the Nuremberg Trials: From Medical War Crimes to Informed Consent*, Houndmills, Basingstoke: Palgrave Macmillan, 2004

15 Informed testimonies

Physicians' accounts of Nazi medical experiments in the context of early Czechoslovak war crimes investigations, 1945–48[1]

Michal V. Simunek

"In Auschwitz gab es keinen hippokratischen Eid"
Dr Hans Münch (1911–2001), 1999[2]

During the Second World War and the German occupation of the Czech Lands, several hundred thousand Czechoslovak citizens were imprisoned in Nazi concentration and death camps, prisons and detention centres throughout occupied Europe.[3] Although there was no extermination camp in the territory of Bohemia and Moravia itself, a significant number of subcamps (*KZ-Außenlager*) were created or relocated here, especially towards the end of the war.[4] There are no indications that coerced medical experiments were conducted in the Theresienstadt ghetto, which was planned as a transit camp (there was consensual experimentation on *Heilgas* (healing gas) for tuberculosis).[5] There is, however, some evidence of experimental, though not systematic, use of the stimulant methamphetamine (Pervitin) in the Prague Gestapo office.[6]

Precise numbers are not available but it may be supposed that among the concentration camp prisoners from Czechoslovakia there were several hundred professional physicians. The top range of a rough estimate stands at about one thousand, a figure that would include not only general practitioners and specialists but also medical researchers. The exact ratio between professional physicians who perished and those who survived also remains unknown, though for instance in physicians of Jewish origin, we could estimate it to be about 4:1.[7]

The end of the Second World War was a time when extermination camps and mass killings committed by the Nazi regime were gradually discovered and exposed. In the aftermath of a military defeat of Nazi Germany, perpetrators could finally be identified, apprehended and punished. However, conditions at the end of the war and immediately thereafter were chaotic, which meant that gathering all the relevant information was exceedingly difficult.

The process of dealing with the horrific Nazi legacy both in legal and moral terms, including the misuse of medicine, had many forms, and was often widely different in the various formerly Nazi-occupied countries.[8]

It should also be noted that a precise definition and understanding of specific crimes against humanity – which came to include also crimes against health and physical integrity of individuals, including medical experimentation – has never been set. This resulted in a lack of clarity in documentation and unfortunately also in subsequent errors in the prosecution of perpetrators.[9]

Attitudes

Representatives of the Czechoslovak government-in-exile participated in the debates and later in the preparation of investigation and prosecution of Nazi medical crimes from the very outset. The government's main representative was Army General JUDr Bohuslav Ečer (1893–1954), originally a lawyer, who had been involved in the efforts to define and punish Nazi crimes for almost the whole time of his exile (1940–45). General Ečer later became the Czechoslovak representative in the United Nations War Crimes Commission (UNWCC) and on 27 April 1944 proposed, among other things, the adoption of the category of "crimes against humanity", which was in the previous year defined by Hersch Lauterpacht (1897–1960, knighted in 1956). On 8 August 1945 at a London conference about the creation of the International Military Tribunal (IMT), crimes against humanity were – alongside crimes against peace and war crimes – adopted as the basic criminal categories recognised by the IMT.[10] In his writing on the category of crimes against humanity, General Ečer explicitly included ". . . murders, extermination, enslavement, deportations, or other inhumane acts committed against any civilian population before or during the war; persecution on political, racial, or religious grounds in the pursuance of or in connection with any crime which falls under the jurisdiction of the tribunal, both in violation or without violating the national laws of the state where such acts were committed".[11] It was also understood that the Czechoslovak state would see the punishment of such acts as an urgent and permanent task.

Evidence from the Nuremberg Medical Trial, which took place from 9 December 1946 until 19 July 1947, were then viewed in this light.[12] This trial not only delivered verdicts against some of the main perpetrators of Nazi medically motivated crimes, such as Karl Brandt (1904–48) and Viktor Brack (1904–48),[13] but also crucially contributed to a shift in Allied priorities away from strategic exploitation and towards evaluation of these acts with focus on criminal and ethical misuse of medicine. Moreover, the Medical Trial also helped reconstruct the genesis and the deepest structures of the Nazi genocide.[14] The prosecution team included a Czechoslovak lawyer Arnost Horlíck-Hochwald, who constructed a well-informed and successful case for "euthanasia", focusing on later phases linked to concentration camps when Allied citizens were among the numerous victims.

Nonetheless, the initial Czechoslovak documentation of Nazi war crimes gathered in 1945–48, which was a necessary precondition of any subsequent criminal prosecution, was due to the nature of the subject matter, the amount of material and numbers of people involved, as well as the brutality of Nazi crimes. In the Czechoslovak case, moreover, we observe a certain relative ranking of Nazi crimes, whereby priorities were determined mainly by current political demand. Emphasis was placed especially on the destruction of the Czechoslovak state in 1938, exploitation of resources during the occupation, crimes committed in Lidice and Ležáky in 1942, and the like.[15] Crimes against health and medical experiments were at this point – and sadly also later – clearly not a high priority. Consequently, they were marginalised and more or less disappeared from collective memory.

The intelligence and information framework

Investigation undertaken by the authorities of restored Czechoslovakia focused from the start at gathering, documenting and evaluating accessible sources of information. More or less from the very outset, it was clear that the Czechoslovak documentation faced certain limitations that would hamper its success. The investigation had to deal especially with the following challenging factors: 1) Nazi crimes were committed within a completely different bureaucratic, administrative, geographic, and general legal framework; 2) they were organised by the state, which is why their preparation, execution and attempts to destroy evidence, but also their reconstruction and interpretation required expert knowledge and special methods; 3) in many cases, these crimes were committed against particular stigmatised groups of population and that did not correspond with the virtual hierarchy of victims of the Nazi regime that was promoted by the official post-war policies; 4) these crimes did not fit the ideologically clearly defined narratives of events of the Second World War and Nazi occupation.

During the immediate post-war period, investigation was carried out almost exclusively by Czechoslovak intelligence services, which were, however, marked by a split reflecting the different politics of Czechoslovak exile representation in Great Britain on the one hand and the Soviet Union on the other hand.[16]

In Great Britain, it was especially the Second Section of the Ministry of Defence in exile headed by Col. František Moravec (1895–1966).[17] A Fourth Section of the Ministry of Defence in exile, dedicated to intelligence work, was created in February 1942. It was headed by Moravec's former subordinate, Lt.-Col. Josef Bartík (1897–1968).[18] His agenda included the gathering of information about the occupation regime, its representatives, collaborators, etc.[19] After the liberation of Czechoslovakia, the work of the Fourth Section was taken up by a new Department for Political Intelligence (Z) of the Ministry of Interior in Prague, which included espionage and investigation.[20] On top of that, however, there also existed Committees for Internal Security, which were in August 1945 transformed into Regional Departments of Security (ZOB II), manned mostly by Communists or their sympathisers.[21] And it was the ZOB II, which were in the Czechoslovak territory responsible for recording "war criminals for all criminal acts" and were supposed to take note of "all suspect persons of any state citizenship".[22] The first general list of such suspects was supposed to be presented in the autumn of 1945.[23] Collection of information focused specifically on German medically motivated crimes officially started only in connection with the Medical Trial in April 1947.[24] It seems, however, that the amount of material gathered during this initiative was extremely small: the relevant authorities limited themselves to in fact just stating that materials created by activities of the German Medical Chamber for Bohemia (*Deutsche Gesundheitskammer für Böhmen*) during the occupation are unsorted and do not permit further investigation.[25]

Czechoslovak activities in the Western occupation zones in Germany were coordinated first from London, where Gen. Ečer was based, from August 1945 from Wiesbaden, where the US Army Europe (USAREUR) was based, and after January 1946 from Bad Oeynhausen, headquarters of the British Army of the Rhein (BAOR), from where the Czechoslovak Liaison War Crimes Groups were sent to search for war criminals. Until these groups were created, only urgent cases were addressed by members of the Czechoslovak military missions.[26] Czechoslovaks closely cooperated especially with the US, in particular with the 7708th War Crimes Group and Col. William Bernan.[27]

The presence of a Czechoslovak mission at BAOR was seen as advisable especially after the experience of the Belsen Trial,[28] which was conducted almost exclusively by Czechoslovak intelligence officers, many of whom had legal education, from Great Britain. So far, however, we know of no participating officer with medical education.[29] Operations aimed at apprehending Nazi war criminals and the process of their extradition to Czechoslovak authorities were conducted in collaboration with Allied forces.[30] Until the summer of 1947, Czechoslovak representatives also participated in compiling the so-called "wanted reports", mainly in cooperation with the Central Registry of War Criminals and Security Suspects (CROWCASS).[31]

Around the Eastern Front, the search for war criminals was conducted by the Military Defence Intelligence Agency (OBZ), which was created as the intelligence service of the First Czechoslovak Army Corps in the Soviet Union in January 1945 and was subordinated to the Soviet secret service NKVD.[32] The intention was that OBZ would not only function as a counterweight to the Czechoslovak intelligence service in Great Britain, but also eventually become an instrument of Soviet influence in liberated Czechoslovakia.[33] It employed mainly well-tested members of the Communist party who had experience especially with political instruction, propaganda and background checking.[34] Alongside the intelligence agenda, it was also entrusted with the execution of security tasks[35] and its "external defence" agenda included, among other things, the identification and apprehension of representatives and collaborators of the Nazi regime.[36] In 1945–50, the OBZ was headed by Bedřich

Reicin (1911–52), an officer of Jewish origin and an experienced propagandist.[37] Currently, it seems that the OBZ was interested especially in the institutes and representatives of the former German Charles University in Prague.[38]

The gathering of documentation including information regarding Nazi medical experiments took place in parallel both in the context of IMT trials and in the context of domestic retribution justice. In Nuremberg, Czechoslovakia was represented by a delegation with the UNWCC headed by Gen. Ečer as the head of so-called "Delegate's Office" and later minister without portfolio. Ečer was already in the spring of 1945 commissioned to represent Czechoslovakia in international negotiations concerning the prosecution, extradition and trial of war criminals.[39] In December 1946, he was appointed as a minister without portfolio in the Czechoslovak government to head the Czechoslovak representation in the subsequent Nuremberg trials.[40] The delegation also included representatives of the Czechoslovak Ministry of Interior and the General Staff, which was appointed by the Ministry of National Defence.[41] In June 1947, this agenda transferred under the Ministry of Foreign Affairs and activities of the delegation ended after the conclusion of Nuremberg trials on 11 April 1949. This had also led to the extinction of the post of a delegate.[42] Results of the Medical Trial had been reported by members of Ečer's team.[43]

Retributive justice in the territory of restored Czechoslovakia was based on presidential decrees No. 16 and 17 of 19 June 1945. Its main goal was supposed to be the punishment of traitors and Nazi collaborators.[44] Priorities reflected in the gathering of surviving written materials of German Nazi origin – a process that basically copied the main trial of representatives of the occupation regime (K. H. Frank, Kurt Daluege and others) and the Protectorate government – did not include crimes against health, which were investigated only in isolated cases.[45] This neglect with respect to medical crimes was aggravated by considerable administrative and executive chaos, which was reflected in the lack of clarity regarding the jurisdiction and authority of various police and intelligence services then active in the liberated Czechoslovakia.[46]

What is evident is the lack of experts whose specialised knowledge of not only Nazi ideology but also the relations and connections between the various German institutions and their representatives may have been used in investigation. The relevant Czechoslovak authorities had been informed of the views of some such experts in 1945 but such proposals remained de facto unanswered. It was especially the October 1945 initiative of Hugo Iltis (1882–1952), a native of Brno, botanist and historian of genetics, who, prior to his emigration to the United States in 1939, systematically studied German academic racism. His efforts aimed at the recognition of a separate category of a "war crime of racism",[47] which he defined as follows: "German science is and has been one of the helpers of German Conquest. German universities, German scientific institutions and German higher schools were not only the shining centres of human progress as pictured by the Germans, but also the breeding places of German megalomania and the arsenals for the fabrication of both chemical and mental poison gas".[48] He distinguished three groups of suspects: 1) A small group of scientists of good standing and even famous who protected and promoted the works and writings of the second and third group although they knew very well that racism is no science but a pseudoscience and political propaganda;[49] 2) A group of popular writers who wrapped in the cover of science and poison to the so-called intelligence[50]; and 3) A great number of coarse or refined politicians who used racism to stir up the people. In addition to Ečer, Iltis also sent his memorandum to Col. H.H. Wade, research officer of the UNWCC, and to Robert H. Jackson (1892–1954) in Nuremberg.[51]

Somewhat later, the Czechoslovak embassy in Bern sent to the Ministry of Interior in Prague a German memorandum by Dr Theo Lang about the activities of some German physicians during the Nazi regime.[52] It stated, among other things, that "the range of activities of the abovementioned persons went far over and beyond the rights and obligations of a physician and aimed at a complete destruction of racially undesirable elements, both by death in concentration camps and by sterilisation".[53] Lang included the names of 13 physicians, especially from the circle of the psychiatrist Ernst Rüdin.[54]

The Medical Chamber for the Czech Lands was eventually contacted only in connection with the "trial of German physicians for experimenting on living persons", i.e., in connection with the Medical Trial. At the request of the Czechoslovak delegate to the American mission, its members who were former concentration camp inmates and direct participants of 12 specifically named experiments in those camps were addressed as potential witnesses.[55] At this point, the Czechoslovak delegation was trying to find especially "physicians, physician's assistants, servants, and other persons forced to assist at those experiments or persons who were subjected to experiments, who experienced them and may be eventually able to identify persons who took an active part in those experiments".[56]

Testimonies

After the war, not all physicians-survivors spoke of their experiences and even fewer gave any sort of written or oral testimony and/or affidavits as part of an official investigation or trial. For understandable reasons (the distribution of prisoners from Czechoslovakia), their testimonies dealt mainly with the conditions in the concentration camps of Mauthausen, Buchenwald, Dachau and Auschwitz.

For the period in question, we have so far been able to find eight such testimonies that concern Nazi medical experiments. Alphabetically ordered, they are the following:

František Bláha (1896–1979) was born in Písek in southern Bohemia. He studied medicine in Prague but also won various study fellowships that took him to Vienna, Strasbourg and Paris.[57] He graduated from the Faculty of Medicine of the Charles University in 1920.[58] In 1924, he started working as a municipal physician in Jihlava. In 1925–38, Bláha was head of the local obstetric department. He was of leftist leanings, joined the Social Democratic Party, and was an active member of the Sokol gymnastic association. After the occupation of Bohemia and Moravia, he was, after several clashes with the Protectorate authorities, arrested in 1939 and imprisoned first in the Špilberk Castle in Brno and later in Breslau and another 21 prisons.[59] In 1941 he was transported to Dachau concentration camp. In summer 1942, Bláha worked as a surgeon in the camp hospital, where he was, among other things, forced to teach students of the SS Medical Academy of the University in Graz.[60] Later, he was transferred to the dissection department, where he stayed until the liberation of Dachau. By that time, according to him he carried out approximately 12,000 autopsies.[61] Over time, he found a way of sending uncensored letters to his family via a neighbouring farm.[62] For instance on 21 November 1943, Bláha wrote: "We who still remain here are just former people. We had taught our senses, especially our hearing, vision, and taste, a sort of mechanical inertia which perceives everything that happens around us but in a kind of subconscious way. . . Otherwise, all our daily waking hours are anything but life and that is surely the most terrible curse for all those who would come back. . .".[63] These letters, however, do not contain substantial information pertaining to his medical activities. After the liberation of Dachau, Bláha was from 3 to 18 May 1945 interviewed several times by the Americans.[64] He stayed in the liberated camp until the end of repatriations and worked as a member of the camp committee.[65] On 24 November 1945, he testified in the Dachau Trial[66] and his testimony was also included in the materials for the IMT in Nuremberg.[67] Bláha testified in Nuremberg and was cross-examined in the trial of the major war criminals on 11 and 14 January 1946.[68] Regarding medical experiments, he spoke especially about Claus Schilling's experiments with malaria and Sigmund Rascher's experiments with changes in pressure, but also about Rudolf Brachtel's liver punctures and about phlegmon (sepsis) experiments, which he linked with the names of Drs Lauer, Babor, Schütz and Kiesswetter.[69] After his return to Czechoslovakia, Bláha published several books based on his testimony in Czech[70] and an extensive study called "Medical Science Run Amok" in English.[71] Bláha is generally considered to have been one of the most important Czechoslovak witnesses for the IMT. Nonetheless, doubts about the relevance of his testimony started emerging soon after the trials. For instance, based on an official Soviet book called *Nuremberg Trial II*[72] an internal analysis was carried out for the Communist Ministry of the Interior, probably in 1955, with the aim of explaining why Bláha testified as a witness for the US even though his testimony involved mainly French and Soviet citizens.[73] In the context of the time, this implicitly hinted that he collaborated with the American intelligence service, which in turn led to doubts being cast on his work in Dachau. The analysis concluded that Bláha's "description of events was distorted or he was truly the 'right' hand of the German doctors who carried out the experiments".[74] Some more recent historical works, too, point to discrepancies in Bláha's testimonies.[75]

Leo Eitinger (1912–96) was born in a Moravian Jewish family in Lomnice. He attended a secondary school and studied medicine at the Faculty of Medicine of the Masaryk University in Brno, where he graduated in 1937.[76] Within the framework of Nansen's relief effort, he was able to leave the Protectorate of Bohemia and Moravia in autumn 1939 and settle in Norway.[77] He worked there as a physician and later lived in the countryside. After the adoption of stricter anti-Jewish measures, he was, on 16 March 1942, arrested in Nesjestranda by Molde and imprisoned in several prisons and camps.[78] A year later, he was included in a transport to Auschwitz (on the ship *Gotenland*).[79] In June 1943, he was placed in the main camp hospital, and later in the hospital of the Monowitz subcamp.[80] At the end of the war, when the liberation of Auschwitz was drawing near, he was, on 16 January 1945, included in a death march. Later in January he arrived at Buchenwald, where he was, on 11 April 1945, liberated by the US Army.[81] He left the camp on 15 May 1945.[82] His first testimonies were recorded ten days later, on 22–23 April 1945.[83] His testimonies dealt mainly with his stay in Auschwitz, in particular with the functioning of the Auschwitz hospital, killing by phenol injections, and the practice of falsifying records of prisoners' deaths.[84] He also named six physicians (Werner Rohde, Heinz Thilo, Bruno Weber, Hans Wilhelm Konig, Helmut Vetter and Eduard Wirths), of whom he said: "They are all guilty of a large number of murders".[85] He explicitly described the role of *SS-Scharführer* Josef Klehr (1904–88), head of the disinfection commando.[86] Regarding prisoners who took part in the killings in the hospital, he noted: "The prisoners who voluntarily participated in the murdering are not alive, they were condemned directly as they got into another camp from Auschwitz".[87] In connection with medical experiments, he mentioned – without giving further details – camp blocks 10 and 11 and the names of Carl Clauberg and Eduard Wirths.[88] He did not name Horst Schumann and referred to him only by his *Luftwaffe* rank.[89] Before leaving Buchenwald, he worked as a physician and opposed a propagandistic use of Nazi medical experiments by the Allies.[90]

Berthold Epstein (1890–1962) was born to a Jewish family in Pilsen, in Bohemia. In 1908–1914, he studied at the German Faculty of Medicine in Prague.[91] During the First World War he served as a sanitary officer at the Italian and Russian front. After the war, he worked as a voluntary assistant in paediatric medicine at the Faculty of Medicine in Berlin. After returning to Czechoslovakia, he worked at the paediatric clinic of the German Faculty of Medicine of the German University in Prague.[92] He received his habilitation at the Faculty of Medicine of the German University in Prague in 1924 and full professorship in 1937, but already in January 1939 he was, due to his Jewish origin, forced to resign from the university. He emigrated to Norway, where he was eventually on 25 October 1942 arrested. He was transported to Auschwitz, where 14 of his relatives had eventually died. In Auschwitz he worked as a doctor for the camp inmates but was also forced to assist Josef Mengele. He received permission to study the epidemic of noma (a gangrenous bacterial disease of the mouth and face).[93] After the liberation of Auschwitz, he joined the First Czechoslovak Army Corps in the USSR as a military bacteriologist and with the Czechoslovak Army he eventually returned to Czechoslovakia.

In early 1946, the JAG's War Crimes Section proposed to the Czechoslovak mission with the BAOR that Epstein should be asked to testify, though not explicitly as a physician who could explain the conditions in Auschwitz and suggest the names of people who ought to be charged.[94] He was named together with Alfréd Milk/Mílek (1899–?) and Ludvík Sand (1910–91), who were referred to as "doctors of the Czech family camp", although Sand was not a physician but a pharmacist.[95]

At the same time, he was in July 1946 accused by several Russian/Soviet former camp inmates, who mistook him for his predecessor, Dr Zenon Zenkteller.[96] He was investigated by the Czechoslovak Military Intelligence Service (OBZ) and its chief, Bedřich Reicin, asked that he be suspended. That, however, did not happen,[97] since several people, including Dr Rudolf Weisskopf/Vítek, testified in his favour.[98] Epstein's own testimony unfortunately does not survive in any records.[99] His testimony in Nuremberg in the end concerned the Monowitz subcamp and was used in the IG Farben Trial.[100] Epstein was supposed to travel to Nuremberg on 13 November 1947.[101] His role, and the position of other physicians who had worked with Mengele, was later brought into doubt. In this particular case, the fact that he himself never published a detailed testimony regarding his experiences in Auschwitz and never published any memoirs no doubt contributed to this view of him.[102] Even in eventual articles published at the occasion of Epstein's jubilees, this chapter of his life remained taboo.[103]

Viktor/Vítězslav Horn (1893–1965) was born in the Moravian town of Třebíč. His father's side of the family was of Swiss origin.[104] He started the study of medicine in 1912, during the First World War he worked in a hospital train, later in a hospital for contagious diseases in Brno.[105] In 1919, he graduated from the Faculty of Medicine of the Czech Charles University in Prague.[106] From 1924 until his arrest in 1939 worked as a physician, later head of surgical department in a hospital in Jihlava/Iglau, where he managed to improve the standard of care.[107] After his arrest, he was kept in Kounic Dormitories and in the Špilberk Castle in Brno, where he provided medical care to prisoners. Later, he was transported to Buchenwald,[108] where he was the first physician to provide surgical care. He survived and was liberated on 11 April 1945.[109] He returned to Czechoslovakia only on 20 May 1945, after he helped fight a typhus outbreak.[110] His testimony was included among so-called "trial documents" in the Nuremberg Medical Trial.[111] It is not known whether he was at the same time also interviewed by Czech investigators. After Horn presented his testimony in Nuremberg, František Bláha accused him of not explicitly charging Dr Hoven with experimenting on prisoners and of defending Nazi physicians.[112] This controversy escalated in 1948, but due to a change of political circumstances in Czechoslovakia (the February 1948 Communist coup d'état) did not lead to any results and petered out.[113]

František Janouch (1902–65) was born in Kamenný Újezd in southern Bohemia. He graduated from the Czech Faculty of Medicine at the Charles University in Prague in 1931.[114] He was active in social medicine and worked in Prague, where he specialised in the treatment of tuberculosis. During the occupation of Czechoslovakia, he became involved in the anti-Nazi resistance movement and on 21 January 1943 was arrested in Prague.[115] From the Pankrác Prison he was sent to Auschwitz, where he worked first as an orderly, then in the Gipsy camp (BIIe) and finally as a laboratory technician in the SS Institute of Hygiene in Rajsko.[116] He survived a death march and presented his testimony for an "international Allied committee, which was investigating war crimes of the Nazi regime" to the Czechoslovak mission for the prosecution of war crimes in London in November 1945.[117] In his statement, it was explicitly noted that it was made "for the trials which would take place in Nuremberg in the coming months, eventually years".[118] His intention was to "describe, using a particular example, how far members of the SS units, in this case officers of the SS Medical Corps, went in their depravity".[119] He described physicians/prisoners who had to work there and focused on the laboratory practice in the abovementioned institute, especially the use of human flesh and the like.[120]

Josef Podlaha (1893–1975) was born in Záhoří near Jindřichův Hradec in southern Bohemia. In 1913–18, he studied medicine at Czech Charles University in Prague.[121] After graduation, he transferred to the newly established Faculty of Medicine of the Masaryk University, where he specialised in surgery.[122] At this faculty, he also received his habilitation in 1927 and full professorship in 1938. During the German occupation, he became involved in military resistance. On 27 November 1941, Podlaha was arrested, imprisoned and subsequently sent to the Mauthausen concentration camp, where he stayed from 3 February 1942 until 1 June 1945.[123] Soon after the camp's liberation, he offered a detailed testimony to members of the American Counter Intelligence Corps (CIC). His interview with this agency took three days.[124] The CIC promised to him "to publish all the documents in Washington and to use them publicly during the coming trial of the war criminals".[125] This in the end did not happen, but in 1946 Podlaha published a detailed report in English on the surgical care received by Mauthausen prisoners.[126] He divided the experiments he viewed as "interesting" in three categories and gave their brief description.[127]

Karl (Karel) Sperber (1910–57) was born in a Jewish family in Tachov in western Bohemia. He graduated from the Faculty of Medicine at the German University in Prague in 1935.[128] In 1939, he managed to leave, bound for Great Britain, where, however, he was not allowed to practice medicine, which is why he took thepost of a ship's doctor.[129] In 1941, he thus worked on the merchant and passenger vessel SS *Automedon*, which was bringing to the British Far East Command important documents from the War Cabinet in London pertaining to Japan's possible entry into war on the side of the Axis powers.[130] On 11 November 1940, Sperber was, together with other members of the crew, captured by the German crew of the auxiliary cruiser Atlantis and placed on a confiscated Norwegian tanker *Storstad*, which served as a floating prison. After disembarking in Bordeaux, Sperber was kept in several POW camps but eventually, due to his Jewish origin and Protectorate citizenship, sent in 1942 to Auschwitz.[131] Here he worked with, among others, Carl Clauberg, Eduard Wirths, Friedrich Entress and finally even Josef Mengele.[132] In 1944 he was transferred to the Monowitz subcamp and from there forced on a death march to Buchenwald, where he was – just like L. Eitinger – eventually liberated.[133] He apparently testified about his experiences in Auschwitz in December 1945.[134] After the war, he received the Order of the British Empire (August 1946) and British citizenship (1948), joined the British National Health Service (1950) and worked once again as a ship's doctor.[135]

Rudolf Weisskopf/Vítek (1895–?) was born into a Jewish family in Pilsen in western Bohemia. During his stay in Auschwitz, he was assigned to work as a physician in the Gipsy camp (BIIe) where he was in close contact with Dr Berthold Epstein (they shared the same room). In March 1946, he testified about Epstein's work. He also spoke of the conditions in the camp hospital, about the falsification of diagnoses in contagious diseases, about Mengele's role in the selection of incoming transports, and the like.[136] His testimony was later used in the IG Farben Trial.[137] His later memoirs are kept in the Archives of the Auschwitz-Birkenau State Museum and in the United States Holocaust Memorial Museum.[138] After the end of the Second World War he changed his surname to Vítek.

In addition to the abovementioned physicians, some other Czech imprisoned doctors also published their testimonies prior to 1948, for instance, the bacteriologist Professor Václav Tomášek (1893–1962) about Auschwitz and Miloslav Matoušek (1900–185) about Buchenwald.[139]

Limitations

The fact that documentation and investigation of Nazi medically motivated crimes in the territory of Czechoslovakia was carried out with limited success can clearly be seen in the case of one group of formerly Czechoslovak citizens of German nationality, in particular the SS camp doctors and other medical personnel serving in the Nazi concentration and extermination camps who came from the German-speaking areas of Bohemia and Moravia. This group, which included at least ten physicians and several medical personnel with the so-called *Sanitätsdienstgrad*,[140] in effect managed to evade the attention of Czechoslovak authorities. Based on current knowledge, the group included the following persons:

1. Dr Otto Adam (b. 28 August 1903, Příchovice/Schumburg, Jablonec n. N./Gablonz a. N.) – Sachsenhausen (1944), Dachau (1945), Flossenbürg (1945).
2. Dr Otto Blaschke (b. 24 September 1908, Obrnice/Obernitz) – Auschwitz (1940–41), Flossenbürg, Ravensbrück, Oranienburg, Mauthausen.
3. Dr Rudolf Adalbert Brachtel (Brachtl; Waligura) (b. 22 April 1909, Kyjov/Gaya) – Dachau (1941–43).
4. Dr Alois Gaberle (b. 30 September 1907, Oelz–Döberney/Debrné–Mostek/Mastig – Sachsenhausen (1943).
5. Dr Wilhelm (Willi) Jobst (b. 27 September 1912, Cheb/Eger) – Groß Rosen, Sachsenhausen, Mauthausen.
6. Dr Othmar Karschulin (b. 1 November 1902, Olomouc/Olmütz) – Buchenwald (1942).
7. Dr Hermann Kiesewetter (b. 7 January 1912, Obora u Kraslic/Hochgarth) – Dachau, Mauthausen.
8. Dr Wilhelm Klimek (b. 29 July 1905, Šumperk/Mährisch Schönberg) – Mauthausen, Buchenwald.
9. Dr Eduard Klug (b. 27 March 1901, Leitmeritz/Litoměřice) – Sachsenhausen.
10. Dr Erich Wagner (b. 15 September 1912, Chomutov/Komotau) – Buchenwald.

Leaving aside the somewhat specific case of Adolf Pokorny (b. 1895) (prosecuted at the Nuremberg Medical Trial but acquitted), at least two of these persons can be directly linked to the execution of medical experiments, namely Rudolf A. Brachtel (1909–88), who was active in Dachau, and Hermann Kiesewetter (b. 1912), who was active in the Gusen concentration camp. One ought to mention, however, that there are extremely few testimonies of physicians, former camp inmates from the Czech Lands, regarding their activities during the war (one such example is František Bláha). Some of these perpetrators, meanwhile, were tried in the Allied courts, especially the Dachau Trials, but only a few were convicted.[141] In these cases, the Allied investigators did not coordinate with the Czechoslovak authorities. This showed clearly the limitations of investigation, which relied mainly on traditional police methods. The names of the Czechoslovak citizens of German nationality who participated in the medically motivated Nazi crimes thus even over 70 years after the end of war remain virtually unknown to the public.

Notes

1 This chapter is published as part of project RVO 68378114. The author is grateful for advice and comments to Tomáš Fedorovič, MA, Museum of Ghetto Terezín, Anna Hájková, PhD, University of Warwick, Šimon Krýsl, MA, Medical Museum Prague, Prof. Paul Weindling, Oxford Brookes University, and Pavel Zeman, PhD, Institute for Study of the Totalitarian Regimes Prague.
2 'Der Doktor und sein Opfer', *Der Spiegel*, 14 (1999), p. 123.

3 In connection with preparations for the Paris repatriation conference, materials sent to central state organs in Aug 1945 mentioned in Part 3 (Human Losses and Damages, Loss of Life or Health, and Injuries to Civilian or Military Casualties of War and Occupation) 244,836 Czechoslovak citizens who were either murdered or lost their lives in the course of the Second World War. See Tomáš Jelínek and Jaroslav Kučera, 'Ohnmächtige Zaungäste. Die Entschädigung von tschechoslowakischen NS-Verfolgten', in Hans G. Hockerts, Claudia Kertts and Tobias Winstel (eds), *Grenzen der Wiedergutmachung. Die Entschädigung für NS-Verfolgte in West- und Osteuropa 1945–2000*, Göttingen: Wallstein, 2006, pp. 813–826.

4 See Wolfgang Benz (ed.), *Der Ort des Terrors, Bd. 1*, Munich: C. H. Beck, 2005.

5 See the forthcoming publication of Anna Hájková, *Medicine and Illness. The Last Ghetto. An Everyday History of the Terezín Ghetto, 1941–1945*, Chapter 4.

6 Prague, Archiv bezpečnostních složek (Archives of the Security Services, hereafter ABS), 305–564–2, report of the Directorate of the National Security (ŘNB) Prague to the Ministry of the Interior Prague concerning the interrogation of Heinz Jantur, 12 June 1945.

7 Based on the kind information of Šimon Krýsl, MA, who is currently working on the general survey of the Jewish physicians from Bohemia and Moravia during the Second World War.

8 Paul Julian Weindling, *Nazi Medicine and Nuremberg Trials. From Medical War Crimes to Informed Consent*, Houndmills, Basingstoke: Palgrave Macmillan, 2004.

9 Ibid., pp. 37–71, 109, 115 and 125. For more on debates preceding the IMT in relation to Nazi medically motivated crimes, their documentation, and punishment, see idem, 'Zur Vorgeschichte des Nürnberger Ärzteprozesses', in Angelika Ebbinghaus and Klaus Dörner (eds), *Vernichten und Heilen. Der Nürnberger Ärzteprozeß und seine Folgen*, Berlin: Aufbau Taschenbuch Verlag, 2002, pp. 26–51.

10 On the IMT, see Gary J. Bass, *Stay the Hand of Vengeance. The Politics of War Crimes Tribunals*, Princeton and Oxford: Princeton University Press, 2000. For the contemporary Czech perspective, see Rostislav Kocourek, *Svět žaluje v Norimberku* [The World Accuses in Nuremberg], Prague: F. Borový, 1946; and Bohuslav Ečer, 'Hlavní materiálně-právní normy norimberského práva [The Main Material and Judicial Norms of the Nuremberg Law]', *Právník*, 85 (1946), pp. 1–10.

11 Ečer, 'Hlavní', p. 2. See also idem, *Jak jsem je stíhal* [How I Prosecuted Them], Prague: Naše vojsko, 1946, pp. 137–161.

12 For the contemporary views see Alexander Mitscherlich and Fred Mielke, *Medizin ohne Menschlichkeit*, Heidelberg: L. Schneider, 1947; Alice Platen-Hallermund, *Die Tötung Geisteskranker in Deutschland. Aus der Deutschen Ärztekommission beim Amerikanischen Militärgericht*, Frankfurt am Main: Verlag der Frankfurter Hefte, 1948.

13 Other persons of crucial importance, such as Philipp Bouhler, Leonardo Conti, or even Adolf Hitler, committed suicide and could not be brought to the IMT.

14 Weindling, *Nazi Medicine*, pp. 93, 250 and 251. See Jürgen Peter, 'Unmittelbare Reaktionen auf den Prozeß', in Ebbinghaus and Dörner, *Vernichten und Heilen*, pp. 452–476.

15 See *Československo a norimberský soud. Hlavní dokumenty norimberského procesu o zločinech nacistů proti Československu* [Czechoslovakia and Nuremberg Trial. The Main Documents of the Nuremberg Trial on the Nazi Crimes against Czechoslovakia], Prague: Orbis, 1946; and Bohuslav Ečer, *Norimberský soud* [Nuremberg Trial], Prague: Orbis, 1946.

16 See Pavla Šimková, *Building a New World. The Czechoslovak Policy of War Crimes Punishment after the Second World War in International Context*, BA thesis, Brno: Masaryk University, 2010. See also Ečer, Norimberský soud, p. 20. On the importance of the prisoners see Paul Weindling, 'Die Opfer von Humanexperimenten im National-sozialismus. Ergebnisse eines Forschungsprojektes', in Insa Eschenbach and Astrid Ley (eds), Geschlecht und "Rasse" in der NS-Medizin, Berlin: Metropol, 2012, pp. 81–99.

The Commission on the Investigation of the War Crimes was established within the Association of the Liberated Political Prisoners (Svaz osvobozených politických vězňů). Its competence in this period, however, remains unclear.

17 On the role and importance of F. Moravec, see Jiří Šolc, *Po boku prezidenta. Generál František Moravec a jeho zpravodajská služba ve světle archivních dokumentů* [On the Side of the President. General František Moravec and His Intelligence Service in the Light of the Archival Documents], Prague: Naše vojsko, 2007.

18 Pavel Kreisinger, *Brigádní generál Josef Bartík. Zpravodajský důstojník a účastník prvního a druhého československého odboje* [Brigadier Josef Bartík. Intelligence Officer and Member of the First and Second Czechoslovak Resistance], Prague: ÚSTR, 2011, p. 92.

19 Ibid., p. 95.

20 Ibid., p. 100.

21 Ladislav Kudrna, 'Vojenské obranné zpravodajství (1945–50). Vývoj, organizační struktury, personální obsazení [Military Defence Intelligence (1945–50). Development, Organization, Personal Staff]', *Paměť a dějiny*, (2008), p. 79.

22 ABS, 315–244–2, circular letter of the Ministry of the Interior No 18639/1945, 30 Oct 1945.

23 Ibid., letter of the ZOB ONV Vrchlabí concerning the CROWCASS, 15 Nov 1945.

24 Ibid., S–416–24, circular letter of the Ministry of the Interior concerning the war crimes of German physicians, 6 Apr 1947.

25 Ibid.

26 Kew, The National Archives (hereafter TNA), WO309/1681, Czechoslovak War Crimes Liaison Mission attached to the Headquarters of the B.A.O.R., 6 Jan 1946.

27 Report of the Deputy Judge Advocate for War Crimes Collection and Development of Evidence – European Command, June 1944 to July 1948, Washington, DC: s. d., pp. 13–21 and 29–31. See also Linda Hunt, *Secret Agenda. The United States Government, Nazi Scientists, and Project Paperclip, 1945–1990*, New York: St. Martin's Press, 1991.

28 TNA, WO 309/1681, Ečer to the Headquarters of the B.A.O.R., 14 Nov 1945.

29 Ibid., correspondence concerning the members of the Czechoslovak Mission (K. Ahar, Z. Arje, K. Čihař, P. Hořecký, V. Hošický, J. Kašák, F. Klein, J. Kováč, H. Kraus, R. Slez), 1945–46.

30 Ibid., list of transfer points on the border between Bavaria and Bohemia, 1946.

31 For information gathering in Czechoslovakia, see ABS, 315–244–2, circular letter of the Ministry of the Interior concerning Crowcass – reporting of the captures war criminals, 30 Oct 1945.

32 Kudrna, 'Vojenské obranné zpravodajství', p. 79

33 Ibid., p. 77

34 Ibid., p. 78

35 Ibid., pp. 77–79.

36 Ibid., p. 78.

37 Ibid., p. 89.

38 See Michal V. Šimůnek and Uwe Hoßfeld, 'The Avantgarde of the Rasse. Nazi "Racial Biology" at the German Charles University in Prague, 1940–1945', *Acta Universitatis Carolinae – Historia Universitatis Carolinae Pragensis*, 54 (2014), p. 94.

39 Prague, National Archives (hereafter NA Prague), 316, b. 82, Application for Military Permit to Enter Germany – Prof. Dr. Bohuslav Ečer, review for the years 1945–1948, 1948.

40 Ibid., b. 8, Ministry of the Interior to the Presidency of the Government, 13 June 1949.

41 Ibid.

42 Ibid., Ministry of the Interior to the Presidency of the Government, 13 June 1949.

43 See Bohdan Donner, *Lékařská věda ve službách zločinu. Jakou cenu měl člověk v rukou nacistických lékařů. Ministerstvo informací* [Medical Science in the Service of Crimes. Which

Worth Had a Man in the Hands of the Nazi Physicians], Prague: Ministerstvo informací, 1948.

44 Benjamin Frommer, *Národní očista. Retribuce v poválečném Československu* [The National Purification. Retributions in the Post-War Czechoslovakia], Prague: Academia, 2010; Norbert Frei (ed.), *Transnationale Vergangenheitspolitik, Der Umgang mit deutschen Kriegsverbrechen in Europa nach dem Zweiten Weltkrieg,* Wallstein: Göttingen, 2006, pp. 31–32; and Karel Kaplan, *Pravda o Československu 1945–1948* [The Truth About Czechoslovakia 1945–1948], Prague: Panorama, 1990, pp. 130–159. See also Jan Eichler, *Mezinárodní aspekty potrestání válečných zločinaů po roce 1945* [The International Aspects of the Prosecution of the War Criminals After 1945], MA thesis, Prague: Charles University, 2010, pp. 30–62; and Dita Sailerová, *Potrestání válečných zločinaů v Československu v komparaci s Mezinárodním vojenským tribunálem v Norimberku v letech 1945–1948* [Punishment of the War Criminals in Czechoslovakia in Comparison With the IMT in 1945–1948], BA thesis, Brno: Masaryk University, 2010, pp. 15–18.

45 ABS, 304–81–1, circular letter of the Ministry of the Interior No Z–XII–3069–31/5–46, 7 June 1946 and No 23669, 9 Oct 1945.

46 See Tomáš Staněk, *Retribuční vězni v českých zemích 1945–1955* [Retribution Prisoners in the Czech Lands 1945–1955], Opava: Slezský ústav Slezského zemského muzea, 2002, pp. 12–15; and Jelínek and Kučera, *Ohnmächtige Zaungäste,* pp. 781–782n13.

47 ABS, Z 38616, Iltis to Ečer, 14 Oct 1945. See Weindling, *Nazi Medicine,* p. 239. Iltis' son Hugh (b. 1925) and later professor of botany at the University of Wisconsin-Madison was as an American officer also involved in the investigation of Nazi war crimes.

48 Ibid.

49 Ibid. The names given by H. Iltis for this group were as follows: E. Fischer, F. Lenz, P. Kuhn, H. Siemens, W. Scheidt, W. Hellpach, A. Bluhm, E. Rüdin, O. Reche, K. Aichel, T. Mollison, O. v. Verschuer, E. Lehmann.

50 Ibid. The names given by H. Iltis for this group were as follows: H. F. K. Günther, B. K. Schultz, F. Kern. L. F. Clauss, M. Staemmler, J. Graf, O. Kankeleit, S. Passarge, E. Ganse, L. Tirala. H. Muckermann, M. Wundt.

51 Ibid.

52 ABS, S–416–24, Ministry of the Interior to the Directorate of the National Security (ŘNB), 18 Mar 1946. On the activities of T. Lang see Weindling, *Nazi Medicine,* pp. 41 and 236.

53 ABS, S–416–24, Directorate of the National Security (ŘNB) Prague, 21 Nov 1946.

54 Ibid.; the names given by T. Lang were as follows: A. Harrasser, K. Thums, E. Longo, R. Formanek, K. Konrad, F. Stumpfel, K.H. Rodenberg, H. Riedel, H. Schroeder, E. Schroeter, K. Greithe, F. Bohn, and K. Hell.

55 NA Prague, 316, b. 45, notice of the Medical Chamber for Bohemia, 14 Nov 14, 1946; ibid., b. 82, Ministry of the Justice to Dr. F. Bouza concerning his question on the Nazi medical crimes, 25 Apr 1947. These camps were especially Dachau, Sachsenhausen, Natzweiler, Ravensbrück, Buchenwald and Auschwitz.

56 Ibid., 316, b. 45, notice of the Medical Chamber for Bohemia, 14 Nov 1946.

57 Prague, Archives of the Charles University (hereafter A UK), Indexes of the Charles University, No 4, Index of the doctors of the Czech Charles-Ferdinand University/ Charles University IV (1917–21), 1824.

58 'The Trial of German Major War Criminals, Sitting at Nuremberg, Germany, 7th January to 19th January 1946', www.nizkor.org/hweb/imt/tgmwc/tgmwc-04/tgmwc-04–33–01.shtml (accessed 2012), p. 204.

59 František Bláha, 'Medical Science Run Amok', in Medical Science Abused. German Medical Science as Practised in Concentration Camps and in the so-called Protectorate – Reported by Czechoslovak Doctors, Prague: Orbis, 1946, p. 16.

60 Ibid., 21.
61 Ibid., 24. See also 'Trial of German Major War Criminals', p. 205.
62 Personal communication of the author with son-in-law of F. Bláha, 2013.
63 Letter of F. Bláha to the family, 21 Nov 1943, kept in private possession of the son-in-law of F. Bláha.
64 Joachim Neander, 'A Strange Witness to Dachau Human Skin Atrocities: Anton Pachelogg a.k.a. Anton Baron von Guttenberg a.k.a. Antoine Charles de Guttenberg', *Theologie Geschichte*, 4 (2009), available at: http://universaar.uni-saarland.de/journals/index.php/tg/article/viewArticle/472/511.
65 Eugen Ost, 'In memoriam Professor Dr. František Bláha', *Rappel*, 34 (1979), pp. 235–241.
66 Neander, 'A Strange Witness', n85.
67 Ibid.
68 'Trial of German Major War Criminals', p. 205. See Weindling, *Nazi Medicine*, pp. 95–96. Actually, F. Bláha was a member of Social Democratic Party, not of the Communist Party.
69 'Trial of German Major War Criminals', 205–206.
70 See František Bláha, *Medicína na scestí* [Aberrant Medicine], Prague: Orbis, 1946; idem, *Zločin a trest* [Crimes and Punishment], Prague: J. Otto, 1946; and idem, *Jací byli* [How They Were], Prague: SBS, 1948. For the Czechoslovak post-war reflections, see also Michal V. Šimůnek, ' "German Science Commited an Offence". German Life Sciences and Czech Post-War Reflections, 1945–1946', in Zdenko Čepič (ed.), *1945 – A Break With the Past. A History of Central European Countries at the End of World War Two*, Ljubljana: INZ, 2008, pp. 293–311.
71 Bláha, *Medical Science*, pp. 14–41.
72 Konstantin P. Gorschenin (ed.), *Norimberský proces II* [Nuremberg Process II], Prague: Orbis, 1953, pp. 777–793.
73 ABS, 52–76–1, analysis of the affidavit of F. Bláha, about 1955.
74 Ibid.
75 Neander, *A Strange Witness*.
76 Magne Skjaeraasen, *Lékař pro život. Příběh Lea Eitingera* [Physician for Life. The Story of Leo Eitinger], Brno: Doplněk, 2012, pp. 10–27. For further detail, see www.eitinger.cz.
77 Ibid., pp. 32–36.
78 Ibid., pp. 48–59.
79 Ibid, pp. 66–78.
80 Ibid., pp. 87–101.
81 Ibid., p. 163.
82 Washington, DC, National Archives (hereafter NARA), RG 549, T 1021, translation of sworn statement of Leo Eitinger, 23 Apr 1945 (confidential). See also Skjaeraasen, *Lékař*, p. 168.
83 Ibid.
84 Skjaeraasen, *Lékař*, p. 2.
85 Ibid.
86 Ibid. See also Hermann Langbein, *Menschen in Auschwitz*, Frankfurt am Main: Fischer, 1980.
87 NARA, RG 549, T 1021, translation of sworn statement of Leo Eitinger, 23 Apr 1945.
88 Ibid.
89 Skjaeraasen, *Lékař*, p. 3.
90 Ibid., pp. 166–167.
91 See Ludmila Hlaváčková and Petr Svobodný, *Biographisches Lexikon der Deutschen Medizinische Fakultät in Prag 1883–1945*, Prague: Karolinum, 1998, p. 61.

92 Ibid.
93 ABS, 302–358–1, testimony of R. Vítek, 11 Mar 1946. On Mengele see Helene Kubica, 'The Crimes of Josef Mengele', in Yisrael Gutman and Michael Berenbaum (eds), *Anatomy of the Auschwitz Death Camp*, Bloomington: Indiana University Press, 1998, pp. 317–337.
94 ABS, 302–358–1, Czechoslovak War Crimes Mission to Ečer, 6 Mar 1946.
95 Ibid.
96 Ibid.
97 Ibid.
98 Ibid., testimony of R. Vítek, 11 Mar 1946.
99 Ibid., Czechoslovak War Crimes Mission to Ečer, 6 Mar 1946.
100 Frankfurt am Main, Archive of the Fritz Bauer Institute (hereafter AFBI), NI–5847, PDB 75 (e), affidavit of B. Epstein, 7 Mar 1947, pp. 168–170.
101 NA Prague, PŘ 1941–51, k. 1937, E 434/8, Association of the Liberated Political Prisoners to Epstein, 15 Oct 1947.
102 See Petra Fischbäck, *Der Todesangel und seine Kollegen. Josef Mengeles Zusammenarbeit mit dem Kaiser-Wilhelm-Institut in Berlin*, Munich: Grin Verlag, 2013.
103 '65 let prof. MUDr B. Epsteina [65 Years of Professor Dr B. Epstein]', *Československá pediatrie*, 10 (1955), pp. 314–317.
104 Vítězslav Horn, *Jak jsem přežil*, Brno: Simon Ryšavý, 2002, p. 13.
105 Ibid., p. 15.
106 A UK, Indexes of the Charles University, No 4, Index of the doctors of the Czech Charles-Ferdinand University/Charles University IV (1917–21), 1674.
107 Horn, *Jak jsem*, pp. 17, 32–33 and 49–50.
108 Ibid., p. 77.
109 'Vítězslav Horn', http://encyklopedie.brna.cz (last modified 2016).
110 Horn, *Jak jsem*, pp. 74 and 95.
111 Klaus Dörner, Angelika Ebbinghaus and Karsten Linne (eds), *The Nuremberg Medical Trial 1946/47. Transcripts, Material of the Prosecution and Defense, Related Documents*, Munich: Saur, 2001, p. 224 (566 – NO-4051, which erroneously states year 1946).
112 Horn, *Jak jsem*, pp. 74–75.
113 Ibid., 75.
114 František Janouch, *Sám Ďábel by se rděl. Otcovy dopisy z nacistických koncentračních táborů* [Even the Devil Himself Would Blush. Father's Letters from the Nazi Concentration Camps], Prague: Akropolis, 2003, pp. 21–22.
115 Ibid., p. 27.
116 Ibid., p. 33.
117 NA Prague, 316, b. 3, testimony of MUDr František Janouch – use of human meal for the experiments in Auschwitz, Nov 1945.
118 Ibid., War Crimes Commission to the Ministry of Justice, 15 Dec 1945.
119 Ibid., testimony of MUDr František Janouch – use of human meal for the experiments in Auschwitz, Nov 1945.
120 See 'Sám ďábel by se rděl [Even the Devil Himself Would Blush]', *Svobodné slovo*, 1 (4 Oct 1945), p. 11.
121 'Josef Podlaha', http://encyklopedie.brna.cz (last modified 2016).
122 Ibid.
123 Ibid.
124 Josef Podlaha, 'Surgery and Medical Care of the Prisoners in the Mauthausen Concentration Camp', in *Medical Science Abused*, p. 62.
125 Ibid.
126 Ibid., pp. 58–75.
127 Ibid., pp. 69–71.

128 A UK, Indexes of the German University, No 5, Index of the doctors of the German University Prague (1931–36), 495.

129 Roger Ryan, 'Dr. Karl Sperber O.B.E. (1910–57)', available at http://mujweb.cz/ipro/ stripky/clanky/sperberen.htm (last modified 1 May 2009); and Claude Romney, 'How all Roads Could Lead to Auschwitz. The Extraordinary Story of Dr. Karl Sperber', *Zachor* (2005), p. 9.

130 See Joseph P. Slavik, *The Cruise of the German Raidar Atlants*, Annapolis: Naval Institute Press, 2003, p. 111.

131 Ryan, 'Dr. Karl Sperber'.

132 Ibid.

133 Ibid.

134 Weindling, *Nazi Medicine*, p. 100.

135 *British Medical Journal*, 117 (1957), p. 888.

136 ABS, 302–358–1, testimony of R. Vítek, 11 Mar 1946.

137 AFBI, subsequent Nuremberg trial, case VI, PDB 75 (e), affidavit of R. Vítek – NI–4830, 3 Mar 1947.

138 See Washington, DC, United States Holocaust Memorial Museum, RG-15.117M, Memoirs, 1945 – Memories on the End of the Gipsy Camp in Birkenau and Henchmen in White Coats, s.d. (the surname is here wrongly given as Bitek). See also ibid., Vol. 232, 179945/1286, 126–141 (under his original German surname Weisskopf).

139 Václav Tomášek, 'Bakteriologie v Mauthausenu a Osvětimi [Bacteriology in Mauthausen and Auschwitz]', *Věda a život* (1945), pp. 402–413; 'Oswieczim', *Medical Science Abused*, pp. 76–89; and Miloslav Matoušek, *Buchenwald*, Prague: Život a práce, 1945.

140 For example in Auschwitz there were at least six such persons, mostly dealing with dentistry. See Stanisław Kłodziński, 'Esesmani z oświęcimskiej służby zdrowia [SS-Men of the Health Service in Auschwitz]', in J. Rawicz (ed.), *Okupacja i medycyna*, Warsaw: Książka i Wiedza, 1971, pp. 339–345.

141 Ludwig Eiber and Robert Sigl (eds), Dachauer Prozesse – NS-Verbrechen vor amerikanischen Militärgerichten in Dachau 1945–1948, Göttingen: Wallstein, 2007.

Bibliography

Archival sources

Czech Republic

Prague, Archives of the Charles University (A UK), Indexes of the Charles University, No 4–5

Prague, Archives of the Security Services (ABS), 52–76–1; 302–358–1; 304–81–1; 305–564–2; 315–244–2; S–416–24 and Z 38616

Prague, National Archives (NA Prague), 316, b. 3, 8, 45 and 82; PŘ 1941–51, k. 1937, E 434/8

Germany

Frankfurt am Main, Archive of the Fritz Bauer Institute (AFBI):
NI–5847, PDB 75 (e)
subsequent Nuremberg trial, case VI, PDB 75 (e)

United Kingdom

Kew, The National Archives (TNA), WO309/1681

USA

Washington, DC, National Archives (NARA), RG 549, T 1021
Washington, DC, United States Holocaust Memorial Museum, RG-15.117M, Memoirs, 1945 – Memories on the End of the Gipsy Camp in Birkenau and Henchmen in White Coats

Literature

'65 let prof. MUDr B. Epsteina [65 Years of Professor Dr B. Epstein]', *Československá pediatrie*, 10 (1955), pp. 314–317

Bass, Gary J., *Stay the Hand of Vengeance. The Politics of War Crimes Tribunals*, Princeton and Oxford: Princeton University Press, 2000

Benz, Wolfgang (ed.), *Der Ort des Terrors, Bd. 1*, Munich: C. H. Beck, 2005

Bláha, František, *Medicína na scestí* [Aberrant Medicine], Prague: Orbis, 1946

—— *Jací byli* [How They Were], Prague: SBS, 1948

—— *Zločin a trest* [Crimes and Punishment], Prague: J. Otto, 1946

Československo a norimberský soud. Hlavní dokumenty norimberského procesu o zločinech nacistů proti Československu [Czechoslovakia and Nuremberg Trial. The Main Documents of the Nuremberg Trial on the Nazi Crimes Against Czechoslovakia], Prague: Orbis, 1946

'Der Doktor und sein Opfer', *Der Spiegel*, 14 (1999), pp. 116–123

Donner, Bohdan, *Lékařská věda ve službách zločinu. Jakou cenu měl člověk v rukou nacistických lékařů. Ministerstvo informací* [Medical Science in the Service of Crimes. Which Worth Had a Man in the Hands of the Nazi Physicians], Prague: Ministerstvo informací, 1948

Dörner, Klaus, Angelika Ebbinghaus and Karsten Linne (eds), *The Nuremberg Medical Trial 1946/47. Transcripts, Material of the Prosecution and Defense, Related Documents*, Munich: Saur, 2001

Ečer, Bohuslav, 'Hlavní materiálně-právní normy norimberského práva [The Main Material and Judicial Norms of the Nuremberg Law]', *Právník*, 85 (1946), pp. 1–10

—— *Jak jsem je stíhal* [How I prosecuted Them], Prague: Naše vojsko, 1946

—— *Norimberský soud* [Nuremberg Trial], Prague: Orbis, 1946

Eiber, Ludwig and Robert Sigl (eds), *Dachauer Prozesse – NS-Verbrechen vor amerikanischen Militärgerichten in Dachau 1945–1948*, Göttingen: Wallstein, 2007

Eichler, Jan, *Mezinárodní aspekty potrestání válečných zločinů po roce 1945* [The International Aspects of the Prosecution of the War Criminals After 1945], MA thesis, Prague: Charles University, 2010

Fischbäck, Petra, *Der Todesangel und seine Kollegen. Josef Mengeles Zusammenarbeit mit dem Kaiser-Wilhelm-Institut in Berlin*, Munich: Grin Verlag, 2013

Frei, Norbert (ed.), *Transnationale Vergangenheitspolitik, Der Umgang mit deutschen Kriegsverbrechen in Europa nach dem Zweiten Weltkrieg*, Wallstein: Göttingen, 2006

Frommer, Benjamin, *Národní očista. Retribuce v poválečném Československu* [The National Purification. Retributions in the Post-War Czechoslovakia], Prague: Academia, 2010

Gorschenin, Konstantin P. (ed.), *Norimberský proces II* [Nuremberg Process II], Prague: Orbis, 1953

Hájková, Anna, *Medicine and Illness. The Last Ghetto. An Everyday History of the Terezín Ghetto, 1941–1945*, Chapter 4 (forthcoming)

Hlaváčková, Ludmila and Petr Svobodný, *Biographisches Lexikon der Deutschen Medizinische Fakultät in Prag 1883–1945*, Prague: Karolinum, 1998

Horn, Vítězslav, *Jak jsem přežil*, Brno: Simon Ryšavý, 2002

Hunt, Linda, *Secret Agenda. The United States Government, Nazi Scientists, and Project Paperclip, 1945–1990*, New York: St. Martin's Press, 1991

Janouch, František, *Sám Ďábel by se rděl. Otcovy dopisy z nacistických koncentračních táborů* [Even the Devil Himself Would Blush. Father's Letters from the Nazi Concentration Camps], Prague: Akropolis, 2003

Jelínek, Tomáš and Jaroslav Kučera, 'Ohnmächtige Zaungäste. Die Entschädigung von tschechoslowakischen NS-Verfolgten', in Hans G. Hockerts, Claudia Kertts and Tobias Winstel (eds), *Grenzen der Wiedergutmachung. Die Entschädigung für NS-Verfolgte in West- und Osteuropa 1945–2000*, Göttingen: Wallstein, 2006, pp. 813–826

'Josef Podlaha', http://encyklopedie.brna.cz (last modified 2016)

Kaplan, Karel, *Pravda o Československu 1945–1948* [The Truth About Czechoslovakia 1945–1948], Prague: Panorama, 1990

Kłodziński, Stanisław, 'Esesmani z oświęcimskiej służby zdrowia [SS-Men of the Health Service in Auschwitz]', in J. Rawicz (ed.), *Okupacja i medycyna*, Warsaw: Książka i Wiedza, 1971, pp. 339–345

Kocourek, Rostislav, *Svět žaluje v Norimberku* [The World Accuses in Nuremberg], Prague: F. Borový, 1946

Kreisinger, Pavel, *Brigádní generál Josef Bartík. Zpravodajský důstojník a účastník prvního a druhého československého odboje* [Brigadier Josef Bartík. Intelligence Officer and Member of the First and Second Czechoslovak Resistance], Prague: ÚSTR, 2011

Kubica, Helene, 'The Crimes of Josef Mengele', in Yisrael Gutman and Michael Berenbaum (eds), *Anatomy of the Auschwitz Death Camp*, Bloomington: Indiana University Press, 1998, pp. 317–337

Kudrna, Ladislav, 'Vojenské obranné zpravodajství (1945–1950). Vývoj, organizační struktury, personální obsazení [Military Defence Intelligence (1945–1950). Development, Organization, Personal Staff]', *Paměť a dějiny*, (2008), pp. 76–89

Langbein, Hermann, *Menschen in Auschwitz*, Frankfurt am Main: Fischer, 1980

Matoušek, Miloslav, *Buchenwald*, Prague: Život a práce, 1945

Medical Science Abused. German Medical Science as Practised in Concentration Camps and in the so-called Protectorate – Reported by Czechoslovak Doctors, Prague: Orbis, 1946

Mitscherlich, Alexander and Fred Mielke, *Medizin ohne Menschlichkeit*, Heidelberg: L. Schneider, 1947

Neander, Joachim, 'A Strange Witness to Dachau Human Skin Atrocities: Anton Pachelogg a.k.a. Anton Baron von Guttenberg a.k.a. Antoine Charles de Guttenberg', *Theologie Geschichte*, 4 (2009), available at: http://universaar.uni-saarland.de/journals/index.php/tg/article/viewArticle/472/511

Ost, Eugen, 'In memoriam Professor Dr. František Bláha', *Rappel*, 34 (1979), pp. 235–241

Peter, Jürgen, 'Unmittelbare Reaktionen auf den Prozeß', in Angelika Ebbinghaus and Klaus Dörner (eds), *Vernichten und Heilen. Der Nürnberger Ärzteprozeß und seine Folgen*, Berlin: Aufbau Taschenbuch Verlag, 2002, pp. 452–476

Platen-Hallermund, Alice, *Die Tötung Geisteskranker in Deutschland. Aus der Deutschen Ärztekommission beim Amerikanischen Militärgericht*, Frankfurt am Main: Verlag der Frankfurter Hefte, 1948

Report of the Deputy Judge Advocate for War Crimes Collection and Development of Evidence – European Command, June 1944 to July 1948, Washington, DC: s. d.

Ryan, Roger, 'Dr. Karl Sperber O.B.E. (1910–1957)', available at http://mujweb.cz/ipro/stripky/clanky/sperberen.htm (last modified 1 May 2009)

Romney, Claude, 'How all Roads Could Lead to Auschwitz. The Extraordinary Story of Dr. Karl Sperber', *Zachor* (2005), p. 9

Sailerová, Dita, *Potrestání válečných zločinců v Československu v komparaci s Mezinárodním vojenským tribunálem v Norimberku v letech 1945–1948* [Punishment of the War Criminals in Czechoslovakia in Comparison With the IMT in 1945–1948], BA thesis, Brno: Masaryk University, 2010

'Sám ďábel by se rděl [Even the Devil Himself Would Blush]', *Svobodné slovo*, 1 (4 Oct 1945), p. 11

Šimková, Pavla, *Building a New World. The Czechoslovak Policy of War Crimes Punishment after the Second World War in International Context*, BA thesis, Brno: Masaryk University, 2010

Šimůnek, Michal V., ' "German Science Commited an Offence". German Life Sciences and Czech Post-War Reflections, 1945–1946', in Zdenko Čepič (ed.), *1945 – A Break With the Past. A History of Central European Countries at the End of World War Two*, Ljubljana: INZ, 2008, pp. 293–311

—— and Uwe Hoßfeld, 'The Avantgarde of the Rasse. Nazi "Racial Biology" at the German Charles University in Prague, 1940–1945', *Acta Universitatis Carolinae – Historia Universitatis Carolinae Pragensis*, 54 (2014), pp. 55–104

Skjaeraasen, Magne, *Lékař pro život. Příběh Lea Eitingera* [Physician for Life. The Story of Leo Eitinger], Brno: Doplněk, 2012

Slavik, Joseph P., *The Cruise of the German Raidar Atlants*, Annapolis: Naval Institute Press, 2003

Šolc, Jiří, *Po boku prezidenta. Generál František Moravec a jeho zpravodajská služba ve světle archivních dokumentů* [On the Side of the President. General František Moravec and His Intelligence Service in the Light of the Archival Documents], Prague: Naše vojsko, 2007

Staněk, Tomáš, *Retribuční vězni v českých zemích 1945–1955* [Retribution Prisoners in the Czech Lands 1945–1955], Opava: Slezský ústav Slezského zemského muzea, 2002

'The Trial of German Major War Criminals, Sitting at Nuremberg, Germany, 7th January to 19th January 1946', www.nizkor.org/hweb/imt/tgmwc/tgmwc-04/tgmwc-04-33-01.shtml (accessed 2012)

Tomášek, Václav, 'Bakteriologie v Mauthausenu a Osvětimi [Bacteriology in Mauthausen and Auschwitz]', *Věda a život* (1945), pp. 402–413

'Vítězslav Horn', http://encyklopedie.brna.cz (last modified 2016)

Weindling, Paul, 'Zur Vorgeschichte des Nürnberger Ärzteprozesses', in Angelika Ebbinghaus and Klaus Dörner (eds), *Vernichten und Heilen. Der Nürnberger Ärzteprozeß und seine Folgen*, Berlin: Aufbau Taschenbuch Verlag, 2002, pp. 26–51

—— *Nazi Medicine and Nuremberg Trials. From Medical War Crimes to Informed Consent*, Houndmills, Basingstoke: Palgrave Macmillan, 2004

—— 'Die Opfer von Humanexperimenten im Nationalsozialismus. Ergebnisse eines Forschungsprojektes', in Insa Eschenbach and Astrid Ley (eds), *Geschlecht und "Rasse" in der NS-Medizin*, Berlin: Metropol, 2012, pp. 81–99

16 Post-war legacies, 1945–2015

Victims, bodies, and brain tissues[1]

Paul Weindling

The making of a critical social history of Nazi medicine

At the close of the Second World War there was a high level of concern with Nazi human experiments. Survivors set out to document and testify, and Allied scientific intelligence officers flagged up the criminality of medical research under National Socialism. Allied occupation authorities were concerned about the holding of victim body parts and required their documentation and removal, whereas many anatomists clung onto their corpses – many headless from the Nazi guillotine or with broken spines from hanging.[2] The Nuremberg Medical Trial (NMT) prosecuted a set of leading perpetrators of human experiments, among whom were 20 physicians and three leading administrators. First accounts were published by the German Medical Delegation at the NMT by Alexander Mitscherlich and his medical student assistant Fred Mielke.[3] Alice Platen-Hallermund, who had dropped out of German psychiatry in 1935 because of its Nazi ethos, published a pioneering account of the "euthanasia" killings.[4] US prosecutors mounted a series of trials at Dachau when further perpetrators were convicted including Claus Schilling for malaria experiments at Dachau, and Helmut Vetter for pharmacological experiments at Mauthausen and Auschwitz with IG Farben pharmaceuticals.[5]

Although the US prosecutors' strategy was to approach medical experiments as hands-on murder, defendants argued that clinical trials were legitimate, in line with international medical procedures, and above all necessary for advancing medical science. The IG Farben Trial at Nuremberg from August 1947 until July 1948 accepted the defence of the necessity of constant clinical trials (despite their being conducted in concentration camps).[6] Accused of experiments at Dachau, the internal medical specialists (and SS officers) Rudolf Brachtel was acquitted in 1947, and Kurt Ploetner evaded justice by working for American intelligence.[7]

Shock at the atrocities resulted in Chancellor Adenauer and his cabinet providing a compensation scheme for experiment victims in 1951, albeit in the belief that there were only few surviving victims.[8] During the 1950s, the initial high level of sensitisation to experiments further diminished. High Commissioner McCloy released the convicted; Allied prosecutions ceased: the

French prosecution of the virologist Eugen Haagen – analysed here by Christian Bonah and Florian Schmaltz – being one of the last Allied trials for coerced experiments. The responsibility for prosecutions passed to the Federal Republic, which was slow to prosecute, and ineffective in securing verdicts proportionate to the crimes; Austria and the German Democratic Republic showed increasing reluctance. Heißmeyer was prosecuted only after his retirement as a chest physician in the German Democratic Republic.[9] After a short but intense set of prosecutions of psychiatrists for "euthanasia" in Austria, increasing Austrian reluctance to prosecute culminated in the scandalous failure to reach a verdict in the prosecution against the brain pathologist Heinrich Gross.[10] Fritz Bauer the energetic Frankfurt prosecutor was constantly thwarted by conservative German judges who were indulgent towards defendants. Collegial physicians would certify that a defendant was too unwell to stand trial, but then the freed defendant would flourish in excellent health. Horst Schumann was responsible for not only "euthanasia" killings but also X-ray sterilisations in Auschwitz: his trial a noted example of a prosecution that collapsed due to his being certified for medical incapacity in 1972, but he lived on until 1983.[11] In 1970 Hans Fleischhacker was not convicted owing to his defence that he did not know that the Jews whom he selected and measured in Auschwitz would be killed for their skeletons. His colleague and fellow anthropologist Bruno Beger received only a three-year sentence for the 86 killings, and was deemed to have served this when in Allied and pre-trial custody.[12]

The experiments were classed as "pseudo-science" by compensation and prosecution authorities, thereby keeping mainstream medical research intact. This led support to the fiction that the experiments involved only a handful of criminal doctors, but mainstream German and Austrian medicine had an impeccable record. In any case – as Henry K. Beecher (professor of anaesthetics at Harvard) and Maurice Papworth (marginalised in British medical circles but influential with his critique *Human Guinea Pigs*) showed, ideas of informed consent were flagrantly disregarded in a Western medicine, which was increasingly scientised.[13]

Scientists managed to deflect the accusation of involvement in killings. A line was drawn between utilising body parts for scientific research, and instigating the killings. Thus leading figures such as Otmar von Verschuer, the eugenicist/human geneticist, and Julius Hallervorden, the neuropathologist, evaded prosecutions by drawing a distinction between the responsibility for killings and what they claimed was passively receiving the body parts of murdered victims for research.[14] Researchers, such as Eugen Haagen, could – as Bonah and Schmaltz show in their chapter – resume their careers. This was similarly true for the neurologist Georges Schaltenbrand in Würzburg.[15]

By way of contrast, there remained a situation of surviving victims of experiments receiving token or no compensation (what they really needed was necessary medical care). Stockpiles of bodies and tissues were held in research institutes for anatomy and for neuro-pathology and brain research. Frankfurt am Main and the Steinhof/former Spiegelgrund "special children's department" in Vienna offer notable cases. Gross was remarkably granted a "Ludwig Boltzmann Institute for the study of the abnormalities of the nervous system" in 1968 to continue researching on the Spiegelgrund victim body parts: the hospital technicians tended the specimens in their hundreds of glass containers beyond his retirement.[16] Sabine Hildebrandt has examined the stockpiling of bodies in anatomical institutes for teaching and research.[17] Similar stockpiling occurred on a massive scale of brain tissues.

It was only during the 1980s that a new critical social history took shape. The history of eugenics developed to cover the era from Imperial Germany to the Third Reich, and beyond in terms of family welfare policies. Robert Proctor analysed how Nazi scientists constructed racial policy.[18] My approach was to show how since 1900 eugenics and racialised forms of medicine penetrated different medical specialisms and public health agencies, culminating in biologically based social policies under the Nazis.[19]

From the late 1970s in Germany there arose a grass roots coalition of critical groups concerned with Nazi medicine and its post-war continuities. At Tübingen a critical group researched Nazi medicine from the perspective of nature therapy, leading to wider concerns with the racialising of medicine.[20] Left-wing radicals argued that the academic establishment held positions of status, power and privilege, drawing on the legacy of National Socialism. Alfons Labisch, Stephan Leibfried and Florian Tennstedt showed how the Nazis destroyed alternative models of a socialised public health, while I indicated how eugenics was already embedded in Weimar social medicine.[21] Labisch and Tennstadt published on the new public health law unifying municipal and state health agencies with an aim to impose coercive sterilisation.[22] The *Gesundheitstag* movement offered a critical alternative as regards health care, and disability rights. Its meetings such as at Berlin in May 1980 and Bremen in 1984 were dominated by heated sessions on Nazi medicine.[23] One issue was that of continuity: Karl Heinz Roth published on the continuity from Weimar eugenics to Nazi medicine. Another view was that Weimar eugenics was authoritarian (in terms of professional power, politics and patriarchy) but it was anti-Nazi.[24] From a feminist perspective Gisela Bock produced a definitive overview of sterilisation along with a new critical wave of historical writing on gender and family policy with abortion and contraception as historical flashpoints.[25] Christian Pross studied the Berlin hospital of Moabit where a plethora of innovative doctors were then removed by the Nazis. Pross then wrote a highly innovative and critical analysis of compensation as a "civil war against the victims".[26] Taken together the above mentioned analyses empirically broke new ground in identifying the importance of medical research for the Nazi state. What was often not appreciated was the sheer difficulty in undertaking research on Weimar and Nazi medicine – until 1987 it involved organising permissions for research in the German Democratic Republic (GDR). Müller-Hill had realised that there were documents on links to Auschwitz that were not in the available inventories in the *Bundesarchiv* (Federal Archives). German

Archives Law has been restrictive regarding research on victims and perpetrators, and archivists vary immensely in their interpretations as regards issues such as defining persons of historical significance. The historian experiences at first hand the German lack of a political culture of accountability and transparency.

While there were disagreements over continuities and reconfigurations, the overall thrust of these studies was to exert a strong impact on interpretations of Germany after 1945. The prevailing narrative of a denazified and liberal social market economy emerging from a *Stunde Null* (zero-hour) in May 1945 giving liberated Germany a fresh start unencumbered by the past began to crumble. The new research on authoritarian elites with profound continuities among the bureaucracy, the professions and business challenged the narrow-minded historical elites concerned with the high politics of Cold War Germany and the post-war economy. Empirically strong, this emergent critical history began to impact on the historical mainstream.

The GDR opened up the history of eugenics from 1983. One can see the new critical social history of medicine as challenging structures of continuity and denial in the two Germanies. The GDR saw concern with technocratic structures of power offering analogies to the Nazi era. The history of eugenics was prioritised along with the history of Nazi "euthanasia" at locations such as the psychiatric hospitals of Bernburg and Sonnenstein near Dresden. In Austria there was a time lag: two Austrians Michael Hubenstorf and Gerhard Baader did much to develop the history of Nazi medicine, but more in the context of a German-oriented approach that does not always fit the peculiarities of the Austrian and especially the Viennese situation. The issue of "euthanasia" victims was opened up by Wolfgang Neugebauer of the Documentation Centre for the Austrian Resistance, and after 2000 a series of studies followed on eugenics, psychiatry and anthropology within a wider Central European context.[27]

The new research on eugenics and racial policies provided the evidence basis for compensation for victims of sterilisation, for "euthanasia" victim families, as well as for persecuted Sinti and Roma, and from the mid-1990s for forced labourers. The results were: apologies (albeit partial), compensation (albeit woefully inadequate and involving waivers whereby victims gave up rights for a small fix-rate amount) and historical programmes of key scientific institutions and professional associations, making science and medicine accountable in terms of past historical conduct.[28] The overall effect was to take the complex of science, medicine and eugenics that was regarded hitherto as marginal, and to make it mainstream in terms of historical significance. At the same time Alfons Labisch and Reinhard Spree took up the agenda of the social history of medicine, so that history of medicine should no longer be a specialist enclave but fully historicised. The social historian Detlev Peuckert developed these essays in a classic analysis of the pathology of social modernity, marking the start that these "outsider" studies in the soft area of health, medicine and gender were no longer marginal but mainstream in terms of their historical significance.[29]

Brain tissues as material continuity

In 1983, Götz Aly, a former *Rote Hilfe* activist was researching towards a Habilitation in Political Science at the Free University Berlin; he applied for access to the collection of brain anatomical slides at the Edinger Neurological Institute in Frankfurt am Main. The slides derived from Julius Hallervorden who had been director of the histo-pathological department of the Kaiser Wilhelm Institute for Brain Research at Berlin-Buch since 1937, and after the war at the Max-Planck Institute for Brain Research (MPIBR) at Giessen until the Institute moved to Frankfurt in 1962. Götz Aly saw direct continuity from the scientific elites in Nazi Germany to those of the Federal Republic. He rightly drew attention to the continued holding of "euthanasia" victim body parts in Frankfurt at what was then a combined MPIBR and Edinger Institute of Frankfurt University.

At first Aly encountered bureaucratic obstructionism in the search for documentation, and then the *Max-Planck-Gesellschaft* (MPG) fiercely denied that the brain specimens were from "euthanasia" victims.[30] The MPG's response to Aly was denial that its senior scientists used either body parts and fluids from concentration camps, or brain tissues from "euthanasia" victims.

In 1989–90 an intense debate erupted in the Federal Republic of Germany over the status of anatomical specimens from the period of National Socialism. Pressure was brought on the German universities and research institutes to remove body parts. The solution was deemed rapid burial of all specimens whose provenance was in doubt. A range of options was considered, and the eventual decision to bury remains was judged the best way to draw a line under an uncomfortable Nazi past when the specimens were obtained. The aim was to achieve closure on this issue by a rapid "cleansing" of scientific collections. However, identification of victims, the circumstances of their death and the ensuing utilisation of their bodies for research and teaching were left unresolved amidst the heated debates at the time. Procedures differed as regards burial – whether the glass slides should be subjected to high heat and essentially cremated (as for the Spiegelgrund in Vienna), or whether the slides should be buried intact in aluminium containers (as for the MPG burial in 1990).

Aly was rightly concerned about provenance of the slides and specimens, and suspected their murderous origins, but his agenda was loaded with controversial political implications. His contention was that medical elites in the Federal Republic sustained authoritarian power structures from National Socialism on into the Federal Republic. As he bitingly wrote, "Die Täter waren vorher und nachher am Werk" (the perpetrators were active both before and after 1945).[31] His request for access to MPG records triggered a long-running discussion as to the status of the Hallervorden collection – whether it was a historical collection that might be considered *Archivgut* (suitable for an archive), or whether it fell under medical confidentiality restrictions?[32] High profile newspapers like *Die Zeit* publicised his findings. The accusations became news stories with significant national and international impact.

Once Aly's permission to view the Hallervorden collection and associated archives was granted, he visited the Edinger Institute on 23–24 May 1984 and researched the documentation on each specimen. His detailed report to the MPG demonstrated that the Hallervorden collection included brains of "euthanasia" victims. He identified a group of 33 children, all killed on 28 October 1940. His verdict was that the brain sections should be destroyed "out of respect to victims of Nazism".[33] Despite Aly's meticulous documentation, his claims were regarded as contentious. Aly searched for further evidence at the Max Planck Institute for Psychiatry (MPIP) in Munich on 1 April 1985, when his research materials went missing. Professor Gerd Peters as Institute Director contested the ensuing publication by Aly.[34]

Aly's strategy was removal and destruction of the brain specimens. His priority of "disposal" arose from concern with the perpetrating elites. In the atmosphere of confrontation and defensive self-justification, the issues of commemoration of the victims, and their identification were lost from sight. At discussions between Aly and myself in 1987, Aly appeared to have given no thought about what should happen to the specimens after their removal. I was left wondering whether burial might not be premature, as determining individual identity seemed to me to be important.

Similar claims to those of Aly regarding a former Kaiser Wilhelm Institute's involvement in murderous research were made by the geneticist Benno Müller-Hill in 1984 about Josef Mengele as the Auschwitz-based assistant to Otmar von Verschuer, Director of the KWI for Anthropology. Müller-Hill pointed out the Institute's role in obtaining blood samples and body parts such as heterochromic eyes of murdered Sinto victims.[35] Müller-Hill's book was in two halves with a documents-based analysis of how human genetics was linked to Nazi authorities, followed by interviews. It showed tellingly how documentation contradicted the stories of denial and evasion told by scientists and their families. Despite the apparent radicalism of their claims, Aly and Müller-Hill only repeated what was known at the time of the Nuremberg Medical Trial of 1946–47 on the basis of extensive documentation, suggesting that in the interim the concern to rebuild science in the Federal Republic had been accompanied by a politics if not of denial then of overlooking provenance of collections and how medical research had taken a key role in the realisation of National Socialist agendas.[36] The MPG authorities were concerned both about the substance of Aly's accusations and their organisation's public image, but considered the claims regarding Nazi victims were exaggerated by left-wing radicals.

Figures like Simon Wiesenthal intensified the hunt for Mengele until his remains were exhumed on 6 June 1985.[37] It was established that Mengele had died on 7 February 1979 near Sao Paolo in Brazil, and was buried under a false name of Wolfgang Gerhard. The announcement triggered renewed interest in Mengele's scientific networks and rationales. In 1985 Karl Heinz Roth and Paul Weindling analysed Mengele's genetics as normal science in the context of the mid-1930s rather than "pseudo-science".[38]

Despite scepticism about links with concentration camps and "euthanasia" killings, the MPG set out to evaluate and verify Aly's documentation. Until 13 October 1989 when the MPG President issued a press statement acknowledging that certain specimens derived from "euthanasia" killings, its position regarding Aly's allegations was that the evidence was not conclusive. Scientists regarded the allegations as unproven, and defended the use of the specimens for research and teaching. In 1989 the position of both sides underwent modification.[39]

Radical medical students took up Aly's accusations, and agitated on the issue of the retention of body parts of victims of Nazi "euthanasia" being used for anatomical teaching and research. The University of Tübingen was a crystallisation point. Here again students and civic activists clashed with the University elite. The historian Benigna Schönhagen documented how the anatomical utilisation of corpses made Tübingen an end point of Nazi extermination.[40] Medical students at Tübingen initiated a series of lectures on "Medicine under National Socialism". The anatomist Professor Ulrich Drews lectured on 17 November 1988 on the problem of the supply of bodies.[41] The students supported excavations at the anatomical burial ground.[42]

The regional television station, *Badische Fernsehredaktion* ran a programme on 19 December 1988 on anatomical specimens of National Socialist victims.[43] Drews now denied that his institute held any remains of Nazi victims.[44] He later reflected on the customary depersonalisation regarding slides, "until now, nobody has thought about histological sections as being part of the body".[45] The issue of provenance became crucial. When the national television station, ARD, broadcast a news item on 2 January 1989 about the use of Nazi victims' bodies for medical teaching, an international furore erupted.[46] The sceptical detachment of the scientific community was overwhelmed by public indignation.

There were demonstrations at the German Embassy in Israel against the use of the body parts of Holocaust victims for teaching. The Israeli Minister for Religion, Zevelun Hammer, petitioned Federal German Chancellor Helmut Kohl. Chancellor Kohl ordered on 11 January 1989 that all state ministries require universities to investigate the matter, and SPD and Green fractions lobbied on the issue.[47] Aly intensified the public shock and horror with an article in the prestigious weekly newspaper, *Die Zeit*, on 3 February 1989 focusing on Hallervorden's request for brains ("the more the better"/"je mehr desto lieber").[48] Aly reflected how the problem related not only to the perpetrators but also to the wider scientific and medical community, "I have not heard of one German anatomist who after the war repudiated Nazi practices and buried his ill-gotten collection".[49]

On 8 February 1989 the Bavarian Ministry for Science and the Arts ordered that all specimens of Nazi victims and those of uncertain origins should be removed.[50] This established a pattern for wholesale and rapid removal of specimens. But it left unresolved questions of provenance of the specimens in terms of whether any were "euthanasia" or concentration camp victims.

These would in turn have raised uncomfortable questions about the involvement of scientists in the Nazi "euthanasia" policies. While the killings of psychiatric patients were acknowledged, the role of researchers in obtaining brains and other body parts was not. The Minister for Science and Culture, Baden-Württemberg on 20 January 1989 and then the Hessen Ministry of Science required anatomical institutes to conduct a survey of their collections. Finally, the German conference of rectors on 25/26 January called for all West German ministers for higher education (*Kultusminister*) to undertake surveys of collections, and to remove specimens of victims of National Socialism and – importantly – those specimens of questionable origin.[51] The period of denial and inertia of the 1980s had become transformed: removal and disposal were seen as a means of offering a final solution to the problem of anatomical body parts. Removal – nothing was recommended as to subsequent handling of the body parts – was prioritised over finding out about provenance.

The University of Tübingen was exceptional and exemplary in its conduct: it rapidly issued a public apology on 11 January 1989, and then convened a full commission on the matter. Anatomist Michael Arnold published in the *Deutsche Ärzteblatt* on 9 February 1989 on the need for transparency.[52] The Commission examined the contents of collections on a university-wide basis, and fully investigated the provenance of each specimen, taking account of earlier Allied post-war investigations, the definition of a National Socialist victim, and associated ethical questions. Within the Commission the Tübingen university institute directors were defensive; they clashed frequently with the medical student representative, the civic figure of the historian Benigna Schönhagen who had just completed her dissertation on *Tübingen im Nationalsozialismus*, as well as the external representative from the law faculty in Basel, Switzerland. The Commission's report was presented on 13 July 1989.[53] Removal was accompanied by identification and full disclosure as to provenance.

The Tübingen model set a standard of best practice. The MPG recognised the importance of the "Tübingen formula", but the MPG adapted the model in two ways. The first was to modify the idea of a public commission to conform to the MPG's internal procedures, essentially that of autonomy and self-administration free from governmental regulation. The MPG President Heinz Staab asked MPG archivist Eckart Henning to examine all relevant documents, patient files and specimen collections from the period 1933–45.[54] Second, in the course of this, the MPG opted for complete removal of all dubious specimens from the period 1933–45. This complied with the requirements of the *Kultusminister* conference, and avoided the time-consuming tasks of tracing provenance and providing identification. This arose from a sense that the pressures of the situation called for prompt resolution, although the wider questions of scientists' complicity in the killings were uncomfortable. Given the location of MPG collections in diverse institutes and their size, it would have taken some time and considerable research to have conducted provenance research and identification of its specimens at a time when public pressure was building up. There were two further factors. First, the MPG understood that opinions might differ on exactly how to define a Nazi victim. The main international sensibilities concerned Jewish victims, and it was primarily in Germany that radicals were concerned with the "euthanasia" killings of the mentally ill and disabled. Second, the hope that removal of all dubious specimens would ensure closure of the issue was an incentive for adopting the solution of rapid disposal.

Thus the MPG did not convene a public commission with external experts but conducted an internal review. The MPG archivist undertook a survey of institute holdings for neurological research, brain research and psychiatry.[55] The MPG was faced with the choice of a wholesale removal of specimens from the Nazi period, or (as Tübingen) instituting a commission to identify those preparations having an unethical provenance. Given that the latter would take time, a wholesale removal of all dubious specimens appeared the better option.[56] In actuality the MPIBR set out to remove all specimens from the Nazi era (although some were overlooked). The Max Planck Institute for Psychiatry (MPIP) attempted to distinguish between "euthanasia" specimens and others. The lack of a comprehensive reference resource identifying the victims of "euthanasia" impeded such a division. The records of Hans Schleussing, the former *Kaiser-Wilhelm-Gesellschaft* (KWG) Prosector at the psychiatric hospital of Eglfing-Haar were not consulted, and became unavailable. Indeed, the MPIP was highly defensive. It is possible that a reluctance of scientists to lose valuable specimens also impeded dispersal. Certainly it appears in retrospect that the decision as to what constituted a specimen from "euthanasia" or other war victims was not done as carefully as it should have been. The Max Planck Institute for Neurological Research (MPINR) in Cologne divested itself of just three specimens out of 2,394 for burial. The declared aim of wholesale removal of specimens from the Nazi era was in practice partial and poorly documented.

What was missing was a commemorative public listing of the names of persons buried, and no inventory of the slides sent for burial was compiled. In 2010 I wrote to the President of the MPG asking for a listing of the persons buried in 1990.[57] It emerged that remarkably no listing was compiled at the time of the burial: in 2015 a partial listing related to Munich eventually surfaced. What emerges is the need to trace slides from the point of killing and the transfer to particular scientists, and then the need to trace the history of the specimen through a maze of transfers and publications.

On 27 April 1989 the MPG decided to follow its understanding of the "Tübingen formula", in that all specimens for which the provenance was uncertain should be cremated. The ashes were to be buried. The initial proposal was that glass slides would be buried as a melted glass block.[58] This led to some disagreements, as not all scientists wished to relinquish slide collections, especially when a Nazi provenance was uncertain. The MPG re-inspected collections and pressed for a removal and collective burial of all slides and specimens of uncertain provenance for the period 1933–45.[59] All documentation was meant to be transferred to the MPG archives. By this time Aly shifted his position from destruction to acquiescing in burial. Thus effectively, both critics and holders of the collection found common ground with rapid removal and burial.

However, not everyone agreed with the burial. Wolfgang Schlote as Director of the Edinger Neurological Institute, Frankfurt am Main stated in a letter to *Die Zeit* that a mass grave was inappropriate.[60] The slides needed to be kept at the relevant institute or in a special documentation centre, taking the view that an anonymised collective burial was undignified. He finally reflected that we could never free ourselves from the past, but remembering was the way that one might live with it.[61]

There was no composite listing issued to the public or kept for reference to the remains, which were buried at the *Waldfriedhof* (Woodland Cemetery). A statement of 25 May 1990 was that the burial consisted of: eight "euthanasia" victims from the Hallervorden collection along with thousands of slides of unknown provenance; from Cologne, three uncertain cases; from Munich 650 cases of which 162 were children killed in "euthanasia" in Haar, and seven executed persons. Overall, 2,940 specimens were removed from the Hallervorden Collection, housed at the Edinger institute. Other specimens came for MPINR (Cologne), and the MPIP (Munich). From the aviation collection (*Luftwaffensammlung*) that had involved the neuro-pathologist Hugo Spatz (who also received one or two brains from Rascher in Dachau) 1,400 specimens and ca. 250 organs were removed.[62] The fate of the brains from the Warsaw Ghetto remains unclear.

The MPG took the burial in the Munich *Waldfriedhof* on 25 May 1990 as the opportunity to stress *Selbstbegrenzung*.[63] The implication of this principle of "self-restraint" was that this was an internal matter for academics to resolve responsibly without political or public interference. The burial tangibly demonstrated MPG autonomy: but it has become clear that the autonomy went with obfuscation, and only partial disclosure. What has emerged is that the lack of clarity over who was buried: confusion over who was a "euthanasia" victim and the circumstances of death means revisiting these issues has become necessary. The MPG takes responsibility for the KWG (there were certainly multiple continuities) and the KWG as a high-achieving scientific organisation. The issues of brain tissues and coerced research leave many open questions unresolved by the rapid burial.

The MPIP examined the provenance of executed victims, drawing a distinction between different categories of criminality. It suggested that only certain persons be accorded burial at the *Waldfriedhof*, as 14 appeared to have been legitimately condemned, whereas six persons were genuine victims of the Nazi *Terrorjustiz*.[64] The evaluation of the MPIP holdings of archives meant that the "genealogical collection Rüdin" was evaluated as extensive – as a gigantic experiment covering the whole of Germany, linking the hereditary records of all hospital patients. This statement would seem to establish the value of its extensive patient and genealogical records. But in the rush to remove potential items of controversy, this collection was declared to be of no academic value and that it should consequently be destroyed.[65] Fortunately, later memoranda endorsed the historical value of the collection. The collection and the extent to which it has survived have an immense historical importance that needs to be fully assessed. Roelcke demonstrated Rüdin's links to research on "idiot" children at Heidelberg. What is needed is to examine Rüdin's research networks so as to reconstruct the extent of coercive experimentation, and to establish whether patient brain specimens were collected. The number of victims, particularly from "euthanasia" killings, remained in dispute – the MPG at first in 1989 conceded responsibility for 33 children. Estimates rose to ca. 700 children as "euthanasia" victims in the Hallervorden collection.[66] The brain pathologist Heinz Wässle has courageously reviewed the situation, and he has raised the possibility that a further thousand brains from the so-called "Series H" derived from "euthanasia" victims.[67]

The memorial ceremony took place on 25 May 1990 at the *Waldfriedhof* Munich. The officiating religious ministers – Roman Catholic, Protestant and Jewish – did not raise the issue of identity and provenance of those being buried. Indeed, one wonders whether any Jewish victims' body parts were buried at the ceremony? At least one French prisoner of war, whose brain tissues were buried, was Moslem. The officiating ministers legitimated a ceremony predicated on the idea of victims as a collectivity rather than as named and identified individuals.

The controversy found resonance abroad. International pressure threatened a boycott of German medical research, and this called for a rapid response. The MPG realised that identification would take considerable time and resources. It preferred complete and wholesale removal in the hope of settling the problem definitively. The international criticism called for identification, but did not offer to participate in what would have amounted to a significant undertaking. Those involved in criticising Nazi science from overseas never thought of making available resources of documentation in locations such as the USA and Canada (where crates of documents on Nazi science and medicine were sent by post-war Canadian scientific intelligence officers). Indeed in the Canadian case, what happened in terms of the seized documentation as part of a policy of scientific exploitation has never been assessed, and what happened to the crates of documents on medicine under National Socialism remains unclear.[68]

The Canadian physician William Seidelman argued forthrightly as regards the anatomical victims: "There must be public documentation of who these people once were, how they died and how institutions representing science, medicine and higher education used their remains for almost half a century after the defeat of the Nazi regime".[69] On 12 September 1989 Seidelman and Arthur Caplan issued "A Call for an international commemoration".[70] They sought to internationalise the understanding of any burials, and to view them as significant in the context of bioethics. Seidelman was shown the burial by Professor Kreutzberg to make the point that the slides matter was now closed.[71]

The student representative body, the *Fachschaft Medizin*, in Frankfurt considered various alternatives. The Frankfurt anatomist Jürgen Winckler, requested that the specimens be retained as both a memorial and a warning to scientists. German universities considered that the reactions in Israel and North America were exaggerated, but they wished to appease their critics in order that current research collaborations should not be disrupted. The reactions showed a high level of sensitivity over Jewish victims, and this led to wider concerns over the high numbers of victims. There was public and political criticism of the medical research establishment on the domestic front. The Hessen Minister for Science and the Arts, Wolfgang Gerhardt (ironically a name also used by Mengele) complained about the reluctance of universities to survey their collections, and that he obtained a response only on the second time of requesting information. Frankfurt and Heidelberg adopted policies of rapid disposal. In the event the search for body parts from Auschwitz that might have been held by von Verschuer did not produce anything, although here the search evidently lacked thoroughness as the evidence is that Karin Magnussen retained the heterochromic eye specimens while working as a schoolteacher in Bremen.[72]

In the Federal state of Baden-Württemberg the SPD presented a petition on 12 January 1989. There was wider unease among rectors and institute directors. The Heidelberg University Rector Volker Sellin phoned through the order for "complete removal" (*vollständige Entfernung*) of brain specimens on 13 January 1989 – "removal" being understood in terms of burial and in the case of glass slides their destruction.[73] On 20 January the state decreed that specimens obtained under National Socialism could no longer be used for teaching and research. Twenty-seven bodies and 12 sets of slides were removed from the anatomical collection, and in October 1990 buried in a collective grave marked to honour them as victims of Nazi justice. Their individual names were not given. It was stated that the remains of children killed for research under the psychiatrist Carl Schneider were removed in the 1960s; around this time specimens of children killed for research at the Psychiatric Institute disappeared.[74]

By August 1990 the Hessen *Wissenschaftsministerium* and Frankfurt University were discussing burial arrangements. Universities in general favoured rapid "disposal" following the MPG's example, rather than any investigative commission on the Tübingen model. For unrelated reasons Minister Gerhardt had to resign with the collapse of coalition in 1991, so that he could no longer contribute to the final report of the conference of *Kultusminister*. The momentum of political pressure was lost.

The victims' bodies were seen as "polluting" German anatomical collections. The rapid disposal of specimens meant that rarely was there any investigation of provenance and identification. The whole "disposal" operation was conducted with little publicly available documentation. The hope was that with burial of the scientific specimens, the controversy would also be finally buried. The burial of body parts from certain universities took place at the Central

Cemetery (*Hauptfriedhof*) in Frankfurt am Main in early December 1990. There were buried: 45 macroscopic specimens, one skull of unknown origins, 30 preparations of tumours and malformations from the Frankfurt obstetrics clinic, 35 histological preparations from the University of Marburg, six specimens of veins from executed persons, ten specimens from the universities of Heidelberg and Leipzig, and a further 2,050 specimens from the Frankfurt neurological institute. Burial was in large aluminium containers, following the precedent of the MPG. Following the MPG precedent, there was no identification of the persons buried.

Medical students complained that their researches into provenance were blocked. The student representative bodies (*Fachschaften Medizin*) of Frankfurt, Giessen and Marburg, and the student council, the ASTA Frankfurt protested that organisations of victims and the persecuted were not invited to the burial of body parts from Hessen universities in the Frankfurt *Hauptfriedhof* in December 1990. Moreover, the students asked why were there no identifications and why was no research project on the topic initiated? With a flourish of heavy-handed irony, the students complained that it was the successors of the Nazi perpetrators who organised the burial.[75] Newspapers like the *Frankfurter Allgemeine Zeitung* (FAZ) publicised these protests. The *FAZ* reporter noted the absence of identifying names for commemoration – who the dead were, men, women or children, how many – all was unknown.[76]

The pattern for most universities was a shift from denial to rapid disposal. The anatomical museum Hamburg was closed down, but resisted scrutiny.[77] Each German institution investigated and disposed of the body parts, as it thought best. There was no national collation of evidence, apart from a perfunctory final report to the *Kultusminister* by the German universities in 1994. The report prioritised removal, but did not inquire further as regards the earlier removals of specimens and documents from the Psychiatric Institute Heidelberg or the Anatomical Institute of the Charité Hospital, Berlin.[78]

The critics stressed the priority of removal and disposal, rather than identification and documenting provenance. In July 1990 the Frankfurt anatomist, Jürgen Winckler made a perceptive comment. He criticised the representative student *Fachschaft* as demanding what amounted to a "posthumous cleansing". He pleaded that these specimens of a traumatic period should be retained by institutes as a *Mahnung*, a warning. Winckler was clearly uneasy with the prevalent parlance – the idea was that victims' remains somehow polluted collections. He was concerned about the mode of thinking that scientific integrity had to be defended, whereas the victims' body parts were deemed extraneous and defiling.

The Tübingen medical student Christoph Rubens went further: he argued that respect for the victims meant that they should not be used as objects of historical research. This position raises a further question – how historical research can serve the interests of commemoration? An alternative view would be that historical research is in the victims' interests in that it restores a sense of human identity and integrity, and explains the reasons for the murderous dissections. The need for independent historical commissions was not yet recognised. However, the Tübingen commission realised a need for new guidelines and – something still not done – the adopting of international standards on how medical institutions should act regarding body parts of victims killed in the context of genocide and political injustice.[79]

The Tübingen commission raised the difficulty of how to define a victim of Nazism. Initially, attention at a national and international level was limited to Jewish and then to "euthanasia" victims. The Tübingen commission worked at first with a definition taken from the German compensation law of 1953. For anatomy it was problematic given the overall rise in executions under National Socialism, excluding certain categories of victims, not least suicides, and persons executed by special courts. The Commission recognised that there were substantial ethical problems regarding so-called "legally acquired bodies". The Commission concluded with admirable reflections on the need for fully open documentation, as well as ethical guidelines as the basis of anatomical collections that would bring Germany into line with other countries.

William Seidelman was now invited to Germany to scrutinise the Commission's findings. Seidelman had reports of undisclosed body parts in Munich, but their existence could not be confirmed. In effect Seidelman took on the role of external scrutineer. The strength of his position was that he was well connected with the North American medical establishment, whom the German Foreign Office and academic interests were anxious to appease. Despite his engaged and committed efforts, his *de facto* role as scrutineer was by no means easy to fulfil, as the German academic institutions wanted closure rather than on-going research and commemoration. A full-scale critical history using archives and institute records did not follow.[80]

The final report of the conference of *Kultusminister* of 25 January 1994 was a summary overview. The report took account of Seidelman's inquiries (although his name was consistently misspelt and universities incorrectly located) and of the inadequate disclosures by universities in the former German Democratic Republic. The University of Jena claimed not to have retained bodies from the era of National Socialism.[81] The actual extent of anatomists' involvement under Nazism was not under discussion.[82] The report came to conclusions that minimised the issue. For in declaring that only two federal states (Baden-Württemberg and Hessen) found with certainty specimens with a Nazi origin; the report conceded that in seven *Länder* there were specimens whose provenance was uncertain.[83]

Overall, the report by the conference of *Kultusminister* was cursory – giving no indications of numbers of victims. The report relied on official notifications by university institutes. The question of individual identification was ignored showing that officials were concerned with removal and burial. The report was not published, again indicating a lack of accountability on the part of the German academic and political establishment. Regrettably from today's hindsight, it is clear that the report contained a number of inaccuracies. It was assumed that if an institute was destroyed in the war that its post-war collections were free from Nazi victims. This need not necessarily be the case given that collections could be out-housed, transferred and amalgamated. Moreover, student claims of confronting decapitated cadavers at institutes as at Giessen were later substantiated.

Austria had to wait for the international furore over the Pernkopf anatomical atlas, when the University of Vienna convened a commission that did investigate provenance.[84] The inclusion of the brain specimens from the Spiegelgrund, and the death of Heinrich Gross, opened the way to the burial of the specimens in 2004.[85] Specimens and face masks of Jews rounded up at the Prater Stadium and (as the chapter by Margit Berner explains) subsequently held at the Natural History Museum were also covered by the commission.[86]

Seidelman took a crucial role in driving forward the issue, as again the prospect of exclusion from North American medical circles caused concern. The University of Vienna conducted comprehensive evaluations of all holdings, and certain other Vienna collections – notably that of the Spiegelgrund children. At first, the City of Vienna decided not to opt for "disposal" or burial of the children's remains, but for an alternative, namely turning the collection into a memorial to itself, thereby avoiding its destruction. It is interesting to note that certain neuro-anatomists had also suggested this for the MPG specimens but that these were deemed not *Archivgut* (suitable for an archive). The report was not published, but remains available on demand.[87] The Vienna Municipality hoped that the public burial and named commemoration would provide an endpoint as regards Nazi body parts, but there is increasing realisation that much further investigation needs to be made of how medical institutions exploited the bodies of Nazi victims for research. Other Austrian anatomical institutes, notably Graz and Innsbruck, have still to resolve these issues.[88]

Clearly, the majority of German universities and research institutes only followed what had become known as "the Tübingen model" in terms of disposal of specimens from Nazi victims or of doubtful provenance, but not their identification. Coming under public, student and international scientific pressure, the solution was that of rapid disposal of body parts. Collective burial in a grave without victims' names appeared to offer closure without any awkward contact with relatives (although the Spiegelgrund burials shows that naming was unproblematic). The German Anatomical Society (*Anatomische Gesellschaft*) took no position on the issue. No thought was given to German anatomical institutes beyond the borders of the Federal Republic. What the situation might have been at the Reich Universities of Strassburg, Posen and Königsberg was not considered. The Strassburg case shows the need to identify victims, as until the victims were identified by Hans-Joachim Lang, all except one – identified from the tattoo of his Auschwitz number – were unidentified.[89] Non-identification of the victims' remains left multiple issues unresolved. The dissenting views of the Frankfurt anatomists Schlote and Winckler show great sensitivity. The idea of continuing responsibility directly contrasted with the policies of rapid disposal and closure.

Towards historical and public accountability

It often remains necessary to identify the victims, the history of research undertaken on the body parts until the time of disposal, the circumstances of the disposal in each institution, the persons with administrative responsibility, and finally the legacy in terms of commemoration and any historical researches. Each victim deserves named commemoration, as well as documentation that is as full as possible.[90] The questions dealt with shows how standards have changed since the 1980s. There is a greater readiness to divulge information on the period of National Socialism, and a far less defensive attitude. The transformation of values coincided with longer-term structural changes of reunification. Here the universities of Berlin, Halle and Jena have shown themselves ready to engage with their past.[91] Identification and burial of victims in Vienna, and a memorial in Heidelberg for victims of brain anatomical research (albeit only partially named) are just two examples of recognition of victims as persons. These innovations represent on-going responsibilities rather than the closure that was strived for in the early 1990s.

In their time, marking the site of atrocity with a collective memorial was an achievement. But names were withheld. How problematic this was can be seen with the MPG memorial in the *Waldfriedhof*, Munich in 1990. When considered against earlier denials, this was a notable commemoration and public admission. But on closer scrutiny the lack of names meant things remained at a very generalised level. Tracing victim life histories from clinic to laboratory was not possible. A commemorative listing was not compiled leaving questions open. The MPIBR in Frankfurt sent specimens comprehensively, and the MPIP in Munich only selectively showed the high level of institute autonomy.

The MPG President Hubert Markl convened a commission on the history of the KWG under National Socialism from 1999, running until 2005. On 7 June 2001 MPG President Markl gave a momentous apology to the Mengele twins and other victims of research. Markl drew on the work of the commission to provide evidence for his apology.[92] The emphasis in the Commission shifted from the Kaiser Wilhelm Institute (KWI) for Psychiatry to the KWI for Anthropology. It was easier for the MPG to accept a critical analysis of an institute that no longer existed (i.e., the KWI for Anthropology) than the MPIP. There was considerable expertise on the commission concerning the history of brain research under National Socialism. Coincidentally, a set of brain slides of about 100 persons were located in the MPG Archives in Berlin-Dahlem in 2001 Remarkably, these further slides were not brought to the attention of the MPG Presidential Commission, which could have identified whether "euthanasia" victims were among the victims. There is a significant distinction between retention of "euthanasia" victim specimens and specimens from patients whose death was clinically unavoidable.

The other shift that occurred following the collective burial in 1990 is the expectation of individual commemoration. The ethic in Holocaust history is increasingly for individual identification and commemoration. This is also the case with respect to victims of other genocides. Whereas the Hallervorden slides were buried anonymously, a group of slides were found among those of the Spiegelgrund in Vienna of two brothers and a cousin from the Kutschke family, whom Hallervorden had had killed because of the research interest in the Pelizeus-Merzbacher genetic disorder. The slides were removed to Vienna by the researcher Franz Seitelberger, who completed his doctorate under Hallervorden and was later Rector of the University of Vienna.

Alfred Kutschke (3 November 1934–6 Apri; 1942), cousin, Günther Kutschke (4 April 1939–18 February 1942), brother and Herbert Kutschke (22 January 1943–24 April 1944), brother, were buried in an individually named grave at the Görden psychiatric hospital in 2003.[93]

The Federal Republic is caught in a debate between the cloaking of "euthanasia" victims under anonymity and permitting a publicly accessible list of names of all "euthanasia" victims. The issue is rendered more complicated in that body and brain of a victim can be in two locations. The finding of 30,000 case files for "T-4" victims among the Ministry for State Security/ *Ministerium für Staatssicherheit* ("Stasi") records in the 1990s has opened new opportunities for research. The Stasi found these records at Pfafferode in Thuringia in 1960, and used them to identify perpetrators, but took no interest in the victims.[94]

The neuropathologist Jürgen Peiffer set out to reconstruct from where brains were obtained and under what circumstances in an ambitious record-linkage based study covering Germany (but not Austria or Poland). He published some statistical evaluations, although the anonymisation means that verification of the statistics in the light of new institutional case studies is likely to mean further modification. In 2015 Bavarian archivists mounted a solid front against historians, victim relatives and numerous psychiatrists against the public naming of victims.[95] Remarkably, also in 2015 the brain pathologist Heinz Wässle found a set of unburied slides in the MPS archive, that had actually been deposited there since at least the time of the President's KWG research programme. This raises further questions regarding the collective burial in 1990.[96] It was for these reasons that in 2016 the MPS has decided to carry out a complete review of its specimens. The way forward for both commemoration and historical understanding is certainly identifying victims of Nazi killings, and reconstructing the fate of their brains and body parts.

There is new recognition that at least names of victims without diagnoses can be publicly released. Assessing the conduct of institutions in terms of the damage that they inflicted is fundamental. The benefits of disclosure are considerable in showing a responsible, accountable and transparent attitude to research. These researches expose a lack of procedure in Austria and Germany regarding the period of National Socialism. First, all documentation needs to be kept. There is no guarantee that further destruction of documents will not occur. Second, files should be accessible to historical researchers. Third, there should be agreement on the need for establishing provenance when it comes to all specimens. The necessity for this is indicated by the destruction of a scientific collection of bones found at the back of the former KWI for Anthropology. That the bones and site are a responsibility of the Free University of Berlin shows the lack of formal procedures regarding the establishing of provenance. The issue as to whether the bones were sent from Auschwitz or were part of the anthropologist Eugen Fischer's African collection remains unresolved. Similarly, the confusion surrounding the burial of slides in a collective grave in 1990 by the MPS can only be resolved by provenance research regarding the identity of persons and the circumstance of death. Post-war Germany and Austria have only reluctantly faced up to surviving victims, the body parts of the deceased and documentation on the killings and scientific exploitation. Where there has been disclosure, it has only been partial; the compensation inadequate. Restrictions on the release of documents and the naming of victims amounts to – if not perpetrator protection – then an excessive protecting of institutions and their reputations. Research on these matters has often been difficult in terms of negotiating access to files. Archivists have varied greatly in access allowed. Constructing an evidence-based documentation on the victims of coerced experiments has been hardest of all in the Federal Republic of Germany.

Notes

1 This is a revised and extended version of: Paul Weindling, ' "Cleansing" Anatomical Collections: The Politics of Removing Specimens from German Anatomical and Medical Collections 1988–92', *Annals of Anatomy*, 194.3 (2012), pp. 237–242. Since 2012 there have been substantial developments regarding body parts and brain tissues from the era of National Socialism.

2 Sabine Hildebrandt, *The Anatomy of Murder. Ethical Transgressions and Anatomical Science during the Third Reich*, New York: Berghahn, 2016, pp. 258–268; Herwig Czech, 'Von der Richtstätte auf den Seziertisch. Zur anatomischen Verwertung von NS-Opfern in Wien, Innsbruck und Graz', *Jahrbuch des Dokumentationsarchivs des österreichischen Widerstandes*, 1 (2015), pp. 141–190.

3 Alexander Mitscherlich and Fred Mielke, *Wissenschaft ohne Menschlichkeit*, Heidelberg: Lambert Schneider, 1949, idem, *Medizin ohne Menschlichkeit, Dokumente des Nürnberger Ärzteprozesses*, Frankfurt am Main: S. Fischer, 1960; idem, *Doctors of Infamy: the Story of the Nazi Medical Crimes*, New York: Henry Schuman, 1949.

4 Alice Platen-Hallermund, *Die Tötung Geisteskranker in Deutschland: Aus der deutschen Ärzte-Kommission beim amerikanischen Militärgericht*, Frankfurt am Main: Verlag der Frankfurter Hefte, 1948; Reinhard Schlüter, *Leben für eine humane Medizin: Alice Ricciardi-von Platen – Psychoanalytikerin und Protokollantin des Nürnberger Ärzteprozesses*, Frankfurt am Main: Campus, 2012; Paul Weindling, 'Alice Ricciardi von Platen', *The Guardian* (13 Mar 2008), www.theguardian.com/world/2008/mar/13/secondworldwar.germany (accessed 18 July 2016).

5 College Park, MD, National Archives and Records Administration (hereafter NARA), RG 549 Records of US Army Europe, War Crimes Case Files 1945–59, 50–2–102 to 50–2–103, Box 322 [Brachtel Trial]; Ibid., RG 153 Records of the Office of the Judge Advocate General (Army), War Crimes Branch, Case Files, 1944–49, 12–226: Vol. 1 Trial Record Part 8 thru 12–226: Vol. 1 Clemency, Box Number 185 [Schilling Trial]; Arolsen, International Tracing Service Archive, Ordner Medizinische Menschenversuche 19, 14 May 1969, 12 page typescript.

6 'Case VI, Decision and Judgment VIII', in *Trials of War Criminals before the Nuernberg Military Tribunals under Control Council Law No.10. Nuernberg October 1946–April 1949. Vol. VII: IG Farben Case*, Washington, DC: US Government Printing Office, 1950, p. 1172.

7 Christine Wolters, *Tuberkulose und Menschenversuche im Nationalsozialismus. Das Netzwerk hinter den Tbc-Experimenten im Konzentrationslager Sachsenhausen*, Stuttgart: Franz Steiner, 2011; NARA [Brachtel Trial]; Ralph Forsbach and Hans-Georg Hofer, *Die Deutsche Gesellschaft für Innere Medizin in der NS-Zeit*, Stuttgart: Thieme, 2015.

8 Stefanie Michaela Baumann, *Menschenversuche und Wiedergutmachung*, Munich: Oldenbourg, 2009.

9 See the chapter by Anna von Villiez.

10 Herwig Czech, 'Selektion und Kontrolle. Der "Spiegelgrund" als zentrale Institution der Wiener Jugendfürsorge zwischen 1940 und 1945', in Eberhard Gabriel and Wolfgang Neugebauer (eds), *Von der Zwangssterilisierung zur Ermordung. Zur Geschichte der NS-Euthanasie in Wien, Teil II*, Vienna: Böhlau, 2002, pp. 165–187

11 'Ausgemustert', *Der Spiegel*, (11.12.1972), pp. 58–59. My thanks to Aleksandra Loewenau.

12 Ernst Klee, *Was sie taten – was sie wurden. Ärzte, Juristen und andere Beteiligte am Kranken- und Judenmord*, Frankfurt am Main: S. Fischer, 1986; Heather Pringle, *The Master Plan: Himmler's Scholars and the Holocaust*, New York: Hyperion, 2006; Hans-Joachim Lang, *Die Namen der Nummern. Wie es gelang, die 86 Opfer eines NS-Verbrechens zu identifizieren*, Hamburg: Hoffmann und Campe, 2004; Paul Weindling, 'Rassenkundliche Forschung zwischen dem Getto Litzmannstadt und Auschwitz: Hans Fleischhackers Tübinger Habilitation, Juni 1943', in Jens Kolata, Richard Kühl, Henning Tümmers and Urban Wiesing (eds), *In Fleischhackers Händen. Wissenschaft, Politik und das 20. Jahrhundert. [Anlässlich der Ausstellung "In Fleischhackers Händen, Tübinger Rassenforscher in Łódź 1940–1942" im Schloss Hohentübingen (24. April bis 28 Juni 2015)*, Tübingen: MUT, 2015, pp. 141–164.

13 Maurice Papworth, *Human Guinea Pigs: Experimentation on Man*, London: Routledge, 1967.

14 Carola Sachse, ' "Whitewash Culture": How the Kaiser Wilhelm/Max Planck Society Dealt with the Nazi Past', in Susanne Heim, Carola Sachse and Mark Walker (eds), *The Kaiser Wilhelm Society under National Socialism*, Cambridge: Cambridge University Press, 2009, pp. 373–399; Hans-Walter Schmuhl, *Grenzüberschreitungen. Das Kaiser-Wilhelm-Institut für Anthropologie, menschliche Erblehre und Eugenik 1927–1945*, Göttingen: Wallstein, 2005, pp. 528–530; Paul Weindling, *Health, Race and German Politics between National Unification and Nazism, 1870–1945*, Cambridge: Cambridge University Press, 1989, pp. 565–570.

15 Thomas Schmelter, Christine Meesmann, Gisela Walter and Herwig Praxl, 'Heil- und Pflegeanstalt Werneck', in Michael von Cranach and Hans-Ludwig Siemen (eds), *Psychiatrie im Nationalsozialismus. Die Bayerischen Heil- und Pflegeanstalten zwischen 1933 und 1945*, Munich: Oldenbourg, 1999, pp. 35–54; Paul Weindling, *Victims and Survivors of Nazi Human Experiments – Science and Suffering in the Holocaust*, London: Bloomsbury, 2015, p. 34.

16 Personal communication, Eduard Gabriel to the author, Mar 2016.

17 Hildebrandt, *Anatomy of Murder*.

18 Robert Proctor, *Racial Hygiene. Medicine under the Nazis*, Cambridge, MA: Harvard University Press, 1988, p. 3.

19 Weindling, *Health, Race and German Politics*, p. 462; idem, 'Die Preussische Medizinalverwaltung und die "Rassenhygiene" ', in Achim Thom and Horst Spaar (eds), *Medizin und Faschismus*, Berlin: Akademie für ärztliche Fortbildung, 1983, pp. 23–35.

20 Walter Wuttke-Groneberg, *Medizin im Nationalsozialismus. Ein Arbeitsbuch*, Tübingen: Schwäbische Verlagsgesellschaft, 1982; Projektgruppe "Volk und Gesundheit" (ed.), *Volk*

und Gesundheit. Heilen und Vernichten im Nationalsozialismus. Begleitbuch zur gleichnamigen Ausstellung im Ludwig-Uhland-Institut für Empirische Kulturwissenschaft der Universität Tübingen, Tübingen: Tübinger Vereinigung für Volkskunde, 1982.

21 Paul Weindling, 'Shattered Alternatives in Medicine', *History Workshop Journal*, 16 (1983), pp. 152–157.

22 Alfons Labisch and Florian Tennstedt, *Der Weg zum "Gesetz über die Vereinheitlichung des Gesundheitswesens" vom 3. Juli 1934. Entwicklungslinien und Entwicklungsmomente des staatlichen und kommunalen Gesundheitswesens in Deutschland*, Düsseldorf: Akademie für öffentliches Gesundheitswesen, 1985.

23 Gerhard Baader and Ulrich Schultz (eds), *Medizin und Nationalsozialismus. Tabuisierte Vergangenheit – Ungebrochene Tradition?*, Berlin: Verlagsgesellschaft Gesundheit, 1980.

24 Karl Heinz Roth (ed.), *Erfassung zur Vernichtung. Von der Sozialhygiene zum "Gesetz über Sterbehilfe"*, Berlin: Verlagsgesellschaft Gesundheit, 1984; Paul Weindling, 'Soziale Hygiene, Eugenik und medizinische Praxis: Der Fall Alfred Grotjahn', *Das Argument. Jahrbuch für kritische Medizin* (1984), pp. 6–20.

25 Gisela Bock, *Zwangssterilisation im Nationalsozialismus*, Opladen: Westdt. Verlag, 1986.

26 Christian Pross and Rolf Winau (eds), *Nicht misshandeln. Das Krankenhaus Moabit 1920–1933. Ein Zentrum jüdischer Ärzte in Berlin, 1933–1945. Verfolgung – Widerstand – Zerstörung*, Berlin: Hentrich, 1984; Christian Pross, *Wiedergutmachung. Der Kleinkrieg gegen die Opfer*, Frankfurt am Main: Athanäum, 1988.

27 Marius Turda and Paul Weindling, *Blood and Homeland: Eugenics in Central Europe 1900–1940*, Budapest: Central European University Press, 2006; Paul Weindling, 'A City Regenerated: Eugenics, Race and Welfare in Interwar Vienna', in Deborah Holmes and Lisa Silverman (eds), *Interwar Vienna: Culture between Tradition and Modernity*, New York: Camden House, 2009, pp. 81–113.

28 Carola Sachse, 'Was bedeutet eine Entschuldigung? Die Überlebenden medizinischer NS Verbrechen und die Max-Planck-Gesellschaft', in Heinrich Berger, Melanie Dejnega, Regina Fritz and Alexander Prenninger (eds), *Politische Gewalt und Machtausübung im 20. Jahrhundert*, Vienna: Böhlau, 2011, pp. 631–649; Paul Weindling, 'Sonstige Personenschäden – die Entschädigungspraxis der Stiftung "Erinnerung, Verantwortung und Zukunft"', in Constantin Goschler (ed), *Die Entschädigung von NS-Zwangsarbeit am Anfang des 21. Jahrhunderts*, Vol. 2, Göttingen: Wallstein, 2012, pp. 197–225.

29 Detlev Peukert, 'The Genesis of the "Final Solution" from the Spirit of Science', in Thomas Childers and Jane Caplan (eds), *Reevaluating the Third Reich*, New York: Holmes & Meier, 1994, pp. 234–252.

30 Götz Aly, ' "Weitere Elaborate Alys verhindern!". Gedächtnisschwund deutscher Hirnforscher', in idem, *Volk ohne Mitte: die Deutschen zwischen Freiheitsangst und Kollektivismus*, Frankfurt am Main: S. Fischer, 2015, pp. 201–239.

31 Idem, 'Der saubere und der schmutzige Fortschritt', in idem (ed.), *Reform und Gewissen. "Euthanasie" im Dienst des Fortschritts*, Berlin: Rotbuch Verlag, 1985, p. 73.

32 Berlin, Archiv der Max-Planck-Gesellschaft (hereafter MPG), E-I-F, Besondere Aufgaben Hirnschnittsammlung, Götz Aly, 'Einsichtsnahme', 4 July 1984.

33 Ibid., E-II-1a 1963, Aly to MPG President Heinz Staab, 17 Sept 1984, letter and report; Aly 'Der saubere und der schmutzige Fortschritt', p. 78.

34 MPG, E-II-1a 1963, Aly to MPG, 22 Jan 1985; ibid., G. Peters, 'Stellungnahme', 1985; Aly, 'Weitere Elaborate'.

35 Benno Müller-Hill, *Tödliche Wissenschaft: die Aussonderung von Juden, Zigeunern und Geisteskranken 1933–1945*, Reinbek bei Hamburg: Rowohlt, 1984; Hans Heese, *Augen aus Auschwitz – Ein Lehrstück über nationalsozialistischen Rassenwahn und medizinische Forschung – Der Fall Dr. Karin Magnussen*, Essen: Klartext, 2001.

36 NARA, Combined Intelligence Objectives Sub-Committee G-2 Division SHAEF (Rear) APO 413, Leo Alexander, 'Neuropathology and Neurophysiology, including Electroencephalography, in Wartime Germany', 20 July 1945; Paul Julian Weindling,

Nazi Medicine and the Nuremberg Trials. From Medical War Crimes to Informed Consent, Houndmills, Basingstoke: Palgrave Macmillan, 2004.

37 Vienna, Simon Wiesenthal Archives, Mengele files.

38 Karl Heinz Roth, 'Die wissenschaftliche Normalität des Schlächters', *Mitteilungen der Dokumentationsstelle zur NS-Sozialpolitik* 1.2 (1985), pp. 1–8; Paul Weindling, 'Blood, Race and Politics', *The Times Higher Education Supplement* (19 July 1985), p. 13.

39 Aly, 'Weitere Elaborate'.

40 Benigna Schönhagen, *Das Gräberfeld X. Eine Dokumentation über NS Opfer auf dem Tübinger Stadtfriedhof*, Tübingen: Kulturamt, 1987, p. 119.

41 M. Walsh, 'Nazi Research under the Microscope', *Time* (27 Feb 1989), pp. 34–35; Ulrich Drews, 'Die Zeit des Nationalsozialismus am anatomischen Institut in Tübingen. Unbeantwortete ethische Fragen damals und heute', in Jürgen Peiffer (ed.), *Menschenverachtung und Opportunismus,* Tübingen: Attempto, 1992, pp. 93–107.

42 Benigna Schönhagen, 'Cemetery X and the Origins of Corpses from Anatomical Institutes under NS: Recollections of Developments at Tübingen', www.pulse-project.org/node/630 (accessed 15 July 2016).

43 MPG, E-II-1a 1963, Badische Fernsehredaktion, *Präparate von NS Opfern*, 15 Dec 1988.

44 U. Völklein, 'Anatomie einer Ente', *Der Stern* (1989), pp. 159–160.

45 Walsh, 'Nazi Research'; Drews, 'Zeit des Nationalsozialismus'.

46 According to Dr Wischnath, formerly Tübingen University archivist, the controversy erupted when a TV camera crew was allowed into the archives: personal communication to the author, 2014.

47 S. Dickman, 'Scandal over Nazi victims' corpses rocks universities', *Nature*, 337 (1989), p. 195; idem, 'Brain sections to be buried?', *Nature*, 339 (1989), p. 498.

48 Götz Aly, ' "Je mehr, desto lieber", Über den Umgang mit Präparaten von Nazi-Opfern vor 1945 und danach', *Die Zeit* (3 Feb 1989), p. 69.

49 Walsh, 'Nazi Research under the Microscope'.

50 MPG, E-II-1a 1963, Bayerisches Staatsministerium für Wissenschaft und Kunst, 'Verwendung medizinischer Präparate von Leichen NS-Opfern', 8 Feb 1989.

51 Bonn, Konferenz der Kultusminister der Länder in der Bundesrepublik Deutschland (hereafter KKLBD), NS 112, AK 25./26. 1. 1989, NS Nr. 1,4, Beschluss der Kultusministerkonferenz vom 25./26. 1. 1989.

52 Michael Arnold, 'Anatomie im Zwielicht?', *Deutsches Ärzteblatt*, 6 (9 Feb 1989), pp. 21–22.

53 Tübingen University, 'Abschlussbericht der Commission zur Überprüfung der Präparätesammlungen in den medizinischen Einrichtungen der Universität Tübingen im Hinblick auf Opfer des Nationalsozialismus', Tübingen: 1989.

54 MPG, E-II-1a 1963, Staab to Hossmann, 28 Feb 1989.

55 Ibid., Staab to Eckart Henning, 28 Feb 1989.

56 Ibid., Eckart Henning, 'Abschlussbericht über die Aussonderung von Hirnpräparaten aus der Zeit des Nationalsozialismus im Max-Planck-Institut für Hirnforschung (Frankfurt/M), Max-Planck-Institut für neurologische Forschung (Köln) und im Max-Planck-Institut für Psychiatrie (München)', 3 Nov 1989.

57 Author to Prof. Peter Gruss, 1 Feb 2011; Felicitas von Aretin to author, 18 Feb 2011.

58 MPG, E-II-1F, 'Ergebnisvermerk Besprechung am 27.4.1989. 11.30 über Hirnpräparate aus der Zeit des Nationalsozialismus', 27 Apr 1989.

59 Ibid., E-II-1a 1963, Eckart Henning, 'Zwischenbericht. Stand der Aussonderungen von Hirnschnitten', 6 Sept 1989.

60 Wolfgang Schlote, 'Einziger Weg', *Die Zeit* (24 Nov 1989), p. 86.

61 MPG, E-II-1a 1963, Schlote to MPG President Staab, 26 Oct 1989.

62 Ibid., Wolfgang Schlote, 'Aktennotiz', 6 Oct 1989; Ibid., Eckart Henning, '2 Bericht', 19 mar 1989; ibid., E-II-1F, 'Ergebnisvermerk Besprechung'; Dickman, 'Brain sections to be buried?'; ibid.,'Memorial ceremony to be held'.

63   'Den Opfern zum Gedenken – den Lebenden zur Mahnung', *MPG Spiegel*, 3 (1990), p. 10.

64   MPG, E II-1a 1963, 'Überprüfung der Hinrichtungsgründe', 13 Feb 1990.

65   Ibid., E-II-1F, 'Ergebnisvermerk Besprechung'.

66   Ibid., 'Medienanalysen', 13 Oct 1989; Götz Aly, 'Hirnforschung im Dritten Reich. Bericht an die Max-Planck-Gesellschaft zur Förderung der Wissenschaften', *Die Tageszeitung* (21 Oct 1989), p. 16.

67   'Hundert Hirnschnitte und das Rätsel der "Serie H" ', *Rhein-Main Zeitung* (21 Apr 2015), p. 36.

68   Paul Weindling, *John W. Thompson. Psychiatrist in the Shadow of the Holocaust*, Rochester, NY: Rochester, University Press, 2010.

69   William Seidelman, 'Legacy of the Nazis', *Nature* (21 Sept 1989), p. 341.

70   MPG, E-II-I-F, William Seidelman and Arthur Caplan, 'A Call for an International Commemoration', 12 Sept 1989; ibid., Generalverwaltung MPG, William Seidelman fax to Edmund Marsch, 19 Sept 1989; William Seidelman, 'In memoriam. Medicine's Confrontation with Evil', *Hasting's Center Report* (Nov/Dec 1989), pp. 5–6.

71   Personal communication, William Seidelman to the author, 25 June 2016.

72   Heese, *Augen aus Auschwitz*, pp. 478–481.

73   Personal communication, Wolfgang Eckart to the author. See also Wolfgang U. Eckart, Volker Sellin and Eike Wolgast (eds), *Die Universität Heidelberg im Nationalsozialismus*, Heidelberg: Springer Medizin Verlag, 2006, pp. 665–666.

74   Christoph Mundt, Gerrit Hohendorf and Maike Rotzoll, *Psychiatrische Forschung und NS Euthanasie. Beiträge zu einer Gedenkveranstaltung an der Psychiatrischen Universitätsklinik Heidelberg*, Heidelberg: Wunderhorn, 2001.

75   Frankfurt am Main, Institut für Geschichte der Medizin, Akten der Medizinischen Fakultät, Verwendung medizinischer Präparate von Nazi-Opfern, Fachschaften Medizin Frankfurt Giessen Marburg, 'Presseerklärung', 16 Dec 1990.

76   R. Schostack, 'Trauergang. Deutsche Szene', *Frankfurter Allgemeine Zeitung* (29 May 1990).

77   Christiane Rothmaler, 'Gutachten und Dokumentation über das Anatomische Institut des Universitäts-Krankenhauses Eppendorf der Universität Hamburg 1933–1945', *1999: Zeitschrift für Sozialgeschichte des 20. und 21. Jahrhunderts*, 2 (1990), pp. 78–95.

78   KKLBD, IIIA 4630/II., 'Abschlussbericht. Präparate von Opfern des Nationalsozialismus in anatomischen und pathologischen Sammlungen deutscher Ausbildungs- und Forschungseinrichtungen. Bonn', 25 Jan 1994.

79   Caro, 'Mit der "Selbstbegrenzung" haben Mediziner ihre Probleme. Diskussion über anatomische Präparate aus der NS-Zeit zeigte Parallelen zu Embryonenforschung und Gentechnologie', *Frankfurter Rundschau* (9 July 1990).

80   William E. Seidelman, 'Dissecting the History of Anatomy – 1989–2010: A Personal Account', *Annals of Anatomy*, 104 (2012), pp. 228–236.

81   Personal communication, Christoph Redies to the author, 2011.

82   Christoph Redies, Michael Viebig, Susanne Zimmermann and Rosemarie Fröber, 'Origin of Corpses Received by the Anatomical Institute at the University of Jena during the Nazi Regime', *The Anatomical Record (Part B: New Anat.)*, 285B (2005), pp. 6–10.

83   KKLBD, IIIA 4630/II., 'Abschlussbericht'.

84   Michael Hubenstorf, 'Anatomical Science in Vienna 1938–1945', *Lancet*, 355 (2001), pp. 1385–1386.

85   Herwig Czech, 'Forschen ohne Skrupel. Die wissenschaftliche Verwertung von Opfern der NS-Psychiatriemorde in Wien', in Gabriel and Neugebauer (eds.), *Von der Zwangssterilisierung zur Ermordung*, pp. 143–163; Waltraud Häupl, *Die ermordeten Kinder vom Spiegelgrund. Gedenkdokumentation für die Opfer der NS-Kindereuthanasie in Wien*, Vienna: Böhlau, 2006.

86 Maria Teschler-Nicola and Margit Berner, 'Die anthropologische Abteilung des Naturhistorischen Museums in der NS-Zeit; Berichte und Dokumentation von Forschungs- und Sammlungsaktivitäten 1938–1945', in Gustav Spann (ed.), *Untersuchungen zur Anatomischen Wissenschaft in Wien 1938–1945. Senatsprojekt der Universität Wien*, Vienna: Akademischer Senat der Univ. Wien, 1998, pp. 333–358; Volkhard Knigge and Jürgen Seifert, (eds), *Vom Antlitz zur Maske. Wien-Weimar-Buchenwald 1939. Gezeichneter Ort. Goetheblicke auf Weimar und Thüringen*, Weimar: Gedenkstätte Buchenwald, 1999; Gershon Evan, *Winds of Life. The Destinies of a Young Viennese Jew 1938–1958*, Riverside, CA: Ariadne Press, 2000.

87 Spann, *Untersuchungen*.

88 Czech, 'Von der Richtstätte auf den Seziertisch'.

89 Lang, *Die Namen der Nummern*, pp. 225–30.

90 Weindling, *John W. Thompson*, pp. 308–12.

91 Redies *et al.*, 'Origin of Corpses'.

92 Hubert Markl, ' "Die ehrlichste Art der Entschuldigung ist die Offenlegung der Schuld" ', in Carola Sachse (ed.), Biowissenschaften und Menschenversuche an Kaiser-Wilhelm-Instituten – Die Verbindung nach Auschwitz. Ansprachen der Eröffnungsveranstaltung, Munich: Presseabteilung MPG, 2001, pp. 7–14.

93 Jürgen Dahlkamp, 'Zeitgeschichte: Tiefstehende Idioten', *Der Spiegel,* 44 (2003), pp. 62–64.

94 Maike Rotzoll, Gerrit Hohendorf, Petra Fuchs, Paul Richter, Wolfgang U. Eckart and Christoph Mundt (eds), *Die nationalsozialistische "Euthanasie"-Aktion T4 und ihre Opfer. Geschichte und ethische Konsequenzen für die Gegenwart*, Paderborn, Schöningh, 2010, pp. 16–17.

95 Gerrit Hohendorf, Stefan Raueiser, Michael von Cranach and Sybille von Tiedemann (eds), *Die "Euthanasie"-Opfer zwischen Stigmatisierung und Annerkennung*, Münster: Kontur, 2014.

96 'Hundert Hirnschnitte', p. 36.

Bibliography

Archival Sources

Austria

Vienna, Simon Wiesenthal Archives, Mengele files

Germany

Arolsen, International Tracing Service Archive, Ordner Medizinische Menschenversuche 19, 14 May 1969, 12 page typescript

Berlin, Archiv der Max-Planck-Gesellschaft (MPG):

E-I-F, Besondere Aufgaben Hirnschnittsammlung

E-II-1a 1963, Hirnforschung. Hirnpräparate (Beisetzung Waldfriedhof München 1990)

Bonn, Konferenz der Kultusminister der Länder in der Bundesrepublik Deutschland (KKLBD):

IIIA 4630/II., 'Abschlussbericht. Präparate von Opfern des Nationalsozialismus in anatomischen und pathologischen Sammlungen deutscher Ausbildungs- und Forschungseinrichtungen. Bonn', 25 Jan 1994

NS 112, AK 25./26. 1. 1989, NS Nr. 1,4, Beschluss der Kultusministerkonferenz vom 25./26. 1. 1989

Frankfurt am Main, Institut für Geschichte der Medizin, Akten der Medizinischen Fakultät, Verwendung medizinischer Präparate von Nazi- Opfern

USA

College Park, MD, National Archives and Records Administration (NARA):

Combined Intelligence Objectives Sub-Committee G-2 Division SHAEF (Rear) APO 413, Leo Alexander, 'Neuropathology and Neurophysiology, including Electroencephalography, in Wartime Germany', 20 July 1945

RG 153 Records of the Office of the Judge Advocate General (Army), War Crimes Branch, Case Files, 1944–1949, 12–226: Vol. 1 Trial Record Part 8 thru 12–226: Vol. 1 Clemency, Box Number 185 [Schilling Trial]

RG 549 Records of US Army Europe, War Crimes Case Files 1945–59, 50–2-102 to 50–2-103, Box 322 [Brachtel Trial]

Literature

Aly, Götz, 'Der saubere und der schmutzige Fortschritt', in Götz Aly (ed.), *Reform und Gewissen. "Euthanasie" im Dienst des Fortschritts*, Berlin: Rotbuch Verlag, 1985, pp. 9–78

—— 'Hirnforschung im Dritten Reich. Bericht an die Max-Planck-Gesellschaft zur Förderung der Wissenschaften', *Die Tageszeitung* (21 Oct 1989), p. 16

—— ' "Je mehr, desto lieber", Über den Umgang mit Präparaten von Nazi-Opfern vor 1945 und danach', *Die Zeit* (3 Feb 1989), p. 69

—— ' "Weitere Elaborate Alys verhindern!". Gedächtnisschwund deutscher Hirnforscher', in Götz Aly, *Volk ohne Mitte: die Deutschen zwischen Freiheitsangst und Kollektivismus*, Frankfurt am Main: S. Fischer, 2015, pp. 201–239

Arnold, Michael, 'Anatomie im Zwielicht?', *Deutsches Ärzteblatt*, 6 (9 Feb 1989), pp. 21–22

Baumann, Stefanie Michaela, *Menschenversuche und Wiedergutmachung*, Munich: Oldenbourg, 2009

Baader, Gerhard and Ulrich Schultz (eds), *Medizin und Nationalsozialismus. Tabuisierte Vergangenheit – Ungebrochene Tradition?*, Berlin: Verlagsgesellschaft Gesundheit, 1980

Bock, Gisela, *Zwangssterilisation im Nationalsozialismus*, Opladen: Westdt. Verlag, 1986

Caro, 'Mit der "Selbstbegrenzung" haben Mediziner ihre Probleme. Diskussion über anatomische Präparate aus der NS-Zeit zeigte Parallelen zu Embryonenforschung und Gentechnologie', *Frankfurter Rundschau* (9 July 1990)

Czech, Herwig, 'Forschen ohne Skrupel. Die wissenschaftliche Verwertung von Opfern der NS-Psychiatriemorde in Wien', in Eberhard Gabriel and Wolfgang Neugebauer (eds), *Von der Zwangssterilisierung zur Ermordung. Zur Geschichte der NS-Euthanasie in Wien, Teil II*, Vienna: Böhlau, 2002, pp. 143–163

—— 'Selektion und Kontrolle. Der "Spiegelgrund" als zentrale Institution der Wiener Jugendfürsorge zwischen 1940 und 1945', in Eberhard Gabriel and Wolfgang Neugebauer (eds), *Von der Zwangssterilisierung zur Ermordung. Zur Geschichte der NS-Euthanasie in Wien, Teil II*, Vienna: Böhlau, 2002, pp. 165–187

—— 'Von der Richtstätte auf den Seziertisch. Zur anatomischen Verwertung von NS-Opfern in Wien, Innsbruck und Graz', *Jahrbuch des Dokumentationsarchivs des österreichischen Widerstandes*, 1 (2015), pp. 141–190

Dahlkamp, Jürgen, 'Zeitgeschichte: Tiefstehende Idioten', *Der Spiegel*, 44 (2003), pp. 62–64

'Den Opfern zum Gedenken – den Lebenden zur Mahnung', *MPG Spiegel*, 3 (1990), p. 10

Dickman, S., 'Scandal over Nazi victims' corpses rocks universities', *Nature*, 337 (1989), p. 195

—— 'Brain sections to be buried?', *Nature*, 339 (1989), p. 498

Drews, Ulrich, 'Die Zeit des Nationalsozialismus am anatomischen Institut in Tübingen. Unbeantwortete ethische Fragen damals und heute', in Jürgen Peiffer (ed.), *Menschenverachtung und Opportunismus*, Tübingen: Attempto, 1992, pp. 93–107

Eckart, Wolfgang U., Volker Sellin and Eike Wolgast (eds), *Die Universität Heidelberg im Nationalsozialismus*, Heidelberg: Springer Medizin Verlag, 2006

Evan, Gershon, *Winds of Life. The Destinies of a Young Viennese Jew 1938–1958*, Riverside, CA: Ariadne Press, 2000

Forsbach, Ralph and Hans-Georg Hofer, *Die Deutsche Gesellschaft für Innere Medizin in der NS-Zeit*, Stuttgart: Thieme, 2015

Häupl, Waltraud, *Die ermordeten Kinder vom Spiegelgrund. Gedenkdokumentation für die Opfer der NS-Kindereuthanasie in Wien*, Vienna: Böhlau, 2006

Heese, Hans, *Augen aus Auschwitz – Ein Lehrstück über nationalsozialistischen Rassenwahn und medizinische Forschung – Der Fall Dr. Karin Magnussen*, Essen: Klartext, 2001

Hildebrandt, Sabine, *The Anatomy of Murder. Ethical Transgressions and Anatomical Science during the Third Reich*, New York: Berghahn, 2016

Hohendorf, Gerrit, Stefan Raueiser, Michael von Cranach and Sybille von Tiedemann (eds), *Die "Euthanasie"-Opfer zwischen Stigmatisierung und Annerkennung*, Münster: Kontur, 2014

Hubenstorf, Michael, 'Anatomical Science in Vienna 1938–1945', *Lancet*, 355 (2001), pp. 1385–1386

'Hundert Hirnschnitte und das Rätsel der "Serie H"', *Rhein-Main Zeitung* (21 Apr 2015), p. 36

Klee, Ernst, *Was sie taten – was sie wurden. Ärzte, Juristen und andere Beteiligte am Kranken- und Judenmord*, Frankfurt am Main: S. Fischer, 1986

Knigge, Volkhard and Jürgen Seifert, (eds), *Vom Antlitz zur Maske. Wien-Weimar-Buchenwald 1939. Gezeichneter Ort. Goetheblicke auf Weimar und Thüringen*, Weimar: Gedenkstätte Buchenwald, 1999

Labisch, Alfons and Florian Tennstedt, *Der Weg zum "Gesetz über die Vereinheitlichung des Gesundheitswesens" vom 3. Juli 1934. Entwicklungslinien und Entwicklungsmomente des staatlichen und kommunalen Gesundheitswesens in Deutschland*, Düsseldorf: Akademie für öffentliches Gesundheitswesen, 1985

Lang, Hans-Joachim, *Die Namen der Nummern. Wie es gelang, die 86 Opfer eines NS-Verbrechens zu identifizieren*, Hamburg: Hoffmann und Campe, 2004

Loewenau, Aleksandra, *Dr. Horst Schumann: The Unpunished Criminal* (submitted for review to Athabasca University Press)

Markl, Hubert, ' "Die ehrlichste Art der Entschuldigung ist die Offenlegung der Schuld" ', in Carola Sachse (ed.), *Biowissenschaften und Menschenversuche an Kaiser-Wilhelm-Instituten – Die Verbindung nach Auschwitz. Ansprachen der Eröffnungsveranstaltung*, Munich: Presseabteilung MPG, 2001, pp. 7–14

Mitscherlich, Alexander and Fred Mielke, *Wissenschaft ohne Menschlichkeit*, Heidelberg: Lambert Schneider, 1949

—— *Medizin ohne Menschlichkeit, Dokumente des Nürnberger Ärzteprozesses*, Frankfurt am Main: S. Fischer, 1960

—— *Doctors of Infamy: the Story of the Nazi Medical Crimes*, New York: Henry Schuman, 1949

Müller-Hill, Benno, *Tödliche Wissenschaft: die Aussonderung von Juden, Zigeunern und Geisteskranken 1933–1945*, Reinbek bei Hamburg: Rowohlt, 1984

Mundt, Christoph, Gerrit Hohendorf and Maike Rotzoll, *Psychiatrische Forschung und NS Euthanasie. Beiträge zu einer Gedenkversanstaltung an der Psychiatrischen Universitätsklinik Heidelberg*, Heidelberg: Wunderhorn, 2001

Papworth, Maurice, *Human Guinea Pigs: Experimentation on Man*, London: Routledge, 1967

Peuckert, Detlev, 'The Genesis of the "Final Solution" from the Spirit of Science', in Thomas Childers and Jane Caplan (eds), *Reevaluating the Third Reich*, New York: Holmes & Meier, 1994, pp. 234–252

Platen-Hallermund, Alice, *Die Tötung Geisteskranker in Deutschland: Aus der deutschen Ärzte-Kommission beim amerikanischen Militärgericht*, Frankfurt am Main: Verlag der Frankfurter Hefte, 1948

Pringle, Heather, *The Master Plan: Himmler's Scholars and the Holocaust*, New York: Hyperion, 2006

Proctor, Robert, *Racial Hygiene. Medicine under the Nazis*, Cambridge, MA: Harvard University Press, 1988

Projektgruppe "Volk und Gesundheit" (ed.), *Volk und Gesundheit. Heilen und Vernichten im Nationalsozialismus. Begleitbuch zur gleichnamigen Ausstellung im Ludwig-Uhland-Institut für Empirische Kulturwissenschaft der Universität Tübingen*, Tübingen: Tübinger Vereinigung für Volkskunde, 1982

Pross, Christian, *Wiedergutmachung. Der Kleinkrieg gegen die Opfer*, Frankfurt am Main: Athanäum, 1988

—— and Rolf Winau (eds), *Nicht misshandeln. Das Krankenhaus Moabit 1920–1933. Ein Zentrum jüdischer Ärzte in Berlin, 1933–1945. Verfolgung – Widerstand – Zerstörung*, Berlin: Hentrich, 1984

Redies, Christoph, Michael Viebig, Susanne Zimmermann and Rosemarie Fröber, 'Origin of Corpses Received by the Anatomical Institute at the University of Jena during the Nazi Regime', *The Anatomical Record (Part B: New Anat.)*, 285B (2005), pp. 6–10

Roth, Karl Heinz (ed.), *Erfassung zur Vernichtung. Von der Sozialhygiene zum "Gesetz über Sterbehilfe"*, Berlin: Verlagsgesellschaft Gesundheit, 1984

—— 'Die wissenschaftliche Normalität des Schlächters', *Mitteilungen der Dokumentationsstelle zur NS-Sozialpolitik* 1.2 (1985), pp. 1–8

Rothmaler, Christiane, 'Gutachten und Dokumentation über das Anatomische Institut des Universitäts-Krankenhauses Eppendorf der Universität Hamburg 1933–1945', *1999: Zeitschrift für Sozialgeschichte des 20. und 21. Jahrhunderts*, 2 (1990), pp. 78–95

Rotzoll, Maike, Gerrit Hohendorf, Petra Fuchs, Paul Richter, Wolfgang U. Eckart and Christoph Mundt (eds), *Die nationalsozialistische "Euthanasie"-Aktion T4 und ihre Opfer. Geschichte und ethische Konsequenzen für die Gegenwart*, Paderborn, Schöningh, 2010

Sachse, Carola, ' "Whitewash Culture": How the Kaiser Wilhelm/Max Planck Society Dealt with the Nazi Past', in Susanne Heim, Carola Sachse and Mark Walker (eds),

The Kaiser Wilhelm Society under National Socialism, Cambridge: Cambridge University Press, 2009, pp. 373–399

—— 'Was bedeutet eine Entschuldigung? Die Überlebenden medizinischer NS Verbrechen und die Max-Planck-Gesellschaft', in Heinrich Berger, Melanie Dejnega, Regina Fritz and Alexander Prenninger (eds), *Politische Gewalt und Machtausübung im 20. Jahrhundert*, Vienna: Böhlau, 2011, pp. 631–649

Schlote, Wolfgang, 'Einziger Weg', *Die Zeit* (24 Nov 19889), p. 86

Schlüter, Reinhard, *Leben für eine humane Medizin: Alice Ricciardi-von Platen – Psychoanalytikerin und Protokollantin des Nürnberger Ärzteprozesses*, Frankfurt am Main: Campus, 2012

Schmelter, Thomas, Christine Meesmann, Gisela Walter and Herwig Praxl, 'Heil- und Pflegeanstalt Werneck', in Michael von Cranach and Hans-Ludwig Siemen (eds), *Psychiatrie im Nationalsozialismus. Die Bayerischen Heil- und Pflegeanstalten zwischen 1933 und 1945*, Munich: Oldenbourg, 1999, pp. 35–54

Schmuhl, Hans-Walter, *Grenzüberschreitungen. Das Kaiser-Wilhelm-Institut für Anthropologie, menschliche Erblehre und Eugenik 1927–1945*, Göttingen: Wallstein, 2005

Schönhagen, Benigna, *Das Gräberfeld X. Eine Dokumentation über NS Opfer auf dem Tübinger Stadtfriedhof*, Tübingen: Kulturamt, 1987

—— 'Cemetery X and the Origins of Corpses from Anatomical Institutes under NS: Recollections of Developments at Tübingen', www.pulse-project.org/node/630 (accessed 15 July 2016)

Schostack, R., 'Trauergang. Deutsche Szene', *Frankfurter Allgemeine Zeitung* (29 May 1990)

Seidelman, William, 'Legacy of the Nazis', *Nature* (21 Sept 1989), p. 341

—— 'In memoriam. Medicine's Confrontation with Evil', *Hasting's Center Report* (Nov/Dec 1989), pp. 5–6

—— 'Dissecting the History of Anatomy – 1989–2010: A Personal Account', *Annals of Anatomy*, 104 (2012), pp. 228–236

Spann, Gustav (ed.), *Untersuchungen zur Anatomischen Wissenschaft in Wien 1938–1945. Senatsprojekt der Universität Wien*, Vienna: Akademischer Senat der Univ. Wien, 1998

Teschler-Nicola, Maria and Margit Berner, 'Die anthropologische Abteilung des Naturhistorischen Museums in der NS-Zeit; Berichte und Dokumentation von Forschungs- und Sammlungsaktivitäten 1938–1945', in Gustav Spann (ed.), *Untersuchungen zur Anatomischen Wissenschaft in Wien 1938–1945. Senatsprojekt der Universität Wien*, Vienna: Akademischer Senat der Univ. Wien, 1998, pp. 333–358

Trials of War Criminals before the Nuernberg Military Tribunals under Control Council Law No. 10. Nuernberg October 1946-April 1949. Vol. VII: IG Farben Case, Washington, DC: US Government Printing Office, 1950

Tübingen University, *Abschlussbericht der Commission zur Überprüfung der Präparate-sammlungen in den medizinischen Einrichtungen der Universität Tübingen im Hinblick auf Opfer des Nationalsozialismus*, Tübingen: 1989

Turda, Marius and Paul Weindling (eds), *Blood and Homeland: Eugenics in Central Europe 1900–1940*, Budapest: Central European University Press, 2006

Völklein, U., 'Anatomie einer Ente', *Der Stern* (1989), pp. 159–160

Walsh, M., 'Nazi Research under the Microscope', *Time* (27 Feb 1989), pp. 34–35

Weindling, Paul, 'Die Preussische Medizinalverwaltung und die "Rassenhygiene"', in Achim Thom and Horst Spaar (eds), *Medizin und Faschismus*, Berlin: Akademie für ärztliche Fortbildung, 1983, pp. 23–35

—— 'Shattered Alternatives in Medicine', *History Workshop Journal*, 16 (1983), pp. 152–157

—— 'Soziale Hygiene, Eugenik und medizinische Praxis: Der Fall Alfred Grotjahn', *Das Argument. Jahrbuch für kritische Medizin* (1984), pp. 6–20

—— 'Blood, Race and Politics', *The Times Higher Education Supplement* (19 July 1985), p. 13

—— *Health, Race and German Politics between National Unification and Nazism, 1870–1945*, Cambridge: Cambridge University Press, 1989

—— *Nazi Medicine and the Nuremberg Trials. From Medical War Crimes to Informed Consent*, Houndmills, Basingstoke: Palgrave Macmillan, 2004

—— 'Alice Ricciardi von Platen', *The Guardian* (13 Mar 2008), www.theguardian.com/world/2008/mar/13/secondworldwar.germany (accessed 18 July 2016)

—— 'A City Regenerated: Eugenics, Race and Welfare in Interwar Vienna', in Deborah Holmes and Lisa Silverman (eds), *Interwar Vienna: Culture between Tradition and Modernity*, New York: Camden House, 2009, pp. 81–113

—— *John W. Thompson. Psychiatrist in the Shadow of the Holocaust*, Rochester, NY: Rochester University Press, 2010

—— '"Cleansing" Anatomical Collections: The Politics of Removing Specimens from German Anatomical and Medical Collections 1988–92', *Annals of Anatomy*, 194.3 (2012), pp. 237–242

—— 'Sonstige Personenschäden – die Entschädigungspraxis der Stiftung "Erinnerung, Verantwortung und Zukunft"', in Constantin Goschler (ed), *Die Entschädigung von NS-Zwangsarbeit am Anfang des 21. Jahrhunderts*, Vol. 2, Göttingen: Wallstein, 2012, pp. 197–225

—— 'Rassenkundliche Forschung zwischen dem Getto Litzmannstadt und Auschwitz: Hans Fleischhackers Tübinger Habilitation, Juni 1943', in Jens Kolata, Richard Kühl, Henning Tümmers and Urban Wiesing (eds), *In Fleischhackers Händen. Wissenschaft, Politik und das 20. Jahrhundert. [Anlässlich der Ausstellung "In Fleischhackers Händen, Tübinger Rassenforscher in Łódź 1940–1942" im Schloss Hohentübingen (24. April bis 28 Juni 2015]*, Tübingen: MUT, 2015, pp. 141–164

—— *Victims and Survivors of Nazi Human Experiments – Science and Suffering in the Holocaust*, London: Bloomsbury, 2015

Wolters, Christine, *Tuberkulose und Menschenversuche im Nationalsozialismus. Das Netzwerk hinter den Tbc-Experimenten im Konzentrationslager Sachsenhausen*, Stuttgart: Franz Steiner, 2011

Wuttke-Groneberg, Walter, *Medizin im Nationalsozialismus. Ein Arbeitsbuch*, Tübingen: Schwäbische Verlagsgesellschaft, 1982

Index